Concussed

Sam Peters is a rugby writer who has been credited with driving cultural change to the sport's attitude towards head injuries and concussion. In 2014 Sam was shortlisted as Sports Journalist of the Year at the UK *Press Gazette* Awards and was runner-up as Rugby Writer of the Year at the 2017 SJA Awards. Sam has written two books: *Broadside,* with England cricketer Stuart Broad, and *The Row to Recovery*.

Concussed

Sport's Uncomfortable Truth

Sam Peters

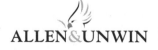

ALLEN&UNWIN

Published in hardback in Great Britain in 2023 by Allen & Unwin, an imprint of
Atlantic Books Ltd.

Plate section photography credits:
Page 3 – middle photograph Warren Little/Getty Images, bottom photograph David
Rogers/Getty Images; Page 4 – top photograph David Rogers/Getty Images, middle
photograph David Rogers/Getty Images, bottom photograph Ben Hoskins/Getty
Images; Page 5 top photograph Cameron Spencer/Getty Images, bottom photograph
Remy Gabalda/Getty Images; Page 6 top photograph Michael Steele/Getty Images,
bottom photograph Gareth Everett/Huw Evans Agency; Page 7 top photograph
Henry Browne/Getty Images; Page 8 top photograph A. Jones/Getty Images; all other
featured images courtesy of the author.

10 9 8 7 6 5 4 3

A CIP catalogue record for this book is available from the British Library.

Hardback ISBN: 978 1 83895 577 9
E-book ISBN: 978 1 83895 578 6

Printed in Great Britain
Page design benstudios.co.uk

Allen & Unwin
An imprint of Atlantic Books Ltd
Ormond House
26–27 Boswell Street
London
WC1N 3JZ

www.atlantic-books.co.uk

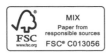

Printed and bound in Great Britain by
TJ Books Limited, Padstow, Cornwall

Concussed is dedicated to Ben Robinson, Cae Treyharn and Jeff Astle, just three of many taken too soon by brain injuries sustained playing sport.

And to mum, dad and Debs, who made this book possible through their enduring love and support.

Foreword

Concussion, and its associated neurological complications, is the single most important issue facing modern rugby. I have been truly shocked reading some of the stories and speaking to some of those now struggling with the debilitating long-term effects caused by the head injuries suffered during their professional playing careers.

During my amateur playing career through the 1970s and 1980s concussion was a constant threat – I suffered several myself – but there's no doubt the crossover into professionalism changed rugby union from a fiercely competitive game requiring bravery, strength and skill into one where power and brute force took precedence.

And while bigger collisions excited fans, there was always a nagging risk they could come at a price for professional players involved in the modern game. Not least players like Steve Thompson, a World Cup winner who I was fortunate enough to coach, who revealed in 2020 he was suffering from early onset dementia.

No journalist has done more than Sam Peters to reveal this painful truth for rugby. His work, which has been balanced but relentless, has forced so many of us to sit up and take notice of a direction of travel many have felt deeply uncomfortable about for many years.

By constantly challenging, probing and being willing to stand alone in the face of hostility from many, Sam has led from the front in exposing an uncomfortable truth. His message has, at times, been hard to hear, but there's no doubt he's done it for the love of rugby and sport more broadly.

Sam, along with many of the campaigners you'll read about in this book, has made sport safer. That will be his legacy.

Sir Clive Woodward

Contents

Three definitions of concussion

Oxford English Dictionary: (1) The act of violently shaking or agitating particularly, the shock of impact. (2) Injury caused to the brain, spine, or other part, by the shock of a heavy blow, fall, etc.

The Congress of Neurological Surgeons, Committee on head injury nomenclature: A clinical syndrome characterized by the immediate and transient post-traumatic impairment of neural function such as alteration of consciousness, disturbance of vision or equilibrium due to mechanical forces.

World Rugby: Concussion is a traumatic brain injury resulting in a disturbance of brain function. There are many symptoms and signs of concussion, common ones being headache, dizziness, memory disturbance or balance problems. Loss of consciousness occurs in less than 10% of concussions but is a clear indication a concussion has been sustained.

Introduction

British Lions v Australia, 6 July 2013.

The look on his face was not one I'd seen up close before. His eyes open yet blank, devoid of expression. That he was physically there was undeniable but at the same time there was a completely vacant look written across his features.

'You OK, mate?' I ask.

'Err, yeah, I think so,' comes the unconvincing reply.

Barely two hours earlier George Smith, one of the most celebrated Australian rugby union players in history, had suffered an injury all too familiar to those of us who worked in the sport, but utterly shocking to anyone operating outside of its tiny bubble.

Four minutes into a match watched by millions on television, Smith had carried the ball into a tackle, only to suffer a brain injury of such significance that, had it occurred in almost any other walk of life, an ambulance would have been called and he would have been blue-lighted to the nearest hospital for an extended spell of observation, tests and treatment.

But the professional rugby field is unlike any other walk of life. Indeed, brain injuries, or concussions as they're also labelled, had become such routine occurrences many involved chose to shrug or laugh them off as simply a 'ding', 'having my bell rung' or a 'head knock'. Well, if you don't laugh...

Gradually, after several minutes, Smith was raised from his stupor and helped gingerly from the field by medics, his left leg trailing alarmingly behind him as the motor function of his brain struggled to control the rest of his body.

After coming out of four years of international retirement to help his already injury-stricken national team, this was not how it was supposed to end for one of Australia's greatest sporting warriors.

'I'd be very surprised if George Smith comes back on the field,' said the Fox Sport commentator, witnessing the evidence in front of him.

His co-commentator agreed: 'He can hardly stand up, hardly walk. He is going to be a very sore man tomorrow.'

'Sore man' is rugby speak for likely to be unable to get out of bed, turn on the lights or walk to the local shop.

To put it more bluntly, 'sore man' meant he was utterly fucked.

Even in a sport where playing on after suffering a concussion had become increasingly normalized, revered as an act of bravery and sacrifice on behalf of the team, by 2013 concern about the long-term risks had prompted a few to call for change. And this one was so bad many assumed Smith would stay off. I didn't for a second and leant across to my colleague in the press box and said, 'He'll be back.' And so he was. Five minutes later, the 32-year-old trotted gingerly out onto the field again and carried on playing.

'That's a massive call,' said the commentator. 'That's a massive call for George Smith's life,' he may as well have said.

*

The Smith case did not happen in isolation. Far from it. Since I'd begun covering rugby union professionally 10 years previously, and in the 20 years before that when I'd played it, I'd witnessed a sport transformed.

From an amateur contact sport played by physically fit, strong and brave young people, rugby had morphed into an extreme version of its former self with players now bigger, stronger and more physically committed than at any point in its 150-year history. The physical consequences for players were becoming increasingly evident.

As money had poured in since the game went professional in 1995, rugby union's injury profile had shot through the roof to a point where I believed, as someone who loved the game to its core, it had become unsustainable. Intolerably dangerous. Reckless even.

Doctors now compared injuries suffered on a professional rugby field to those normally witnessed in road traffic accidents. Biceps and hamstrings torn off the bone, knees obliterated, collarbones crushed. Brains battered. As collisions got bigger and more frequent, so too, of course, did concussions.

Everyone knew the sport was far more dangerous than ever before. And I mean everyone. The players. The doctors. The coaches and the media. We all knew it. Even the administrators and advertising folk, many of whom had never laced a pair of boots in their lives. In some people's eyes rugby had become 'beautifully brutal'. But beauty is in the eye of the beholder.

As the collisions increased and head injuries got worse, so too did the pressure to get players fit and back on the pitch faster than ever. Previously accepted medical norms were dispensed with, unthought-of treatments practised, untold pain managed. And training was sometimes worse than matchdays as players vied against each other for contracts, and coaches made it up as they went along.

Worse still, the more players suffered concussions the more they were returned to the field by compliant medical staff, often directed by coaches who cared little for tomorrow. Get up, get going and go again.

Bodies and brains were being damaged in the long term, I had no doubt. And as stories began to emerge of former American footballers dying prematurely, sometimes choosing suicide over living with the depression, anxiety and violent mood swings associated with the effects of repeated blows to the head, I became increasingly convinced rugby's authorities were doing irreparable damage to a generation of young professional players.

And while everyone knew rugby had outgrown itself, few were prepared to say so in public. Silence pervaded. A dangerous *omertà* we all accepted. Somehow rugby union convinced itself to turn a blind eye to the increasing damage being inflicted on a cohort of young athletes who knew no better and were not being protected from themselves. The data the corporate doctors presented in defence of the sport told us there was nothing to see and to look the other way. I refused.

And when I spoke to the players and their families away from the cameras and followed their injury stories, I became more convinced a light needed shining on rugby's injury crisis. An uncomfortable truth needed telling. Rugby had morphed into something it was never meant to be.

*

Since becoming a sports journalist, I'd written for almost every national newspaper while in my twenties and early thirties but now here I was, rugby correspondent for the *Mail on Sunday*, in a stadium where 12 years earlier I'd been a fan in the stands wearing a Lions shirt and screaming my team on for victory.

Over the past decade I'd written more about rugby's injury crisis than any of my colleagues and been told time after time I was looking in the wrong place.

That was all about to change. Over the course of the next few years I would embark on a journey I never thought possible. A journey which would see me labelled a 'pariah', a 'rugby hater' and a 'rogue journalist'. I'd be physically threatened, verbally abused and whispered about behind my back. Time and again I'd ask myself if I was doing the right thing reporting what was right before my eyes.

But the more I dug, the more I realized the problem was far more severe than I'd ever imagined. Before I knew it, my worst fears about players developing dementia in their thirties and forties would come true.

For many, the campaign I launched would come too late. For them, I am truly sorry. Perhaps this book may do something to help those players and their families who don't know what may be lying in wait in the future while forcing the authorities to act and face up to the truth. Perhaps it may inform professional players today who hear what they want to hear from people paid to protect them, paid by the very organizations whose interests are best served by telling them 'there's nothing to see here'.

I'll be accused by many of reopening old wounds by writing this book. I'll be accused of being a sport hater. Being soft. Being woke. Whatever. I've been accused of a lot worse. But one thing I haven't been accused of yet is losing my moral compass. My sense of what's right and wrong. And it's my deeply held belief that rugby has got it badly wrong since the game went professional. I've long since stopped caring if that makes me unpopular.

And besides, I promised some good people I'd help them. People like Peter Robinson and Karen Walton, who lost their 14-year-old son Ben to a brain injury suffered on the field in 2011. People like Althea Trayhern, whose 36-year-old son, former Pontypool captain Cae, committed suicide in 2016. People like Dawn Astle, who lost her dad, former England and West Bromwich Albion striker Jeff, to early onset dementia in 2002.

I promised them all I'd help tell their loved ones' stories. To uncover the truth, however uncomfortable it may be for those of us who love sport.

1

A love affair begins

From as early I can remember, sport was my life. Rugby union and league, football, cricket, horse racing, golf, tennis, Formula One, motocross, wrestling, boxing, golf, athletics, squash, BMX, skiing (on TV – Dad would never actually take us). Anything. You name it, I watched it. Or even better, I played it. I lived for sport, breathed sport. Sport got me out of bed in the morning, kept me sane in the classroom. It kept me fit, strong and largely healthy, minus the odd broken finger, black eye or sprained ankle. I loved sport.

As an adult I watched sport live or in the pub, played it with my mates, wrote about it for a living and even, on occasion, got paid to talk about it on television or the radio. Sport has been in my life from the moment Dad hung me up in a bouncer in the living room doorframe and let me gurgle at England playing in the Five Nations on TV. In fact, sport's not just been in my life. It has been my life.

I first played rugby when I was four. I'd insisted on joining my big brother Tom in his first game for our local club Richmond against rivals London Welsh. Too little to be thrown straight in, I spent most of the morning shivering on the touchline. It was freezing. I cried and told Dad I wanted to go home. It was the only time in my childhood I can recall ever not wanting to be near a sports field.

I soon forgot about the discomfort and the following season pulled my tracksuit on again and never looked back.

If it was on TV, we watched it. If it was on the field, we played it. As we grew older, if it was in the newspapers, we read it. The back pages were our happy place, as were the fields, parks and pavements where we lived out our sporting fantasies.

TV was big too. Wrestling on a Saturday morning, followed by *Saint and Greavsie* and *Grandstand* or *World of Sport* with Dickie Davies, then out to watch Old Meadonians play rugby or cricket with Dad in the afternoon. Mini rugby on Sunday mornings followed by lunch and an afternoon watching *Ski Sunday* and *Rugby Special.* Perfect.

Watching was good but playing was better. Obviously. Even being diagnosed aged four with a blood disorder – idiopathic thrombocytopenic purpura – which my eagle-eyed nurse mum spotted and insisted the GP refer me to a specialist, hardly slowed me down.

Thanks to Mum, I recovered, and soon had sport coursing through my veins again.

My dad, Roy, was born at Quintin Boat House by Chiswick Bridge in 1944 just before it was bombed by the Luftwaffe (fortunately, the family were in a coal cellar next door). His dad, Tom, had taken over as a boatman from his own father, Freddie, in 1934. Dad never rowed. Rugby, football and cricket were his great loves. Quintin, like most sports clubs in those days, was governed by class and social status. Dad's mum was a stern, upright Victorian lady called Elsie who made amazing fruit cakes and cut the crusts off fishpaste sandwiches to keep the committee men sweet. Incidentally, one of her relatives, Charlie Dorey, was the fruit chairman of Brentford Football Club.

Dad's two brothers, Eric and John, were keen sportsmen too. John, a junior international class oarsman, is still President at Quintin, whereas Eric was captain. Their elder sister Gwen, a PE teacher, taught them cricket.

The boat house was the family home where Grandpa Tom, a Queen's Waterman who rowed the royal barges and was Great

Britain's official boatman at the 1960 Rome Olympics, kept the place in good order.

But the Peters family's undisputed claim to sporting fame was Dad's second cousin, Martin, who scored 'the other goal' in England's 4–2 World Cup final win over West Germany in 1966. Nicknamed 'the Ghost' for his uncanny ability to run untracked from box to box, he made more than 700 professional appearances for West Ham, Tottenham Hotspur, Norwich City and Sheffield United before a brief, unsuccessful stint as Sheffield United manager in 1981. He was the first ever £200,000 transfer and also won 67 caps for England, scoring 20 goals. Martin died in 2019, aged 76. He was the third from that team to die from dementia.

By all accounts, Dad was an excellent amateur rugby player and cricketer. He captained, played full back for Southern universities and Middlesex and, so he still reminds us, once hit England fast bowler John Snow for two fours in an over. Dad's rugby career ended aged 27 when a specialist at Moorfields Eye Hospital told him he'd go blind if he took another blow to the head. He's still only partially sighted in his right eye.

My mum, Jennie, was not so into sport but kept fit cycling to and from her shifts at Queen Mary's Hospital, Roehampton, where she worked in the plastic surgery unit. She also made sure we always had clean kit to wear and sandwiches to eat, and was forever on hand to patch up the endless bumps, bruises, grazes and cuts we picked up along the way.

My maternal grandmother, Alma – Nanny – also trained as a nurse in her fifties after divorcing my grandfather Bill, a head teacher and active figure in the Derby trade union movement. She would play football with me and Tom in the fields behind her bungalow in Littleover, Derby, where we spent many happy summer holiday breaks with our cousin Jonathan.

Tom and I competed fiercely. It was a classic sibling rivalry and our friends knew to steer clear if we had a grump on with each other.

If there was a flattish piece of road, grass or track, we'd turn it into a cricket, football or rugby pitch and get playing. Or fighting.

When we were very young, Dad fashioned a tackle bag out of old carpets tied together with string, which meant we could practise tackling at home. We'd often get the bag out when our friends came round to play. What our neighbours made of us hitting the bag at full tilt every Sunday morning I'll never know. We just wanted to play. All the time.

Dad worked long hours, meaning it was often left to Mum to ferry us to the various sports clubs and after-school activities we were desperate to be involved in.

Weekends were our time with Dad, who would take us to Dukes Meadows in Chiswick in the rugby season to watch his beloved Old Meadonians (now Chiswick RFC) or Chiswick House in the summer to watch the cricket. We'd go in our tracksuits and play for hours in the dead ball area while Dad caught up with his old team-mates over a pint of Fuller's in the rickety old clubhouse with a corrugated iron roof. At full time the players would enjoy half pints of bitter shandy, lined up on a tray by the steps of the clubhouse. One day, when I was 8 and Tom 10, we drank three halves each while no one was looking.

The players changed in the boat house across the road and I'll always remember the excitement of hearing the studs chattering on the tarmac behind the hedge before they charged into view and out onto the pitch, accompanied by the inescapable waft of Deep Heat. We'd watch for a bit and then play until darkness fell before shuffling back into the clubhouse, caked in mud, waiting for what seemed like hours for Dad to finish up in the dark, smoky bar. A meat pie with watery mash and vinegary ketchup would stave off the hunger until we'd convinced Dad it was time to leave before he got in trouble with Mum.

I first went to Twickenham Stadium in 1985, aged seven, when Dad got us tickets for London Welsh against Bath in the John Player

Cup final. Tom's maths teacher Kevin Bowring was playing No.8 for Welsh and we were close enough to the pitch to get a sense of how physical the game was. The bravery of the players and ferocity of the contest took my breath away.

Just a couple of months later Dad, an avid Brentford fan, got us tickets to Wembley with our uncle Eric and cousin Ewen, to watch the Bees lose 3–1 to Wigan Athletic in the final of the Freight Rover Trophy. My heart nearly thumped through my chest when we entered the stadium.

At school I'd spend lessons staring out of the window, desperate for the haven of the sports field. I was quite good too. One cricket season, aged 12, I averaged 332, out once in seven innings, before scoring my first century against Caldicott the following year on my way to a first XI school record of 430 runs in seven innings at an average of 107.5. I was obsessed with statistics and kept all our team's scores and averages in a notebook.

Growing up, mini rugby on a Sunday morning was a ritual. After that first freezing cold introduction, I fell in love with everything about the game and, with Dad as coach, we were all conquering. Richmond went unbeaten for two seasons in the Under 11s and Under 12s, culminating in a win over arch-rivals Chiltern in the final of the London Irish tournament, which we won 6–0. The game was played in front of a full grandstand and a crowd several rows deep around the pitch. That's how I remember it anyway. For us, the win was our first ever over our fiercest rivals; for Chiltern, their first ever loss in their final game together after five years unbeaten. They'd even made their way into *The Guinness Book of Records*. At the final whistle, we all cried.

On 4 November 1988, Dad took me, aged 10, to my first international at Twickenham. England's team contained the core who would go on to reach the World Cup final three years later. The back row of Dean Richards, Dave Egerton and Andy Robinson tore up the Wallabies, while RAF flying officer Rory Underwood shredded them out wide. I drank in every second of the game, captivated from first whistle to last as Will Carling's unfancied England pulled off a famous 28–19 victory. Wallaby legend Michael Lynagh, who played fly half that day, would later describe it as the day 'England got serious at rugby.' It was the day I did, too.

The journey home to Sheen felt like we were travelling on air. I pored over every inch of the programme, asking Dad questions. How heavy was Paul Rendall and how fast was Andy Harriman? Was Will Carling actually in the Army? How much did you weigh when you played, Dad? What would the players be doing tonight?

I continued to study the programme all weekend and took it to school on Monday to show my friends. I was fascinated by players' weight, height, number of caps and career points scored. When it came to sports stats, I couldn't get enough.

I must have watched that game 200 times on our home VHS recorder over the next few years. I'd fast forward and rewind Rory Underwood's two brilliant tries, while Tom and I tried to recreate one of his left-handed touchdowns by piling pillows on Mum and Dad's bed and diving endlessly until Dad stormed up, worried that we were going to crash through the ceiling.

From that day forwards, rugby became my obsession, with a short summer recess for cricket.

In 1990, I witnessed my hero Jeremy Guscott score a stunning solo try at Twickenham when England beat Ireland 23–0 on their way to what looked sure to be a first Grand Slam since 1980. But David Sole's Scotland, playing with their eyes on stalks, sank them at a politically charged Murrayfield. I never did like Maggie Thatcher after that.

We watched the game at home on TV and, while devastated by England's loss, I remember being captivated by the commentary of Bill McLaren. He was so evidently Scottish, but at the same time unfailingly impartial. I loved his voice. It gave me comfort even when England were losing. Tom and I would spend hours fizzing passes to each other while chanting 'it's chocolate bar service from a slot machine' in a faux McLaren voice. Looking back, they were gloriously innocent days.

As a teenager, I played fly half in a decent Middlesex Under 16 team in which my Richmond team-mate Michael Swift, who would become Connacht's all-time most capped player with 269 appearances, was the linchpin of our pack. In the backs, Wayne Andrews stood out for his footballing abilities and pace on the wing. I'd just fling it wide and invariably Wayne would be on the end to run it in from 50 metres. In the end, Wayne pursued a career in professional football and made 190 league appearances as a striker for a variety of clubs including Watford, Coventry City and Crystal Palace.

I made it into the London & South East Under 16 side that year, forging a decent half back partnership with a young scrum half from Eastern Counties, Peter Richards, who would go on to play 13 times for England. I narrowly missed out on full England selection that same year when Richards and I inexplicably split up in the final trial. Richards made the cut. I didn't. I'll get over it. One day.

Undeterred, I ended up captaining my school first XI at cricket and first XV at rugby, dropping a goal to win the game against fierce rivals Wellington College in September 1995. That year we faced a Dulwich College XV containing three future England internationals, Andrew Sheridan at No.8, Nick Easter at blindside and David Flatman at tighthead. Jon Dawson, who went on to play for England Under 21s, Bath, Saracens and Harlequins, propped the other side of the scrum. We lost. On reflection, I probably shouldn't have sulked for a week.

At school I was lucky with injuries. I suffered a few concussions – almost everyone did – but never missed a game through injury. On one occasion, aged 14, playing in an Under 15 game against Wellington, I hadn't even noticed I'd taken a blow to the head. But when I got home I realized I had no recollection of the coach journey and felt nauseous and drowsy. I ended up spending the evening in bed with the lights out, vomiting occasionally and feeling disoriented. I slept through the night and felt fine the next morning and didn't mention anything at school on Monday. I played the following week. That was normal.

Aged 16, against Dulwich, I dived for the corner attempting to score a try and the tackler's head crashed into mine, pinning my head against the corner flag as we hit the ground. I heard a high-pitched ringing in my ears and saw flashing lights. As I attempted to stand up, I stumbled and fell to the ground. Our coach, former England player Dave Rollitt, attended me, along with one of our substitutes who had the water bucket and 'magic sponge'. Within a few minutes I felt OK and carried on playing.

After school, I spent my gap year in the Army with the Royal Fusiliers, playing lots of rugby, and drinking lots of beer while learning how to iron a shirt and fire a semi-automatic rifle. I turned up for the Freshers trial at Edinburgh University, where I'd secured a place reading Politics and Economic & Social History, in distinctly average shape. Somehow I managed to impress and found myself on the first XV bench that weekend. I started against Berwick the following week and played several games for the 'Ones' before a shoulder injury I'd suffered playing rugby in the Army became altogether more troublesome.

I'd play for the university every Saturday and most Wednesdays but also occasionally turned out for a very handy college team, captained by a big character called Robbie Aarvold, who was the grandson of legendary British Lion Sir Carl Aarvold.

In one game, on a freezing late January day, I took the ball blind from a midfield scrum only to look up and see their 17 stone blindside flanker heading straight for me. Instinctively, I stuck out a hand but just as I attempted to push out for the hand off, he hit me, effectively driving the ball of my shoulder through the joint and out the other side. Just for extra spice, I dislocated my acromioclavicular joint and fractured my collarbone at the same time. It was, to put it mildly, sore.

Some kind soul drove me the 2.5 miles to Edinburgh Royal Infirmary, where it took the doctors another hour to pop my shoulder back into place.

The specialist advised I could avoid surgery by sticking to a strict regime of strengthening exercises. I took the non-surgical option and, despite missing the rest of the season, was picked for the university's first XV tour to Australia that summer where we were scheduled to play five matches. I lasted one game before my shoulder dislocated again. I'll save the tour diary for another book.

Two years, one more tour to New Zealand, roughly 30 dislocations and three operations later, I was close to calling time on rugby and a career in the Army. A new life plan was needed.

*

While at Edinburgh, I'd surprised myself with how much I enjoyed the social history element of my course.

In particular, I was fascinated by the origins of formalized sport. The class divides. The social dynamic at play. The use of sport as an establishment tool to control workers while affording them the 'privilege' of downtime and leisure. I was fascinated by the anachronistic class-based notion of 'gentlemen and players', amateurs and professionals, and the Corinthian Spirit, the intertwining of Church, State and education, and the role played by the country's major public schools, one of which, St Paul's, I'd attended, in formulating codified rules.

I'd always been proud of my family's working-class roots and didn't always feel comfortable with rugby union's historic association with class and privilege.

I studied the central role the Church played in England, Scotland and Wales in driving notions of patriotism, especially at times of war, while preaching 'manliness is close to Godliness' through Christian teachings where sacrifice, subjugation, the advancement of righteousness and the protection of the weak were central pillars in the cult of 'Muscular Christianity' imagined and pursued by Dr Thomas Arnold of Rugby School.

The notion that rugby union existed on a higher moral plane than other sports would be actively perpetuated by those seeking competitive commercial advantage after rugby turned professional, with the global governing body World Rugby's own slogan by 2013 proclaiming 'Rugby, building character since 1823'. The association between 'character' and a willingness to tolerate physical punishment fascinated me.

I was interested in the role the printed press played in how sports presented themselves, especially when it came to calling on clubs and players to 'do their duty' with the formation of pals battalions at the start of the First World War. My dissertation, 'Attitudes Towards Professional Sport During the First World War in England and Scotland', explored the role sports authorities played in Britain's recruitment drive and the growing societal tensions presented by the commercialization of sport set against the class-based societal order.

So while my time at university taught me about the fragility of my own body and limitations on a sports field, I also learned about the history of organized sport and understood that politics and sport definitely mix. When I left, I still loved sport, but my understanding of its commercial and cultural role within society had grown significantly. On reflection, perhaps I'd already begun to doubt some of the establishment pillars upon which rugby union had been built.

Having completed our finals that summer, I embarked on the trip of a lifetime with my old friend Matt, flying to Australia to follow the Lions on their 2001 tour. After watching the first game in the Walkabout pub in Edinburgh, starring 21-year-old Simon Taylor, who only a week or so before I'd played alongside for the Sambuca

Guzzlers in an intra-college Sevens game, we flew to Sydney for the start of an incredible adventure.

We watched the second game against the New South Wales Waratahs, when Aussie Duncan McCrae was sent off for repeatedly punching Ronan O'Gara on the floor, travelled up country by train via Coffs Harbour, where we watched the Lions demolish the New South Wales Country Cockatoos, before heading to Brisbane for the eagerly anticipated first Test.

What we witnessed that night at the Gabba, along with roughly 40,000 other fans proudly wearing red, was one of the greatest Lions performances. The atmosphere was electric from the first whistle and the Lions, who scored after just three minutes courtesy of rugby league convert Jason Robinson, delivered a performance to match.

We drank long into the early hours and the next morning boarded a plane, along with a load of other bleary-eyed Lions tourists, for the short flight to Canberra. Sitting behind us were three faces I recognized. One was *Sunday Times* rugby correspondent Stephen Jones; the second was former England fly half Stuart Barnes, who I'd first watched play for Bath at Twickenham in 1985, and the third, Paul Morgan, then editor of *Rugby World* magazine, to which I subscribed.

'Imagine being paid to write about sport. I'd love to do that,' I said to Matt.

'Why don't you, then?' he replied.

A few months later, back in England, I was at midweek training with Rosslyn Park, where I'd picked up a few games, and hit a tackle bag with my right shoulder only for my left one to pop out of its socket. I hardly even felt it. It still came as a shock when the surgeon suggested it was probably time to concentrate on more sedate pursuits.

I moped for a few days before thinking back to my conversation with Matt. If I couldn't beat them, I'd try to join them.

There was a snag. Apart from obsessively reading the sports pages for the past 15 years, and being fascinated by the life of Donald Woods, the white South African newspaper editor who exposed the death in police custody of black human rights activist Steve Biko, and who the 1987 Richard Attenborough film *Cry Freedom* was based upon, I hadn't shown any actual interest in being a journalist. A letter published in the *Cricketer* magazine complaining about Ian Botham being picked for England's 1992 tour to New Zealand after missing the start because of Christmas pantomime commitments, and a solitary feature in the school magazine which Matt edited, headlined 'Carling, Back and Able', supporting Will Carling's return as England captain after labelling the Rugby Football Union (RFU) committee '57 old farts', hardly constituted a CV.

Somehow, City University offered me a deferred place on their post-graduate diploma course in newspaper journalism, on condition I spent a year gaining work experience to prove my commitment.

Unpaid stints on the sports desks of various newspapers including the *Richmond & Twickenham Times*, the *Daily Telegraph* and the *Scotsman* followed, but it was a two-week spell at the *Independent*, under the tutelage of sports editor Paul Newman, which really engaged me, provided my first by-line and, crucially, the all-important first paid work, as the Sunday PA on the news desk.

England won the Rugby World Cup in 2003, which for a trainee sports journalist, and a rugby-loving one at that, was rather good timing.

About 50 of us watched the final in the Pig & Whistle in East Sheen, drinking our first pint when the doors opened at 7am on Saturday and our last, some of us anyway, well into Sunday.

On Monday, I gave a presentation to my class at City titled 'The Cult of Jonny Wilkinson'. The 24-year-old who, in Ian Robertson's words, had just 'kicked England to World Cup glory' was on the front and back page of every paper and was the talk of every radio and television station. Rugby union had gone mainstream.

Goodwill towards rugby had, in England at least, never been greater and, after gaining my diploma, I secured a place on the Press Association's sports traineeship programme, based in Howden, East Yorkshire.

While at City, I'd watched on television as Wasps took on Gloucester in an all-English Heineken Cup quarter final at the Causeway Stadium, High Wycombe. Midway through the first half Lawrence Dallaglio and Paul Volley were involved in a sickening clash of heads in which both players were knocked unconscious attempting to make a tackle. Gloucester prop Phil Vickery was so alarmed by Volley's state he placed his opponent in the recovery position to prevent him swallowing his tongue.

Following extensive treatment, Volley was hauled back to his feet, still clearly unsteady, before, to everyone's astonishment, both players were allowed to carry on playing. When the half-time whistle blew, several minutes after the incident, Dallaglio needed assistance to reach the tunnel.

I thought to myself, 'That doesn't look right,' but, like pretty much everyone else, assumed they would not have been allowed to play on if it had been unsafe to do so.

2

Growth, growth, growth

To understand how radically and rapidly rugby union changed after becoming the last major participation sport to turn professional, you only had to watch it.

Almost overnight following the conclusion of the 1995 World Cup, rugby union, after more than a century of systematically denying payment to players, turned from a sport played for fun and a break from the day job into, well, the day job.

*

Historically fiercely resistant to players being paid to play, which debased Victorian notions of valour and fairness associated with playing sport purely for the love of it, or the 'Corinthian Spirit', as it was known, rugby union had been increasingly commercialized throughout the 1980s as formalized leagues in England made games more competitive and attractive to television audiences.

The inaugural 1987 World Cup, won by New Zealand, coincided with the formal acceptance of a league structure in England.

With the success of the second World Cup staged four years later in England and won by Australia, the move towards professionalism gathered pace. South Africa, Australia and New Zealand led the calls for rugby union to 'go open' almost 100 years after the so-called great schism had seen the establishment of rugby league in northern England. It was a move which essentially divided the sport along geographic and socio-economic lines.

For decades, league players, coaches and pundits derided their union counterparts for their lack of preparation, athleticism, skill, organization and physicality. And they had a point.

Conversely, union clung on blindly to its Corinthian values while avoiding the uglier face of professionalism, including a win-at-all-costs culture where head-high tackles, or hits, were commonplace, staying on the field with a brain injury had become normalized and coaches were undisputed top dogs.

Speaking about her first experience as a physiotherapist with Dewsbury, Lisa Hodgson, who in 2000 would become the Rugby Football League's first head of medicine, told the website Women in Rugby League:

> It was a first team fixture at Huddersfield and Sir Alex
> Murphy was the coach. And he knew it was my first game.
> The other two physiotherapists I was shadowing were away
> on conferences. One of the players went down. Alex Murphy
> grabbed me by the scruff of the neck, and he said, 'You don't
> bring that player off,' and then he looked me straight in the
> eyes and said, 'Unless he's —ing dead.' And then he pushed
> me onto the field. Well, I was shaking and then I went to the
> player, 'You look to be hurt.' He replied, 'Of course, I'm hurt!'
> I remember thinking, I can't do this. Once I was back off the
> field in the dug-out Alex Murphy turned and just winked at me,
> he said, 'Welcome to rugby.'

As television money poured in, union's amateur players, denied payments despite increasing demands on their time, became frustrated by the governing bodies' ideological resistance to paying them. Something had to give and, in August 1995, rugby union went pro.

'After the success of the World Cup in South Africa there had been almost an air of inevitability about it [going professional],' wrote former England captain Bill Beaumont in his 2017 autobiography. Beaumont retired in 1983 on the advice of neurologists and would go on to become chairman of the International Rugby Board (now World Rugby). He continued:

> The only problem was that we in England were ill prepared for it and rather caught with our pants down,
>
> Those who were determined to retain the game's almost unique amateur ethos were really backing a loser. It was no longer a game played purely for recreation. Events like the World Cup, increased television coverage and massive media interest had raised its profile to such an extent that the opportunities for making serious money out of the game seemed limitless.

In an earlier autobiography, *Thanks to Rugby*, Beaumont had written: 'I have always firmly believed no one should ever receive any money for actually playing rugby. The game, in that sense, must remain strictly amateur. If players were ever to be paid for playing, it would ruin the game itself and the whole structure of rugby in Britain.'

Almost in the blink of an eye, the shape of the players visibly changed and, inevitably, so too did rugby's physicality and risk profile. Once promoted as a game played by 'all shapes and sizes', professional rugby began to edge out the small guy. And one player was largely responsible: Jonah Lomu.

At 6ft 5in tall, weighing 18 stone and able to run 100 metres in under 11 seconds, Lomu's impact on the rugby landscape in 1995, aged 20, when he scored seven tries in five World Cup matches, is impossible to overstate.

The image of the marauding New Zealand All Black winger running directly over the top of England full back Mike Catt in the semi-final, eschewing any notion of a swerve or sidestep to trample over the 14 stone defender, is iconic.

After the game, which his side lost 45–29, England captain Will Carling said: 'He's a freak and the sooner he goes away the better.'

But Lomu didn't go away. Not for a while anyway. He would earn 73 international caps and score 43 tries, and his legacy would live on long after he died tragically young, aged 40, from a chronic kidney condition.

From 1995 every coach on earth wanted their own version of Jonah Lomu. He was rugby union's first, and arguably only, global icon.

'He was huge, he was quick and he was skilful,' said former Springbok Joel Stransky. 'To play against him was more stressful than you can imagine. Not just because one would need to tackle Jonah, which was not an inviting thought, but he drew defenders to him, which left other great players around him in space. Jonah's presence changed defensive structures and strategies forever.'

Previously, in the amateur game, the thought of a player of Lomu's dimensions playing anywhere other than the second or back rows was unthinkable.

In 1993, England head coach Geoff Cooke tore up the rule book by playing three No.8s in his back row, picking Dean Richards (6ft 3in, 17st 12lb) at No.8, alongside Ben Clarke (6ft 5in, 17st 5lbs) and Tim Rodber (6ft 6in, 17st 12lb) on the flanks to face New Zealand at Twickenham. It was the biggest international back row ever selected, but while all three were high-class international forwards, none of them had Lomu's speed of foot or sleight of hand. The thought of any of them playing in the three-quarters, positions traditionally reserved for players smaller, faster and nimbler than the ball-winning forwards, would have been absurd.

But while that trio's selection indicated rugby's direction of travel, Lomu's arrival two years later significantly upped the ante. Single-handedly he reframed rugby's optics and kicked off an arms race based on power and pace which no one in the new professional game could afford to ignore.

Players were free to lift weights and pop as many protein tablets as they could fit into a day's training while coaches had charge of their players for the full working day. And boy, did they work them.

Former Leicester and England captain Martin Johnson would later write in his autobiography:

> We were all crammed in together, craning our necks to see Bob [Dwyer] and his assistant, the former Wallaby prop Duncan Hall, and hanging on his every word. His message was simple and to-the-point: 'Being professional is not about being paid to play rugby, it's about the way you behave, the way you train, and the way you play. I'll see you all at the gym for weight training at 7a.m. on Monday.' There was a sharp intake of breath and a few people exchanged glances, but we all turned up as commanded the following Monday...
>
> We trained our backsides off in that first year. From meeting up two or three evenings a week and playing on the Saturday, suddenly we were all at the club twice a day.

But while many could see that the demands being placed on players were increasingly extreme, little was done to rein in potentially dangerous practice. Former England prop Jason Leonard wrote in his autobiography: 'There was much talk in the papers of the increasing pressures on players, and how unfair it was on them to have to train harder, but there was no real talk of anything ever being done about it.'

In 1987, when the first Rugby World Cup was held, the average weight of the New Zealand team in the final was 14st 7lb with their three-quarters averaging 12st 9lb and the forwards 16st 2lb. By the 2019 final, 24 years into professionalism, South Africa's average player weighed 16st 12lb with their three-quarter line averaging 14st 5lb and forwards a massive 18st 8lb each.

England's fly half George Ford, his side's smallest back at 13st 10lb, would have been the second heaviest player in New Zealand's 1987 backline.

With livelihoods now on the line, winning became the be all and end all. And teams spent a lot of time working out how to win.

According to the RFU's injury figures between 2002 and 2004, the teams finishing in the top four in the Premiership lost an average of about 600 player days per season through injury. The next four lost closer to 800. The bottom four lost around 1,000. Teams established that the fewer hours you lost to injury, the more games you won. Returning players faster than ever from injury became a commercial necessity and was culturally normalized.

With television money flooding in, laws were constantly tweaked to speed up the game and improve the spectacle. Rugby became a 'product', players 'assets', countries where it was played 'markets'.

A sport already demanding extreme bravery bordering on foolhardiness took on a new dimension. Players became fitter, faster, stronger. Collisions replaced contacts, hits replaced tackles. Passes became offloads.

Tackles were more frequent, scrums reduced, hits got bigger. Money rolled in. Audiences grew. This was boom time, rugby's goldrush. And there were cowboys everywhere.

With time to train, formerly amateur coaches made it up as they went along. With little or no regulation, some directors of rugby, many of whom had only just hung up their boots themselves, instituted extreme training regimes at club level.

Critically, before 2002 there was limited data on how the shift to professionalism had changed rugby's injury risk. In 2002/03, amid concerns over mounting injuries, the joint RFU and Premiership Rugby injury surveillance audit was launched to build the database.

The first year of the audit would therefore become rugby's injury baseline, although it was entirely probable this baseline had already shifted dramatically in the previous seven years.

Of course injuries became more severe as collisions intensified and became more frequent. But while it was possible to strengthen necks, shoulders and other parts of the human anatomy to withstand greater impacts, there is no means of strengthening the skull or the gelatinous brain inside.

As professional rugby's juggernaut got rolling, England's Rugby Football Union effectively parked in a lay-by, closed their eyes and hoped it would all go away by imposing a 12-month moratorium on professionalism. Meanwhile, players followed the money. Finally, after a year of absent leadership, the RFU lifted their moratorium and English professional rugby was allowed to proceed, albeit severely compromised. Steve Bale wrote in the *Independent*:

> All of a sudden money, with which rugby union has had an
> equivocal relationship ever since it started coining the stuff in
> sponsorships while denying players these fruits of their labours,
> talks. Those clubs who do not have enough, quite possibly
> including some of the giants of the game, are about to find that
> out the hard way. For an innately conservative sport, this is
> unalloyed Thatcherism.

Some clubs, like Richmond, played the get rich quick card, backed by former City trader Ashley Levett, who proceeded to lose an estimated £6 million in four years before pulling out in 1999. Once insolvent, Richmond were relegated seven divisions by the RFU in an act of unheralded spite. Richmond were far from the only English rugby club to get their numbers spectacularly wrong.

Why? Too much, too soon. At the advent of professionalism clubs scrambled for their 'best' players and salaries rocketed. Clubs agreed contracts for one, two, three years without detailed knowledge of their first year's income. In some cases unrealistic business plans were put in place and in others hearts ruled heads. Many club administrators and officials simply did not have enough expertise to administer annual payrolls of between £1 million and £2 million.

Many players had good occupations outside of sport but were pushed by their clubs into becoming full-time professionals. They were told they needed to train every day or they would not be picked.

'We all knew it would happen but the actual announcement caught everybody by surprise,' said former England fly half Rob Andrew in 2015. 'Soon everyone was running around trying to sign us up. No one had a clue what we were worth: I was a chartered surveyor working in London but within a few weeks I was on my way to Newcastle in a big leap into the unknown.'

Immediately, there was tension between the commercially aspirational clubs, who had signed up the players, and the uneasy defenders of financial good governance, the RFU, who were now not only in charge of the amateur game but also possessed a major stake in the newly formed professional game, out of which Premiership Rugby emerged as the commercial vehicle responsible for England's top league. Now, in sponsorship and TV rights terms, both organizations were fighting for the same pie. They had set themselves up as rivals and the players were the pawns. The RFU's failure to offer central contracts would prove a disaster for the health and wellbeing of England's top players.

*

For the players and a new breed of agents who emerged, it was time to cash in. As many former union stars who'd crossed codes for financial reasons in the late 1980s and early 1990s returned 'home', including the greats Alan Bateman, Scott Gibbs, Alan Tait, Scott Quinnell, Dai Young and John Bentley, union embraced their more professional approach. Soon, rugby league coaches also began to enter the rival code many had formerly mocked.

In October 1996, tragedy struck. Oxford University centre Ian Tucker died at London's National Hospital for Neurology and Neurosurgery two days after sustaining catastrophic brain damage attempting a try-saving tackle in a friendly game against Saracens.

This was a hellish scenario for a newly professional sport attempting to trade on an image which combined physicality, bravery, skill, but, above all, safety. The incident led some to raise concerns about where rugby was heading.

'Ian Tucker's death was caused by a freak accident, but it once more brought into focus how dangerous a collision sport can be,' wrote rugby journalist Ian Malin in his 1997 book *Mud, Blood and Money: English Rugby Union Goes Professional*. 'The 21-day rule for resting players is still abused and needs to be constantly monitored. Hopefully coaches and directors of rugby will be responsible enough not to flout it, even if it means resting key players for vital games.'

I have spoken to sources who told me Tucker had suffered a previous head injury less than a month before he died, while a report published in 1999 by Dr Jennian Geddes of the Royal London Hospital titled 'Neuronal cytoskeletal changes are an early consequence of repetitive head injury' examined the brains of 'two boxers, an amateur footballer and a mentally subnormal man who habitually banged his head'.

The 'footballer' was described as 'a 23-year-old man, a keen amateur footballer, who regularly "headed" the ball while playing.'

The report added that:

He was reported to have been previously well with no history of neurological disease, although he had had a single severe head injury in the past, from which he had made a full recovery (no further details available). He sustained a head injury while playing in a football match and developed an acute subdural haematoma and brain swelling, from which he died.

The report identified a specific gene, 'apoE', associated with poorer outcomes from repetitive head injuries while also finding that 'chronic mild repetitive head injury, such as that sustained by boxers, leads at an early age to subclinical but definable pathological changes'.

The report also stated: 'Similar neuropathological findings are present in all the cases: we believe that they are early changes caused by chronic head trauma, and as such represent a prelude to the fullblown pathology of dementia pugilistica.'

Through researching this book, I have read a footnote in a research paper published in 2015 by Professor Ann McKee which states: 'Although often referred to as a *soccer* player, the young subject with CTE described by Geddes et al. 1999 as the "keen amateur footballer who frequently 'headed' the ball while playing", was an amateur *rugby* player (personal communication, T. Revesz).' Chronic Traumatic Encephalopathy (CTE) was not a term which had, to my knowledge, ever been described in the British media. Certainly not in the sports pages. In fact, at the time, even the NHS had no reference to it on their website. This would soon change. CTE was essentially the rebranding of an old and established neurodegenerative disease caused by repetitive head injuries called *dementia pugilistica* and first identified in deceased boxers by Harrison Martland almost a century earlier. One expert would later describe it as 'akin to a crack in the windscreen of a start where over time it gets progressively worse and you need to replace the entire windscreen. But you can't replace a brain.'

How this apparent mistake in identifying this unfortunate individual occurred remains to be seen. But it is my understanding that this rugby player, wrongly identified as a footballer, was Ian Tucker.

*

The 1997 British and Irish Lions tour broke new ground as manager Fran Cotton, a seven-time former Lion turned successful entrepreneur, teamed up with Ian McGeechan, the coach of the 1989 Lions who won the series 2–1 in Australia, to form a strong coaching partnership with a shared vision of combining the old with the new. Their squad selection was radical, with several players who had barely featured at international level since returning from league, including Tait, Bentley, Young, Quinnell and Gibbs, alongside a core of established union stars including incumbent England captain Lawrence Dallaglio and bruising Leicester lock Martin Johnson, who was a surprise choice as captain.

That tour opened many people's eyes, including my own, to the realities of professionalism, with groundbreaking fly-on-the-wall documentary *Living with the Lions* charting a largely harmonious tour off the pitch with heightened physicality on it.

The image of young England centre Will Greenwood's head snapping back on the ground before he lay motionless, attended by increasingly fraught medics after he swallowed his tongue and stopped breathing for several minutes, was captured on film in graphic detail.

Clive Woodward took over from Jack Rowell as England coach in 1997 and he too recognized the value of tapping into rugby league and other sports outside union to gather valuable insight into what it took to be truly professional. Ultimately, Woodward was interested in winning and he set about systematically overhauling England's training methods, diet and overall outlook. He was a risk taker, empowering players to make their own decisions on the field and, with the financial clout of the RFU behind him, providing a backroom set-up unrivalled in world rugby, including taking his team away from their historical pre-match hotel the Petersham, a five-minute walk from Richmond's town centre, into the more serene and luxury environment of Pennyhill Park, 20 miles away. One of Woodward's first appointments, and arguably his best, was former Great Britain rugby league head coach Phil Larder as England's first full-time defence coach.

Larder had been introduced to Woodward by Cotton, who had read out a message to the entire Lions squad before the first Test in South Africa that summer titled 'Defence wins championships', signed by the Great Britain players.

After the tour Larder met Woodward, who sold him on the vision of beating the southern hemisphere's big three, notably Australia.

A strong coaching partnership emerged. But while league had long since recognized and responded to the need to look after players during the week to ensure their readiness for matchdays, union's training methods were Neanderthal by comparison.

'The first training session I observed [before England played New Zealand] was taken by the forwards coach John Mitchell. It was long, drawn-out and often barbaric,' Larder described in his autobiography *The Iron Curtain.*

> As an ex-All Black coaching against his own country 'Mitch' was determined to make a statement to the England squad about the level of commitment needed to be successful… I can still remember him saying 'Phil, what you don't understand is how tough the rucks are in union; for players to perform well in an international on Saturday, training must be tougher than the game. They have to understand how tough international rugby is, and the only way to prepare them is to make training tougher.'

But while this attitude was entrenched early on in professional union, with a default setting of 'work harder' rather than 'work smarter', Larder brought a more enlightened perspective.

> Frankly I felt that this kind of beasting belonged in the coaching stone age. With the advent of full-time professionalism, league training sessions had concentrated more on skill development and decision-making and had

tended to become shorter and less brutal. The game itself had become far more physical as the impact of collisions between the ball-carrier and the tackler increased. The opinion of the British Medical Association was that the human body could no longer handle more than one game a week and the RFL [governing body of rugby league football in England] had made a concerted effort to remove all midweek fixtures so as to reduce the number of injuries. Prolonged contact sessions were therefore a thing of the past.

Mitch certainly worked the forwards hard and was well respected by them because of it. That was the way in union at that time.

Larder's influence helped tone down England's training sessions under Woodward, making them more focused on skill, technique and thinking clearly under pressure. At the same time, England got serious about defence.

Phrases like 'line speed', 'offload', 'winning the collision' and 'dominating the tackle' entered union's lexicon. With the game speeding up, coaches recognized that the faster the ball was recycled, the less time opponents had to organize defences. Conversely, defence coaches recognized there was often no need to commit more than a couple of players to the breakdown.

Where previously young rugby union players were taught to tackle passively, now the tackle was seen as a potential weapon with which to 'hit' an opponent, potentially dislodging the ball in the process. Players started to aim tackles higher up the torso, not at the waist or just below, as had been traditional in the sport for the best part of a century. Highly risky two-man 'double' tackles also entered union.

Under Woodward, and in direct response to Lomu, England were among the teams who experimented by picking backline players who previously would only ever have been picked up front. England's last-gasp defeat to Wales at Wembley in April 1999 should not only be remembered for Scott Gibbs's brilliant match-winning try, but also as the game in which England winger Steve Hanley (6ft 4in, 16st 8lb) and centre Barrie-Jon Mather (6ft 7in, 16st 4lb) both made their first and last appearances for England.

While neither Hanley nor Mather played internationally again, the direction of travel for the sport was set. In 2001, a promising Northampton Saints front-row forward called Steve Thompson was selected for England's summer tour to North America. At 6ft 2in and close to 19 stone, Thompson was significantly taller and heavier than any England hooker ever previously selected. By contrast, England's hooker in the 1991 World Cup final against Australia, Brian Moore, was just 5ft 9in tall and weighed 14st 9lb, while Jeff Probyn, England's tighthead prop in the same game, stood 5ft 10in tall and weighed under 16 stone.

Thompson was not just significantly bigger than both – indeed he was bigger than any England front player to be selected before the professional era – but he was also faster, more athletic and more dynamic. Having started his career in the back row, he had moved through the second row and into the front row as the game had rapidly evolved in the post-Lomu late 1990s. Australia's Tommy Lawton had set the bar for giant hookers in the 1980s, with Argentina's Federico Méndez and Wallaby Phil Kearns following, and Thompson's emergence consolidated that upward trend. His rise to prominence in the front row symbolized the changing face of rugby union almost as much as Lomu's appearance in the three-quarters had done six years earlier. Undeniably, rugby's top players were getting bigger across every position.

Naturally, as players grew bigger, faster, stronger and laws were tweaked to attract new audiences, the game also started to speed up which meant more tackles, more rucks and more collisions. Even those of us with the most basic grasp of physics have some kind of handle on Newton's laws of motion, especially the second, which can be simply expressed as: 'Force equals mass (weight) times acceleration.'

It stood to reason that as players got bigger and faster, and with more ball-in-play time and more collisions through rucks and tackles – which was certainly happening by the start of the 21st century – the impacts on the field increased in volume and ferocity, leading inevitably to a greater number of injuries. Critically, training sessions, became longer, more frequent and intense, with injuries increasing as a result too.

Coaches looked for every edge to gain competitive advantage. 'You'd get told to use your head to clear out. That's what you got told to use. "It's the best weapon you've got. Look at the size of your head. Use it",' Steve Thompson told the BBC in 2022.

> At the end of the week you'd just think to yourself 'how on earth am I going to play this game'.
>
> There were many more impacts and they were faster and harder. At hooker the pressure on my head was relentless and enormous. There were scrum sessions where the scrum machine would be pegged into the ground so it wouldn't move.
>
> There'd be so much pressure the scrum machine would be bending up as it wouldn't give. The pressure would go all the way through your body and as everyone broke off you'd just pass out.
>
> I'd have a few seconds to come around and then just do it again. You'd have burst blood vessels all round your eyes. It was madness.

*

In rugby union it had been mandatory since 1977 for any player diagnosed with concussion to be stood down for three weeks and only return to play when cleared by a neurologist. Early on in professionalism it was obvious head injuries were on the rise but with rugby evolving so fast and the quest for growth so all-consuming, concussions were often laughed off while directors of rugby habitually pressured players to stay on the pitch. Many players needed no convincing. Playing on with a concussion was normal practice.

But what if we had been told more of the historical work which had established the link between repetitive head injuries and longer-term neurological damage? What precisely was known and when of the long-term effects of concussion?

A brief history of concussion

(With special thanks to Professors Tony Collins and Stephen Casper) Stephen Casper, professor of the history of medicine at Clarkson University in New York State, explains:

> It has been recognized for a long time that concussions are dangerous injuries with potentially life-changing consequences, ranging from permanent symptoms to degenerative neurological states. The intellectual history of medicine and science from 1870 to the recent past shows both a continuity of clinical observations about head injuries and a steady, incremental accumulation of knowledge refining our understanding of those observations from a remarkably wide sphere of scientific disciplines.

Concussion has been observed since ancient times. It is mentioned in Ancient Greek medical texts as 'commotion of the brain'. The 10th-century Persian physician Razi was the first to distinguish concussion from other head injuries, and his definition of the condition as a transient loss of function with no physical damage was the standard medical understanding of concussion for centuries.

Until the 17th century a concussion was usually described by its clinical features. But after the invention of the microscope physicians began to understand there were underlying physical and structural mechanisms involved.

In 1839, Guillaume Dupuytren described brain contusions, which involve many small haemorrhages, as contusio cerebri and showed the difference between unconsciousness associated with damage to the brain and that due to concussion, without such injury.

Traumatic dementia, caused by head trauma, was described in research papers as early as the 1890s (Kramer), while traumatically induced motor neurone disease and Parkinsonian syndrome were identified in 1911 (Woods) and 1934 (Grimberg) respectively.

In 1905, surgeon William Bennett noted that concussions can occur even when 'no loss of consciousness occurs at all' and can 'have far graver results' than concussions which are immediately treated due to loss of consciousness. Bennett noted that symptoms of impartial recovery from concussions included criminal inclinations, ill-temper, proneness to suicide and insanity.

Also in 1905, the *Journal of the American Medical Association* editors noted that American football players risked being left a 'lunatic for life', mentioning 'brain injuries resulting in insanity'.

In 1928, neuropathologist Harrison Martland described the clinical features of the neurodegenerative disease chronic traumatic encephalopathy (CTE) caused by repeated blows to the head when he performed autopsies on traumatic cerebral haemorrhage cases among boxers.

The haemorrhages Martland found were microscopic in nature and he proposed a connection between these and boxers who experienced neurological symptoms, or 'punch-drunk syndrome', after suffering repetitive head trauma.

In 1934, Dr Harry Parker built on Martland's thesis and presented more evidence of CTE's existence, noting that 'punch drunkenness' can present as a 'medley' of symptoms through different symptomatic time courses.

In 1936, Dr Edward J. Carroll Jr published 'Punch Drunk' in the *American Journal of the Medical Sciences*. Carroll stated: 'No head blow is taken with impunity, and each knock-out causes definite and irreparable damage. If such trauma is repeated for a long enough period, it is inevitable nerve cell insufficiency will develop.'

In 1937, J. A. Millspaugh published an article presenting more examples of cognitive dysfunction in naval boxers suffering from dementia and disorientation. Millspaugh also renamed 'punch-drunk syndrome' as 'dementia pugilistica'.

In 1952, Augustus Thorndike, chief of surgery at Harvard, recommended that American football players should retire after three concussions.

In 1955, Elisha Gurdjian and colleagues noted cellular damage to the brain caused by 'sub-concussive' blows.

In 1962, Sir Charles Symonds described patients with 'punch-drunk syndrome' who gradually developed mental and physical signs of diffuse brain damage despite concussion never having been severe but where it had been repeated and there had been frequent sub-concussive blows.

In April 1975, the Irish Rugby Football Union organized the 'International Congress on Injuries in Rugby Football and Other Team Sports'. Scotland coach Bill Dickinson told the conference: 'I am also concerned about head injuries. There seems to me, and this is only impression, there are more of these injuries going about. Collisions are more likely because it is "fluid", the pace of these collisions are more likely to increase, and this also gives me some concern.'

At the same congress, Peter Carey, a consultant neurosurgeon at Dublin's St Lawrence's Hospital, presented a paper titled 'Brain Injuries in Sport' in which he stated: 'The most constant feature of primary damage to the brain in blunt head injuries is diffuse neuronal injury, that is injury to the nerve cells of the brain. Even after relatively mild injuries such as a boxing knockout many brain cells die and are never replaced. Repeated injuries of this type have a cumulative effect and are responsible for the syndrome known as "punch-drunk".'

In 1975, the *Lancet* published a paper by D. Gronwall and P. Wrightson entitled 'Cumulative Effect of Concussion' in which they presented their findings that the effects of concussion seemed to be cumulative and noted the implications for sports where such injuries were common.

In February 1976, the *Lancet* published an editorial on 'Brain Damage in Sport' which, although focused on the dangers of boxing, also acknowledged the potential for 'punch-drunk syndrome' in rugby.

Also in 1976, a paper in the *Lancet* entitled 'Brain Damage in National Hunt Jockeys' by J. Foster, R. Leiguarda and P. Tilley revealed that 'Five National Hunt jockeys have been found to have post-traumatic encephalopathy – three with epilepsy and two with significant intellectual and psychological deterioration.'

In his paper 'Diagnosis of Concussion on the Field', Geoffrey Vanderfield, a neurosurgeon who would later become the medical advisor to the Australian Rugby Union, argued that 'the player who has had a severe concussion should not play for at least three weeks and until a medical clearance'.

Vanderfield's recommendation was adopted by the International Rugby Board (IRB) in 1977 when it set up its Medical Advisory Committee. The IRB stance would be articulated in its Resolution 5.7: 'a player who has suffered definite concussion should not participate in any match or training session for a period of at least three weeks from the time of injury and then only subject to being cleared by a proper neurological examination.'

In 1980, the *British Medical Journal* published a paper entitled 'Serious Head Injury in Sport'. The authors noted that it had already been demonstrated that the effects of repeated minor injury are cumulative and had been shown to cause traumatic encephalopathy in boxers and jockeys, and it had been posited that a similar encephalopathy may occur in other sports, including rugby football.

In August 1985, the official journal of the RFU, *Rugby World & Post*, noted that 'in recent years there has been increasing concern amongst medical workers who see the long-term effects, that concussion is one of the most serious injuries that can be sustained by any participants in sport'.

In a 1993 article, 'Risks and Injuries in Rugby Football', Donald Macleod, a medical advisor to the Scottish Rugby Union (SRU), stated:

> The essential feature with concussion is to recognize it is associated with brain damage. The player may appear to make a rapid and complete recovery in a very short time but there is a sustained and ill-defined period during which the brain has a reduced ability to process information. In addition the severity and duration of the functional impairment is increased with repeated concussions.

Macleod stressed that 'the accepted recommendations in modern rugby are that any player having a second concussion in a single season should avoid all contact sport for three months; if a third concussion is sustained within the same season he should avoid all contact sport for six months'.

In March 1997, *The Lancet* reported on the American Academy of Neurology's newly published guidelines on concussion in sports, explicitly naming rugby and American football. It stated that 'over time, athletes who have been concussed can develop mental dysfunction, sleep disturbances, light-headedness and tinnitus'.

In 1999, Oxford University Press published *Mild Head Injury: A Guide to Management* by D. Gronwall and P. Wrightson. They reiterated their previous findings and stated: 'It is well known that people who have been concussed a number of times – rugby footballers and boxers in particular – change in character and lose some of their abilities.'

In 2001, Stephen Marshall and Richard Spencer published the paper 'Concussion in Rugby: The Hidden Epidemic', which concluded that the incidence of concussion in rugby was probably much higher than previously suggested.

In 2002, in Zurich, the First Consensus Statement of the Concussion in Sport Group (CISG) – a cohort of experts organized by international sports federations (including, since 2008, the IRB/ World Rugby) who meet approximately every four years to establish a consensus on the scientific understanding of concussion in sport – made no specific mention of the long-term impact of concussion, other than that further research was needed.

The same year, a post-mortem examination of Mike Webster, a former NFL player, confirmed that he had died from chronic traumatic encepalopathy (CTE).

Also in 2002, the initial post-mortem and inquest concluded that the degenerative brain disease that led to the death of former English professional footballer Jeff Astle had been caused by his repeated heading of footballs.

In 2005, a University of Turin study of 7,325 male professional football players in Italy found a 'highly significant relationship playing professional football and ALS [amyotrophic lateral sclerosis, a form of motor neurone disease] in a large retrospective cohort' and proposed a range of possible football-related contributory factors including heading, increased exposure to fertilizers and herbicide or use of performance-enhancing drugs.

In 2009, the CISG's Third Consensus Statement acknowledged the suggested association between sports concussions and late-life cognitive impairment. It was agreed clinicians 'need to be mindful of the potential for long-term problems in the management of all athletes'.

In the same year, the NFL acknowledged that 'it's quite obvious from the medical research that's been done that concussions can lead to long-term problems'.

A 2012 retrospective cohort study of 3,439 former NFL players found their risk of dying from neurodegenerative causes was three times higher than the general US population, and their risk of dying from motor neuron disease or Alzheimer's disease was four times higher.

*

By the dawn of the millennium, discussions about the long-term risks associated with repeatedly banging your head in sport appeared to be intensifying. US military veterans who survived blasts from Improvised Explosive Devices in Iraq and Afghanistan subsequently demonstrated significant behavioural changes during their lifetimes, while post-mortem examinations of their brains discovered similar pathologies to those which would soon be found in the brains of deceased NFL players.

The first Concussion in Sport Group meeting was held in Berlin in 2001, chaired by a man who had already established himself as one of the 'go to' doctors for contact sports. Having spent 15 years as the team doctor at high-profile Australian Football League club Collingwood, Paul McCrory had significant experience in managing and treating head injuries pitchside and understood the dynamic that existed between players, coaches and doctors involved in professional contact sports.

In early 1999, McCrory had published a paper in the *British Journal of Sports Medicine* (*BJSM*), titled 'The Eighth Wonder of the World: the Mythology of Concussion Management', in which he highlighted the lack of coherent thinking when it came to the pitchside management of athletes who'd suffered head injuries but, naturally, wanted to return to the field of play. He argued:

In sports medicine, doctors and others providing athletic care recognise and manage a spectrum of brain injury. Unlike severe brain injury, however, the management of concussion is mostly derived from anecdotal experience. In many cases current management practices have more in common with mythology than science.

There is no universal agreement on the standard definition of concussion. The most widely accepted definition in sports medicine is that originally proposed by the Congress of Neurological Surgeons, a professional association representing neurosurgeons, neurosurgical residents, medical students, and allied health professionals. It states that 'concussion is a clinical syndrome characterised by the immediate and transient post-traumatic impairment of neural function...'

McCrory went on to pinpoint ten 'myths' around concussion while reiterating a player had to be knocked unconscious to have suffered a concussion. Much of the paper was common sense, although it tiptoed into controversial ground by appearing to cast doubt on a rare but widely recognized phenomenon known as second impact syndrome (SIS) which informed a lot of concussion thinking, due to the widely held view that the risk of fatal brain damage was increased once an initial trauma had been sustained. Children were known to be especially vulnerable.

From 1980 to 1993, the National Center for Catastrophic Sports Injury Research, based in North Carolina, identified 35 'probable' cases of SIS in American football players.

In 2011, 14-year-old Ben Robinson would become the first British rugby player to be formally diagnosed as having died from Second Impact Syndrome, while in 2013, Canadian 17-year-old Rowan Stringer's cause of death was also found to be SIS; she was captain of her high school rugby team.

But McCrory challenged the very existence of second impact syndrome, citing a study he had conducted two years earlier. Under a subheading, 'The myth of second impact syndrome', McCrory stated:

> Diffuse cerebral oedema is a rare but recognised complication of mild brain injury in sport, which occurs in children. It has been postulated that a form of diffuse brain swelling may be the consequence of a repeated minor head injury, the so-called second impact syndrome. Belief in this concept rests on the interpretation of anecdotal reports. In such cases the evidence that repeated concussion is a risk factor for this entity is not compelling.

The paper becomes progressively less sympathetic towards the idea that players who have been diagnosed with concussion should necessarily be stood down for an extended period – while also casting doubt on other conditions which had become associated with head injuries, including epilepsy. Under a subheading, 'The myth of post-traumatic epilepsy', McCrory declared: 'Concussive convulsions are an uncommon but dramatic association of minor head injury. Although often assumed to be epileptic in origin, a recent study [which McCrory authored] has delineated their benign nature. From a clinical standpoint, late seizures do not occur, anti-epileptic treatment is not indicated, and prohibition from collision sport is unwarranted.'

Most tellingly, McCrory insisted it was a 'myth' that players who had suffered a concussion were at greater risk of suffering further injury if they carried on playing, while also stating that the idea of cumulative damage caused by multiple head injuries was another 'myth': 'It has become a widely held belief that having had a concussive injury, one is more prone to future concussive injury. Although suggested by retrospective studies, recent prospective studies have not supported this concept but show that the subsequent injury rate reflects the amount of time playing the sport rather than any inherent risk.'

In 2001, soon after taking over as editor of the *BJSM*, McCrory published another article, titled 'When to retire after concussion?', in which he stated: 'There is no scientific evidence that sustaining several concussions over a sporting career will necessarily result in permanent damage.' He went on to describe other previously accepted science around head injuries as 'neuromythology'. This was of course music to sport's ears.

Meanwhile, in England, club versus country tensions were superficially eased by the Elite Player Squad agreement between the RFU and Premiership clubs which gave England's head coach a limited amount of access to 40 top stars. The deal, agreed in June 2004, was an unsustainable fudge. But with clubs wanting their players to peak at certain key points in their fixture calendar, conflict between club and country was baked into the deal. England's elite players were caught in the impossible position of having to serve two masters. And two increasingly demanding ones at that.

Under the agreement, a total of 59 players (40 senior squad, 15 Senior National Academy and four Sevens players) came under the direction of the England head coach, National Academy manager Brian Ashton, and Sevens coach Mike Friday. The process would be centrally managed by the RFU's performance director Chris Spice.

Elite Player Squad players received individual playing, training and rest programmes, planned jointly by the RFU and their clubs with an upper limit of 32 on the number of 'matches', defined as 40 minutes of play or more, a player could play for their club and country and an 11-week off-season period of preparation.

It looked good on paper but was not adequately policed. In 2012/13, England and Leicester prop Dan Cole featured in 41 games before requiring surgery on a bulging disk in his neck the following year.

In 2022, a study by Bath University would find that players who played more than 31 games a season faced a 'significantly higher injury burden'.

The off-season break was also routinely ignored. Indeed, the so-called guaranteed 11-week break was chipped away so routinely that by 2017 the Rugby Players' Association (RPA) 'celebrated' a new deal guaranteeing five weeks off between seasons. There is a concept in the environmental movement called 'shifting baseline theory' where, as the environment is degraded on a local, regional and global scale, people's tolerance of this degradation grows. People's accepted thresholds for environmental conditions are continually lowered and their acceptance of degradation increases with each passing generation. The shifting baseline theory could be applied to rugby: the players struggled to notice, but in every way things were getting worse for them.

Two years earlier, in 2002, two more very significant developments took place. Firstly, the RFU and Premiership Rugby, in a rare public display of unity, and amid growing concern at what appeared to be a significant spike in serious injuries, jointly commissioned the first comprehensive injury surveillance study across the Premiership and England teams. The study, then known as the professional rugby injury audit, was organized, administered and reported on by the RFU and Premiership Rugby, with assistance from Bath University, in an initiative which was widely welcomed as an important development in player welfare. The second development occurred in the United States and few would know about it for three years. An American neuropathologist performed an autopsy on NFL hall of famer Mike Webster, who had died of a heart attack aged 50, having spent his final years living out of a pickup truck or in doorways in train stations between Wisconsin and Pittsburgh. Webster suffered terrible neurological problems after ending his 16-year playing career, in which he'd suffered countless head injuries and battled amnesia, depression and chronic insomnia. Towards the end, Webster took to electrocuting himself just to get to sleep.

That single detailed medical examination in a Pittsburgh mortuary would change the course of sport forever.

The timing of the launch of the rugby injury audit was not directly related to Webster's autopsy. But it is reasonable to surmise that, with growing unease in the United States about the possibility of lasting damage to those exposed to the contact sport for an extended period, senior figures within rugby would have been keeping a very close eye on developments.

*

An article in *The Times* stopped me in my tracks in April 2002. In it Dean Ryan, the former England, Wasps and Newcastle No.8, said the cause of his recently diagnosed epilepsy had been mismanaged concussions at the end of his career.

Having been knocked out three times in a week while playing for Newcastle Falcons, Ryan, who was Bristol's head coach in 2002, ignored official guidelines, which at the time instructed any player suspected of having concussion to stand down for a minimum of three weeks, and continued playing.

'Who was going to tell me not to play in a title run in?' he said.

The article described scans revealing bruising around Ryan's brain and went on to promote a 'revolutionary test' developed by a doctor in Melbourne, Paul McCrory, to be introduced by England's leading clubs in the following months.

The new system of psychometric testing known as CogSport was reportedly being analysed by the RFU, which would send new guidelines to clubs to deal with concussed players.

A deal with the RFU, debt free and with net assets at the time of £30 million and the most commercially influential union in the world, had the potential to be hugely lucrative.

The idea behind CogSport was that, through eight computer-based card games, taking about 15 minutes each to complete, players' 'baseline' psychometric score could be established before each season and then compared after a suspected concussion. Players were tested for decision-making, memory, reaction times, problem-solving and other cognitive functions.

'How long can bigger, fitter players who are playing more games in a season and have less recovery time continue to take the big hits?' asked Dr Graeme Wilkes, who helped draw up the new RFU concussion guidelines along with their head of medicine Dr Simon Kemp.

> That is potentially a recipe for disaster unless concussion
> is managed optimally. If boxing is in the premier league for
> concussion, rugby along with ice hockey, American football
> and Aussie rules are in the first division, vying for promotion.
>
> The game today is faster, stronger, with bigger impacts. The
> concern is what effect this will have on players in the future.
> It might be that Dean Ryan's plight is the first in a series of
> problems we will see in ex-players. We really do not know.
> We must do the research and we must, in the meantime, ensure
> optimum care for today's players. What we are doing is trying
> to get across the concept of a rehabilitation process for the
> brain, as players do with, say, a hamstring injury.

*

All the while, professional rugby continued to speed up, as collisions grew bigger and more frequent. In 1987, when the first World Cup was played, there were on average just 94 tackles per match. With no tactical substitutions in those days, this meant, give or take, an average of three tackles per player, per match. With international male players averaging around 14st 2lb in the late 1980s and tackle techniques still very much focused on the passive 'rolling' technique which used the ball carrier's momentum to fell the player around the legs, rugby union was still very much a 'contact' rather than 'collision' sport. By 1995, the year rugby turned professional, this figure had risen by 19 tackles per game to an average of 113.

In November 2002, England played South Africa at Twickenham in a game which saw Springbok lock Jannus Labuschagne sent off for a late tackle on Jonny Wilkinson after 23 minutes. The game, which England won 55-3, was notable for the extreme violence enacted largely, although not solely, by Springbok captain Korne Krige.

Dawson, the England scrum half, was one of four England players concussed, with Wilkinson, Jason Robinson and Phil Christophers the others, when Krige's swinging arm caught him flush in the face before continuing on to knock out his own player, fly half Andre Pretorius.

Dawson was attended through the game by team doctor Simon Kemp, but allowed to play on.

Afterwards, Woodward said: 'We have got to be very careful as a sport. In the cold light of day everybody in the game has got to look at what went on. There were a lot of cheap shots. The players won't say anything, because they're not that sort of team, but I can.'

In 2018, Dawson would tweet 'I'd love to say I remember it well but he [Krige] knocked me in to the next day…. I played on for 10/15 mins calling all my club moves… unfortunately I do fear there'll be plenty of consequences in the long term for me. #brutalgame #notformykids' prompting Krige to admit he had been 'ashamed' of his actions that day.

By 2003, however, when Woodward's team won the World Cup, the average number of tackles per match had more than doubled to a staggering 189 per game.

A small mitigating factor was that tactical substitutions allowed for 22 players each side per match. This would increase to 23 players, or eight substitutes each team, in 2009. This slightly reduced the overall number of tackles made in a match for each player, although there is a strong argument that tactical substitutions make rugby even more dangerous as fatigued players face off against fresh players late in the game.

In many ways Jonny Wilkinson was the embodiment of change. For the best part of a century the fly half, rugby's equivalent of the star quarterback in American football, was not expected to tackle effectively on top of their duties as main playmaker. Indeed, I recall watching Les Cusworth, weighing around 11 stone, play against Wales at Twickenham in 1988 and barely attempting a tackle all game.

By 2003, this had all changed. Wilkinson, a fiercely driven competitor whose dedication to training was revered by team-mates, opponents and coaches alike, was at the vanguard of change. One hit he made on France's experienced and notoriously powerful winger Emile N'tamack in Paris during the 2000 Six Nations was so eye-wateringly physical it almost defied belief. As N'tamack cut a line from the blindside wing to take a trademark switch pass inside from France fly half Freddie Michalak, he met the muscular shoulder of England's young No.10 which hit him around his sternum. N'tamack was lifted up and dumped several feet backwards on the floor. It was, and still would be today, an entirely legal tackle, demonstrating near perfect technique.

Sky Sports commentator Miles Harrison was not alone in being shocked by the force of the tackle.

'And it's Wilkinson again,' Harrison said. 'He's flattened N'tamack. The half-time whistle goes but N'tamack will wish it was the full-time whistle. Just treated like a tackle bag. Brilliant.'

That tackle, perhaps more than any other between 1995 and 2003, encapsulated rugby union's rapidly evolving face. A 6ft 2in, 14st 7lb winger 'treated like a tackle bag' by a brutally physical fly half making tackles which would make an NFL linebacker wince.

It was evident, to anybody watching, that rugby union had changed forever.

3

Someone's going to have to die

I moved north in the summer of 2003 to begin life at the Press Association (PA). My starting salary was £11,000 a year and I rented a small semi-detached house on the outskirts of York with a friend from City University, Mike McGrath.

We worked shifts across weekends and bank holidays, with the Christmas Day 7am to 3pm one to avoid. There were early starts and late nights, inputting sports-related data to service PA's myriad commercial tie-ins including Teletext and the Six Nations and Premier League websites. Accuracy and speed of copy were prized. What happened? To whom? When? Where? How? Now.

With so much competition, the opportunities for aspiring football journalists like Mike to get out on the road and cover games, especially the big ones, were limited.

Rugby union games, by contrast, were in less demand. So I set about making North of England rugby my 'patch'.

Newcastle was a short train ride from York. The Falcons had, like Richmond, been among the first clubs to embrace professionalism, with Sir John Hall essentially buying the club's first Premier League title in 1998, having signed seasoned England internationals Rob Andrew and Dean Ryan from Wasps, along with former rugby league stars Inga Tuigamala, Alan Tait and John Bentley, and Scotland internationals Doddie Weir and Gary Armstrong. In the same season a certain Jonny Wilkinson made his debut, aged 18.

By the time I started at PA, Wilkinson's 'brand' had gone global. His name on a team sheet guaranteed attention from the national press, although this was infrequent as Wilkinson's injury struggles over the next four years brought rugby's physical nature into focus.

Sale Sharks, playing at Stockport County's Edgeley Park ground, were the coming force in English rugby under former France winger Philippe Saint-André. With England World Cup winner Jason Robinson, rising star Mark Cueto and Jos Baxendell alongside Charlie Hodgson in the midfield and a youthful Ben Foden out wide, Sharks had a top-class backline and brutish pack including Sébastien Chabal, Andrew Sheridan, Ignacio Fernández Lobbe and Scotland's Jason White.

Leeds Tykes were the poor relations of the three, seemingly always struggling for form and commercial relevance under the personable former Wales No.8 Phil Davies. But even Tykes, living in the shadow of an uncomfortable ground share with rugby league giants Leeds Rhinos, had a host of promising English youngsters, including Tom Palmer and Tom Biggs, playing alongside another World Cup winner experiencing a career-threatening injury run, Iain Balshaw.

I was always happiest out on the road reporting and I'd routinely arrive at grounds and pinch myself that this was now my job. But despite the elation at being paid to cover the sport I loved, a constant theme kept emerging in my reports: injuries. To start with at least, I parked my concerns. I had a living to make and a career to forge.

Mum occasionally used to bring a copy of the *Daily Mail* back from a hospital shift but otherwise I never read it growing up. So, while I knew of most of the broadsheet rugby writers before I got to PA, I'd never heard of the *Daily Mail*'s rugby correspondent Peter Jackson. That would soon change. The first time I found myself in a press conference 'huddle' with Jackson, I was immediately taken by his self-confidence, style and razor-sharp questioning. In a media landscape increasingly driven by quotes 'Jacko' invariably got the line. He was polite but relentless. Assured but not arrogant. And boy did he have his finger on the pulse. There was no one in rugby Peter Jackson couldn't pick the phone up to. The more I read what he wrote, the more I realized how good he was.

I observed Jackson closely. He would often detach himself from the 'pack' and slink off without anyone noticing. Heads would spin twitchily when his rivals realized he wasn't in the room. He'd be off hiding in the shadows ready to pounce on an unsuspecting subject to garner information no one else had or grab an exclusive quote. He was normally the last to leave the ground and never seemed flustered. I admired him enormously.

In September 2004, less than 10 months after leading England to World Cup glory, Sir Clive Woodward quit. Jackson, of course, was all over the story.

It had been clear for some time that Woodward was frustrated at the Elite Player Squad agreement made that June between the RFU and Premiership clubs, which permitted strictly limited periods of access for England's coaches to their top players.

England had got across the line by the skin of their teeth in Australia to win the World Cup. With Martin Johnson, Matt Dawson, Neil Back, Richard Hill, Jason Leonard and Will Greenwood nearing the end of their careers – and rugby's schedules and physical demands set to get even more gruelling – Woodward saw a chance, with rugby buoyant, to repair the damage done by the RFU's failure to act in 1995 by centrally contracting the country's top players. Woodward wanted England's biggest stars fit for the biggest games.

Leading up to 1998, the Rugby Players' Association was formed by a collective of former players, among them recently retired Wasps and England centre Damian Hopley, who were growing increasingly concerned about the physical toll the sport was taking on the top players, while also recognizing the need for representation in disputes over salaries, match fees and commercial rights.

According to Michael Aylwin in his book *Unholy Union: When Rugby Collided with the Modern World*, 'Player collectives in America and Australia are legally bound to be independent from the governing bodies they negotiate with – and are ferociously so. When proper collective bargaining agreements are hammered out, industrial action, including lock-outs, is common.' But the RPA was most certainly not independent.

In 2004, the RPA became the exclusive commercial representative of the England team, performing the following duties on their behalf: negotiation with the RFU over the Elite Player Squad contract, England and Saxons (the men's second team) match fees, England team win bonuses and image rights payments.

But with the vast majority of the organization's funding coming directly from the RFU and Premiership Rugby, the players' union was compromised. The very organizations their members needed protecting from controlled their purse strings. How could they drive the hardest bargain for England players, not just in terms of appearance fees but also around rest periods and in-season breaks, when they were negotiating with the people who had the power to withdraw their principal source of funding?

With the huge uplift in media interest, player participation and general feelgood factor around English rugby promising more investment in early 2004, Woodward convinced RFU chief executive Francis Baron to find the budget to centrally contract a core of top stars. He knew the only way to achieve sustained success, with so many competing interests, was to have control of when, where and how much his best players trained and played. It made both commercial and ethical sense.

Midway through 2004, Woodward believed he had made a breakthrough in his discussions with Baron in freeing up a sizable increase in England's playing budget to compensate clubs for relinquishing their most valuable playing and marketing assets.

Everything pointed to a deal. Woodward, for one, believed it was done. But the fat lady was not singing. Without the head coach's knowledge, and apparently contrary to perceived logic, the England team doctor Simon Kemp assured Baron that England's medical department could work in harmony with club doctors to ensure the players were looked after. It was, of course, nonsense. But it came as music to Baron's ears and he pulled the deal.

Following Kemp's intervention, Woodward resigned, and the best chance English rugby had of creating a genuinely manageable landscape for its top stars disappeared overnight. 'We have gone backwards,' Woodward said at the time.

> If I had far more control of the players and I could do my job then I would be staying.
>
> We won the World Cup by inches. You cannot compromise. But agreements have taken place between the RFU and clubs that on paper look great. They're not. We had a clear plan of how we were being successful, and that has been watered down. We sat around the negotiating table with people who, with respect, have no idea about elite performance.
>
> When you see your top players dropping out because they are absolutely run-down you have to say 'enough is enough'. Players today play too many games. To be an elite performer you have to control the athlete all the time – and the England head coach has to have more control of his players. You can't control them through directors of rugby. It's like trying to run a business without a workforce.

By December 2006, the war between Baron and Woodward showed no sign of abating, with any hope of delivering a programme truly in the players' best interests fading fast. Woodward told the *Sunday Times*:

> It is personally shattering for me to say this, but winning the World Cup was the worst thing that ever happened to the England team.
>
> Everyone said at the time that we won the World Cup because of the system. The truth is that we won the World Cup in spite of the system. We won it because we had an awesome group of players.
>
> I hate to copy other countries but look at what New Zealand are doing. They're putting the player first, the team first. And we're trying to put out a team to play against these people.
>
> All I want is for the players to be given a fair chance. We're now seventh or eighth in the world and would be complete outsiders to beat New Zealand. So something's not right. The players are playing too much rugby. If you are a top player, you can only play so many games.

In the meantime, he backed his second in command Andy Robinson to succeed him, adding, 'Andy thinks he can work within this compromise.' Unsurprisingly, Robinson could not. The next two years were a disaster as England lost 13 out of 22 games under Robinson, who stood down in 2006 before he was pushed. His replacement, Brian Ashton, hardly fared any better.

In November 2014, in the wake of yet another England injury crisis in the run-up to an international series, Woodward would tell me for his column in the *Daily Mail*:

> Post World Cup my first major disagreement with the RFU came about when the current RFU head of medicine Dr Simon Kemp argued strongly that he could ensure players were well

looked after at their clubs by working closely with the club doctors. I totally disagreed with that philosophy. You can only have one boss in any business.

At the time rugby had all the cards in its favour. It wasn't a case of contracting players but it was about giving more money to clubs to make sure that ultimately the England coach had the final say on when a player played. That didn't happen and we now have the situation we have now.

England and the RFU have accepted the current playing structure so there can be no excuses but the injury rate is now a serious cause for concern. The question needs to be asked: why are they happening? The toll has gone beyond simple bad luck.

*

In sports journalism, the exclusive is king and Peter Jackson got more than most. Following his lead I took to grabbing a quick word with a player, administrator or coach, away from the main press pack. The higher the profile the better, and I was chuffed when World Cup winner Iain Balshaw agreed to talk to me when I collared him after Leeds played at home in late 2004.

Balshaw had endured an horrific injury run and seemed disconsolate. He rattled off injury after injury he'd suffered since making his international debut four years earlier. He was hollow. Weary. And clearly feeling sorry for himself.

My first time interviewing one of my World Cup-winning heroes proved a sobering experience. Not because Balshaw wasn't polite and generous with his time – he was. But because it dawned on me there were serious consequences for these guys from the big hits and brutality I'd spent the last decade drunkenly cheering. Getting injured was more than just a sentence on a page. Their livelihoods and families' futures depended on their bodies working.

Balshaw and I were similar ages and by the end of the interview all I wanted to do was give the bloke a hug. I didn't, of course, but that interview, in the gantry at Headingley, troubled me.

In the early years of reporting, I had mixed feelings watching men I'd played with and against running out in front of packed stands. But soon I realized, even if I had made the grade, life as a professional rugby player was harsh, high risk and fraught with pitfalls. Worse still, there was no one in their corner.

In March 2005, Matt Hampson, a 20-year-old prop forward apparently destined for international honours, broke his neck when a scrum collapsed during an England Under 21 training session.

Hampson survived, just, but the force of the impact had severed his spinal cord and left him tetraplegic, wheelchair bound and reliant on a ventilator for the rest of his life. Only the presence of referee Tony Spreadbury, a trained paramedic, saved the young prop's life.

Playing or watching sport you get used to injuries. You must or you'd never lace up your boots or walk into a ground.

When I was 14, I stood barely 10 feet away when St Paul's School winger John Shimmin, playing for the first XV against Wellington, suffered a compound fracture of his lower leg in a ruck. I'll never forget the anguish on his face, or the sight of his fibula poking out through his sock like something from a Vietnam war film.

But a broken leg was recoverable. What happened to Hampson felt unimaginably cruel. I pictured him in my mind, unable to move on the hospital bed, terrified.

During the 1995 World Cup, Ivory Coast winger Max Brito had been left paralysed, with only limited use of his arms, when his spinal cord was severed in the first minute of his team's pool game against Tonga in Rustenburg. Brito was heard to call out to his captain Jean Sathicq, 'It's over,' seconds after the initial crushing collision. Twenty years later Brito would tell the *i* newspaper's Hugh Godwin he spent the next 14 to 15 years in a 'fog' but bore no resentment towards rugby which, in truth, had done nothing to encourage a reduction in collisions or improvements in player welfare. Had the 'rugby family' really looked after him?

While Matt has since gone on to become one of Britain's most inspirational people, establishing the Matt Hampson Trust, helping others affected by spinal injury and holding no grudge against the sport, at the time he had no public profile. And while his injury gained some coverage in rugby circles, I couldn't understand why it wasn't back page news. If he had been a footballer, it would have been. But rugby, if it wasn't the international game, was hidden away on the periphery of the media. It was another sobering moment.

And while these incidents were always referred to as 'freak', with next to no reliable data to examine at this time, it was impossible to establish if this was actually true.

In the three years since the RFU and Premiership Rugby professional rugby injury audit began, and with clubs initially highly reticent about sharing sensitive injury information, little useable data had been generated. But with what was available, in 2005, RFU head of medicine Simon Kemp co-authored a paper with Colin Fuller, a consultant in sports risk management, titled 'Epidemiology of Head Injuries in English Professional Rugby Union'. It was an influential piece of work.

The study tracked 757 professional players over three years, collating data around matchday injuries, and the results showed the overall incidence of match concussions was 4.1 concussions for every 1,000 playing hours, resulting in 13 days lost on average. However, 'A large proportion of players (48%) were allowed to return to play safely within seven days.'

The report, which acknowledged the 'dearth of information' around risk factors in rugby, found the overall incidence of training ground concussions to be 0.02 per 10,000 playing hours while also stating: 'Head injury and its prevention are critical issues facing many contact and collision sports because of the potential for both acute catastrophic head injury and *longer-term neuro-psychological sequelae* [my italics] resulting from repeated mild head injury.'

So in 2005, the RFU acknowledged a long-term association between head injuries and longer-term problems.

*

That summer of 2005 will be remembered by most English sports fans as the summer we got our cricket team back. Michael Vaughan's men recorded a magnificent 2–1 Ashes triumph in what will go down as one of the greatest Test series of all time. But on the other side of the Atlantic an altogether more sombre and important development was playing out.

Dr Bennet Omalu, who three years earlier had examined Mike Webster's battered brain on an autopsy table, published the results of what he'd found in collaboration with doctors at University of Pittsburgh Medical Centre. The paper was titled 'Chronic Traumatic Encephalopathy in a National Football League Player' and set out to 'present the results of the autopsy of a retired professional football player that revealed neuropathological changes consistent with long-term repetitive concussive brain injury'.

Omalu found that before his death Webster had been suffering symptoms including 'cognitive impairment, a mood disorder, and parkinsonian symptoms'.

Omalu found 'Chronic Traumatic Encephalopathy was evident with many diffuse amyloid plaques as well as sparse neurofibrillary tangles and tau-positive neuritic threads in neocortical areas.' The neuropathologist concluded: 'This case highlights potential long-term neurodegenerative outcomes in retired professional National Football League players subjected to repeated mild traumatic brain injury… We recommend comprehensive clinical and forensic approaches to understand and further elucidate this emergent professional sport hazard.'

The findings were dynamite but completely passed most of us in the UK media by. I don't recall reading a word of copy or watching or hearing any coverage of the case at the time.

In April 2006, another significant development passed most of us by too when Dr Michael Turner, chief medical advisor to both the British Horseracing Authority and the Lawn Tennis Association, co-authored a paper titled 'Neuropsychological Dysfunction Following Repeat Concussions in Jockeys' which found:

> Multiple concussions were associated with clear decrements in high level executive/attentional functioning. Younger athletes were more at risk.
>
> Our results are consistent with those of previous reports suggesting that uncomplicated cases of concussion may not necessarily lead to negative long term consequences. However, multiple concussions appear to be associated with worse long term outcome.
>
> Individuals with two or more concussions performed below those with a single concussion on the Stroop colour-word interference task, and, to a less robust degree, on Trails 2. This suggests that multiple concussions may interfere with executive skills, including response initiation/inhibition, divided attention, and concentration. This supports previous reports that attention/executive difficulties may follow multiple concussions.

In November 2006, Turner was awarded the Institute of Sports Medicine's Robert Atkins Award for 'consistently valuable medical service to sport'. Tony Goodhew, the Horseracing Regulatory Authority's director of racecourse licensing and standards, who oversaw the Medical Department, said:

> This award is due recognition for Michael's tireless work not only in racing but also in sport overall... Most recently, Michael

has introduced a concussion management system which means that following a concussive incident, the length of suspension is now clinically evaluated rather than relying on a fixed period of suspension relating to the time the jockey was unconscious. Gone are the days of a fixed 21 days off for a jockey after concussion, so often the bane of a jump jockey's working life.

Across sport, the three-week minimum stand-down was being challenged.

*

In November 2005, I covered my first international, Scotland's 19–23 defeat to Argentina at Murrayfield, and following another busy season which saw me report on more than 40 games, in August 2006, I returned to London, ready to try my luck as a freelancer.

In truth, I was hopelessly ill-equipped as I realized that a contacts book containing the names of about 30 current players, a couple of coaches and a handful of PRs and administrators wasn't going to cut it if I was going to swim with the big fish.

Fortunately, I landed a chance exclusive interview with former Australian cricket captain Kim Hughes, in which he tore shreds off the current Aussie team and cast doubt on some of their key performers. The *Daily Mail* took 700 words, my first by-lined page lead. A few days later I received a call from Dean Wilson at Hayters Sports News Agency and he offered me a job as cricket and rugby reporter. It was my passport to the international beat, where all aspiring sports journalists want to operate. Or at least think they do.

The following September, four years after I'd watched the final in a pub, I packed my bags and headed to Paris to report on the 2007 World Cup.

As an agency reporter, I was in the privileged – although often fraught – position of technically being able to file for every newspaper going. No one begrudged me that freedom because I could act as an insurance policy for them, attending every press conference humanly possible in order to gather as many quotes and titbits of useful information to distribute to other reporters or desks, normally for a fee paid to Hayters.

I was primarily reporting for the *Daily Star* and *Sunday People*, who didn't staff their rugby coverage, although I also filed variously for the *Sun*, *Daily Telegraph*, *London Paper*, *Daily Express*, *Rugby World* and *Daily Mirror*. Even the *Daily Sport* took some copy on occasion. If people would pay for it, we would file it.

There was plenty of work and good money to be made, especially after England, missing their injured talisman Jonny Wilkinson, had been thumped 36–0 by South Africa in the pool stages yet somehow found their way to the final.

My friends thought I had the dream job. Mostly, I agreed. Interviewing players and uncovering stories was great, but matchdays were when the job really came to life. The ground was where the magic happened. Where dreams came true and nightmares unfolded. Where stories were written and names made.

I'd usually get to the ground at least an hour and a half before the start of play. This was the time to catch up on gossip, ensure you weren't missing a big news story, or just chew the fat with friends, colleagues and contacts.

On a good day, I'd have another article to file, hopefully a news story to ruffle some feathers when the first edition went out later that night, or a big feature interview with a high-profile current (preferably) or former player, coach or administrator with something juicy to say to make a decent headline.

For the bigger games, especially the internationals, there was a frisson of excitement among the reporters, most of whom, like me, had originally been fans. I never thought I'd be good enough to hold a candle to the lead rugby writers of their day; people like Peter

Jackson (*Daily Mail*), Stephen Jones (*Sunday Times*), Paul Ackford (*Sunday Telegraph*), Chris Hewitt (*Independent*), Ian Stafford (*Mail on Sunday*), Alex Spink (*Daily Mirror*), Andrew Baldock (Press Association), Tony Roche (*Sun*), Steve Bale (*Express*), Chris Jones (*Evening Standard*), Rob Kitson (*Guardian*) and Mick Cleary (*Daily Telegraph*), even though I aspired to write 'seriously' about rugby. Since the age of about 11, in fact probably ever since that famous England win over the Wallabies in 1988 which really ignited my rugby passion, I had devoured the sports pages of national newspapers, especially the rugby columns.

Some of the reporters I now found myself sitting alongside in the press box or socializing with in the evenings were writers I'd looked up to for many years. I'd only really been 'at the coalface' for a couple of years and aged 29 was the youngest national reporter regularly on the England beat by some distance during the 2007 World Cup. I felt a constant sense of 'imposter syndrome' working alongside and occasionally competing against some of the big beasts of the industry.

Jackson was especially intimidating because he was so bloody good. So it was a thrill when I managed to get hold of the news of Jonny Wilkinson's long overdue return to the fold the night before England officially named their side to play Tonga in the second game of the tournament. I filed the story to the *Daily Star*. While others may not have been scouring that paper's rugby coverage for scoops, Jackson was.

'You had the whole team, Sam. Man for man,' he said as I walked into the team announcement press conference. 'Where did you get that from then?' he followed up with a grin, knowing full well I wouldn't tell him.

Gradually, over the course of the six weeks or so I was in France, I began to establish myself within English rugby's press pack.

But while this was the tournament where I started to find my feet as a national reporter, it was also where my initial concerns about the injury toll faced by players in the Premiership began to morph into a wider concern about the risks faced by international players.

*

One of those players whose commitment to the cause had become legendary since he made his debut in November 2002 was Lewis 'Mad Dog' Moody. The Leicester flanker's extra-time tail of the lineout catch of Steve Thompson's throw in the World Cup final in 2003 is arguably the most important lineout take in English rugby history. He was a softly spoken, gentle soul off the pitch who would morph into a whirling dervish when he crossed the whitewash.

Moody was feared by opponents and respected by team-mates and, as it happened, by the media. Not that Lewis would have been too worried about the latter. His main focus, whenever he took the field, was to demonstrate his absolute commitment by throwing his not inconsiderable 6ft 4in, 16st 7lb frame around the field with, it seemed, total disregard for his own safety. Moody wore that reputation with pride. If he could give nothing else, he would give his body for the cause.

Moody had chosen to play rugby instead of a career in the Army, where he no doubt would have made an outstanding officer, and his leadership credentials came to the fore during the 2007 World Cup, when head coach Brian Ashton effectively lost control of the dressing room following that catastrophic, injury-plagued defeat to eventual tournament winners the Springboks.

That tournament's England v Tonga game at Parc des Princes, Paris, was the first time I had been seriously concerned that a player might die in front of my eyes.

Lewis was knocked out twice. First by a knee to the head charging down a kick, and the second when he was hit high by the Tongan captain. On both occasions he was attended by pitchside doctor Simon Kemp and allowed to play on.

Moody recalled the incident in his autobiography *Mad Dog: An Englishman*, ghost-written by Ian Stafford, in which he said:

> [The game] was almost over for me inside the first five minutes.
> In attempting to charge down a clearance by Vungakato Lilo,
> I received an accidental knee to my head and was knocked
> clean out. I was unconscious for nearly five minutes. All I
> can remember is the distant sound of Matthew Tait saying,
> 'Moodos, Moodos'. Simon Kemp, the team doc, suggested I
> should come off. I told Kempy where to go. I'd waited this
> long to get my chance in the World Cup, and there was no
> way I was walking off after five minutes. A lineout followed
> and I had no idea what was going on. Cozza went through the
> move beforehand and, a minute or so later, I had come round
> properly. Ironically, I was knocked out for a second time in the
> second half, although not for as long. This time my head was
> jerked back by the force of an arm smashed into my face by Nili
> Latu, the Tongan captain. I think he was attempting to kill me!
>
> A trip to Euro Disney followed the next day. This was
> optional but, of course, I went and Annie came along, too.
> The problem was my head was spinning from the double blow
> I'd received the night before. Midway through my first ride –
> Aerosmith's Rock 'n' Roller Coaster – I felt so sick I thought
> my head was going to explode. Annie had been under orders
> from the medics to check up on me every hour during the night
> until she gave up on me at 5 o'clock in the morning. Now, in
> my wisdom, I was lurching around a fast, indoor roller coaster
> with flashing lights and heavy rock music blasting. Every loop
> the loop was torture. Every jerk of my car was like having a
> needle shoved through my head.

While the failure to remove Moody from the field at the time caused some consternation in the press box, with several of us questioning privately why he had not been taken off after the first knockout, let alone the second, we were assured, as always, that player welfare was the RFU's priority and Moody was being afforded the very best medical care available. Little did we know this involved a trip to Euro Disney barely 12 hours after the double knockout.

Instinctively, the whole thing looked wrong. But ultimately we were being told by medical people and high-level representatives of the unions that there was no problem. Certainly, nothing presented by the RFU from the injury audits suggested a problem, while the line 'they receive the best possible medical care' was almost as ubiquitous from official channels as 'player welfare is our number one priority' would become. Who were we, a group of rugby hacks, to question their position? And, it has to be said, it was convenient for us to believe them.

Kemp would later tell me the incident was a driving force in him pushing for the Head Injury Assessment – or Pitchside Suspected Concussion Assessment as it was originally called – which would cause so much controversy when it was first introduced in 2012. But at the time, no one within the RFU's medical department was directly challenged over the incident.

Anyhow, England had won and were, against the odds, on course for a World Cup quarter final in Marseille the following Saturday. While some mentioned Moody's knockouts in their match reports, no one to my recollection, including me, took a public stance against their handling. And it came as absolutely no surprise when he was picked to face the Wallabies the following week.

Despite my concerns, I was far too new on the scene to cause a fuss or swim against the tide and I was relieved not to have done so when I arrived in Marseille to discover I had been booked into the same hotel as the England players and backroom staff.

Besides, despite the criticism we sent England's way in defeat to South Africa, it was only fair to reflect on a gutsy performance in seeing off Tonga. To add to England's new-found buoyancy was the news Jason Robinson was back. He had suffered a hamstring tear of such significance against South Africa, it was thought unlikely he'd play again in the tournament.

Within the England squad, Robinson's unexpected return was viewed as a triumph for the medical team. Returning a player to the field as soon as possible had become the holy grail for professional rugby's doctors, and Kemp advocating a homeopathic injection of Traumeel – perceived as a lower risk alternative to corticosteroids – apparently paid dividends after Robinson agreed to be injected.

Kemp would tell the *Financial Times* in 2009 in an article titled 'How economists tackle sports injuries':

> We're dealing with people whose priorities are very different from the man on the street. While I might advise an amateur to try conservative treatment, which will still let him lead a pretty active life, professionals can't get by with that. Besides, they're used to injury... We're on the cutting edge and we have a very small window. We'll try new things, so long as the science suggests they'll help, and we think they're not dangerous.

Several players who played during that era would subsequently tell me they had been injected by Kemp before matches and, on occasion during the half-time interval in England internationals, without any knowledge of what they were being injected with.

During the course of me writing this book, Steve Thompson told me:

> I was injected countless times before and during matches. I had no idea what I was being injected with but it was normal practice. I'd get taken off into the showers to be given a jab, especially for a rib injury I suffered playing for Northampton. Lots of people knew it was happening but would look the other

way. As far as I was concerned if it would get me back on the field faster, I'd let them do it.

And Kemp was not alone in delivering painkilling injections before matches. The use of either painkilling injections or tablets was, and still is, commonplace throughout rugby. I should know: in 1999 while at university I developed a stomach ulcer and regularly spat blood after overdosing on ibuprofen, which I took habitually before matches to mask the pain in my shoulder.

'When it came to the pills they'd just be left out before matches for everyone to take,' Thompson told me. 'The doctors knew we were going out there to get the shit kicked out of us so thought it was better to get the pain relief done in advance so they could get off to their practices afterwards. My stomach suffered as a result of the ibuprofen. It's still not right today.'

The practice was by no means confined to adult teams. In his 2015 autobiography *Man and Ball*, former Ireland and Ulster flanker Stephen Ferris wrote about his treatment for a shoulder injury during the 2005 Under 21 World Cup: 'Samoa are next up and I need Eanna Falvey, our team doctor, to inject me with painkillers before each remaining game. At half time too.' In 2020, Falvey succeeded Martin Raftery as World Rugby's chief medical officer.

The pressures on professionals to mask, ignore or play through pain was immense. It still is. Saracens and Namibia flanker Jacques Burger told *Rugby World* in 2017:

In my last three years, every day I took painkillers. It was a way of life. It was mostly paracetamol and ibuprofen, but that can be hard for the stomach. Some guys take co-codamol but it made me sleepy. Celebrex is an anti-inflam that is easier on the stomach. I took them every day, but not every day now. In the last year I cut down a bit because the danger is it can lose its effect.

At Saracens the club docs were very wise and looked after you. I'll not name names but there are some places where they take everything out of you.

Lewis Moody, who in 2005 had been diagnosed with chronic inflammation of the colon, ulcerative colitis, told *Rugby World*:

> I was taking drugs so I could play, like ibuprofen and diclofenac. It was like I was a walking medicine cabinet. I don't think I'd change much about my life, but I would probably change my lax approach to this.
>
> I remember once, we were on a bus. It was almost a kind of challenge to see how many 'smarties' we could take. Around then I was 27 or 28, in 2008, and I would be s****ing myself, essentially. Losing blood, losing weight. I certainly didn't understand that. I didn't ask questions then.

Dan Cole, a team-mate of Moody's at Leicester and with England, would later tell the BBC:

> You struggle to get a good night's sleep after a game on a Saturday afternoon because your ear's hanging off or your shoulders hurt. You get to three o'clock on a Sunday and you start feeling worse. Normally Monday is the worst day for stiffness, tiredness, pain.
>
> What hurts most depends which way you've been lying, but usually you'll have a stiff neck or a stiff shoulder. You're creaky in your lower limbs, but you still get going. You have to get going. Usually by Thursday you're close to 95 per cent. I'd never say you're 100 per cent fresh.

Back in France in 2007, the criticism of England's team and management had been scathing following the crushing, albeit injury-afflicted, 36–0 defeat to South Africa in the second game of the tournament. It was by some distance England's worst defeat of the professional era. And the early criticism of their performances by the press had clearly stung. After the team pulled off a shock win over Australia to move through to the semi-final against France, No.8 Nick Easter, who'd emerged as one of England's leading players of the tournament, thanked the gathered press 'from the heart of my bottom'. Nice one, Nick.

That evening a few of us made our way down to Marseille's attractive harbour, along with several of the England players, and watched on the big screen with thousands of passionate French fans as the hosts saw off favourites New Zealand in a match still remembered, unfairly, for English referee Wayne Barnes's failure to spot a forward pass in the build-up to France's try in a famous 20–18 win in Cardiff. No one at Marseille harbour seemed to care as a balmy late summer's evening turned into one of the most jubilant celebrations of rugby I had ever witnessed. I remember taking time out at one point to smoke a cigarette away from the crowd and thinking how utterly blessed I was to be doing this job. My career was only going in one direction and England were into the World Cup semi-final. Best of all, I'd be covering it.

England beat France in the semi-final but finally ran out of luck against South Africa in the final when Mark Cueto had his sliding doors moment which, sickeningly for him and England's travelling fans, saw television replays deny him a first-half try which would have set his team on course to victory and changed his life forever. In truth, South Africa were worthy winners.

Personally, the tournament had been a massive step forward. I'd filed for every national paper, covered as many games as any other reporter and was now firmly part of the UK rugby press pack.

As we filed out of one last press conference in the basement of England's Paris hotel, home beckoning after a long trip, Peter Jackson looked over and nodded at me. 'See you soon, Sam.'

4

Bloodgate, statistics and damned lies

For me, the Lewis Moody incident in Paris played on my mind. The injury attrition rate we'd witnessed during the World Cup had been truly shocking and consideration for the players' welfare limited at best. Although everyone agreed players were getting 'bigger, stronger, faster' in the quest for ever more powerful and physically confrontational athletes, it felt as if every pre-match or competition press conference was dominated by conversations around injuries, with next to no serious discourse about what could be done to change the course rugby was now on. Trying to look at it dispassionately, I really didn't like what I was witnessing.

After the World Cup, all the talk among senior IRB administrators seemed to be about the need to grow the game to attract new audiences, or markets as they were now called. We were bombarded with press releases telling us the latest tournament was the biggest and best, with more television viewers than ever before. Syd Millar, IRB chairman, said in the wake of the tournament that the game needed speeding up to increase its appeal. There was no mention of players being protected.

All I could see, evidenced by cases such as Moody in the game against Tonga, was players not being protected from themselves. No self-respecting professional, or amateur for that matter, would ever voluntarily leave the field; the idea of putting the onus on the player to make the call was beyond silly. Moody had suffered a brain injury and was in no fit state to decide if he should carry on. To me, medics needed empowering and somehow separating from management.

I sensed the injury toll becoming normalized in the eyes of players, coaches, medics, administrators, media and fans.

The data was beginning to come through on injuries, if not concussion, but with nothing to compare it to, there was no way of knowing how fast the sport was changing other than by listening to players and trusting our eyes.

One study, 'The Impact of Professionalism on Injuries in Rugby Union', conducted by Alvie Epidemiology Associates with the University of Edinburgh, which I only discovered upon researching this book, suggested the frequency of injuries actually doubled between 1993/94 and 1996/97. The study, involving more than 800 players, both amateur and professional, found:

> The proportion of players who were injured almost doubled from 1993–1994 to 1997–1998, despite an overall reduction of 7% of the playing strength of participating clubs. Period prevalence injury rates rose in all age specific groups, particularly in younger players. This translated into an injury episode every 3.4 matches in 1993–1994, rising to one in every 2.0 matches in 1997–1998. An injury episode occurred in a professional team for every 59 minutes of competitive play.

The study's authors concluded: 'The introduction of professionalism in rugby union has coincided with an increase in injuries to both professional and amateur players. To reduce this, attention should be focused on the tackle, where many injuries occur.'

By anyone's measure, a doubling of the proportion of injuries in four years is highly significant. As was the identification of the tackle as the highest-risk action.

When it came to concussion, it was only when a high-profile incident occurred that people paid any attention. And while it's been highlighted since, the Moody incident received very little coverage at the time and was not called out as another example of a sport completely failing in its duty of care to the players. It was easier for all of us to believe everything was OK.

In boxing, a sport most perceive to be far more dangerous than rugby, Moody would not have been allowed to continue fighting following the first knockout he suffered against Tonga.

*

I returned home from France exhausted but satisfied at a job well done. I had my first World Cup campaign under my belt as a reporter and my career was moving in the right direction, even if rugby wasn't.

The start of the Six Nations in 2008 saw another high-profile injury when Mike Tindall suffered two fractured ribs, a punctured lung and badly lacerated liver when he felt the force of an accidental Lee Byrne boot in England's game against Wales at Twickenham. Unable to breathe, Tindall required lengthy treatment on the field with oxygen before being taken to hospital, where he spent several days in intensive care.

It is often said that football's beauty is in its simplicity. The rules of the sport have essentially not changed since they were formalized at Cambridge University in the late 1800s. Rugby union's laws, on the other hand, have been in near constant flux, even before the onset of professionalism. Even for those of us who have followed the game closely, it has been almost impossible to keep up.

The laws on substitutions changed dramatically with profession-alism. Previously, only injury replacements were permitted, following their introduction in 1968. Three tactical substitutions were introduced in 1996 and within a few years this had risen to eight. At the time of writing, this number remains highly contentious, with many arguing that fresh players entering the fray against tired players late in the game have increased injury severity and concussions.

In the years following the introduction of professionalism, the need for rugby to appeal to a wider audience became, in my view, an unhealthy obsession. There was a general acceptance from most within the game that endless mauls and reset scrums did not appeal to the masses, despite the protestations of those who harked back to a bygone era when a 6–3 fight in the mud followed by 10 pints down the Dog and Duck was the height of ambition. But the major challenge, it seemed to me, was that the more you sped up the game and the more ball-in-play time, the bigger and more frequent and intense the collisions inevitably became. This could only mean one thing: greater risk of injury.

The marketing folk loved collisions and 'big hits' which got clicks online and meant rugby matches could be promoted like something akin to monster truck events. But the difference between massive trucks smashing over things and human beings is that there are physical consequences for the latter.

While the technical understanding of defensive structure and technique evolved rapidly as a result of the influx of rugby league influences on union, another aspect which saw radical change, with more unintended consequences, had been the scrum.

During the late 1990s and early 2000s, as a direct result of technical input from professional scrum coaches, a new phenomenon emerged: the hit. This was the moment both sets of forwards engaged to begin what had historically been a battle for possession and trial of strength with both hookers required to 'hook' the ball backwards while the other seven forwards used all their strength to drive forward. Critically, neither set of forwards was allowed to gain unfair advantage by pushing before the ball had been put into the scrum by the scrum half.

Something that had previously involved both sets of front rows leaning into each other rapidly morphed into a seismic collision of two giant packs, by now averaging between two and three stone per player more than in the mid-1980s, with six front-row players taking the equivalent weight through their necks and shoulders. While the number of scrums per match was reducing as the result of laws designed to speed up the game, the force involved in each scrum was skyrocketing.

Head-on-head collisions were common and actively encouraged by some coaches.

'I was once told to use my head to clear out at the ruck,' former England captain Dylan Hartley would tell the *Mail on Sunday* in 2022. 'When I started out, there was an opposition hooker who would look me in the eye before every scrum and head-butt me at the engage. It intimidated me. Naturally, young Dylan Hartley thinks, "Well, that was horribly effective, I'm gonna go and do it to the next young guy I face".'

Meanwhile, collapsed scrums, boring for television viewers and, much more importantly, where catastrophic injuries were most likely to occur, were on the rise.

But it should be acknowledged as a first triumph for the injury audit that, by demonstrating where injuries were occurring through data analysis, change could be made to the laws to reduce them. In 2007, with the enactment of the 'touch, pause, engage' sequence, rugby removed the hit from the game overnight. The negative response generated by this player welfare-driven change was fierce. Despite the hit being a new phenomenon, there was a powerful lobby who defended it and accused rugby's authorities of 'going soft' for legislating to remove it. It was total nonsense, of course.

But while the changes to scrum laws were welcomed by anyone who did not believe guaranteed spinal damage was a reasonable expectation for people doing their jobs, there was little else to cheer about when it came to protecting players in those days. Another increasing concern was the breakdown, which along with the contest for the ball at the restart, separated union from league or American football.

Before the onset of professionalism the 'jackal', effectively stealing the ball at the breakdown in play following a tackle, basically didn't exist. But by the mid-1990s, intelligent back-row forwards, including New Zealand's Josh Kronfeld, England's Neil Back and France's Laurent Cabannes, realized the tackle presented an opportunity to 'turnover' possession.

With the coaches searching for every competitive advantage, stealing the ball at the breakdown became an artform requiring skill, strength, opportunism and, above all, extreme bravery. The few who could execute it regularly were treasured by coaches and admired by fellow players. If you were prepared to 'put your head where it hurts', simultaneously spreading your legs wide to form a strong base, you had a chance of effecting a 'jackal'. This inevitably increased risk. The defending player contests over the ball with their head, neck, shoulders and knees exposed and vulnerable to being recklessly 'cleared out' by an opponent. It was next to impossible to referee and examples of dangerous 'clear outs' were commonplace. So were neck injuries.

While the medical facilities at Twickenham by now resembled a small, well-equipped A&E department, that was just English rugby's shiny showcase. Medical provision, even at Premiership level, was often basic at best, while further down the leagues, where theoretically the risk of injury was reduced, the picture was even bleaker.

In 2018, Coventry and Hartpury universities undertook the first ever study to investigate whether amateur rugby clubs' medical provisions met the requirements outlined by RFU regulations. The results were shocking but received almost no coverage in the national media.

Researchers found that only a quarter of the 91 clubs surveyed were compliant, while nearly a third of the clubs were unsure if their medical personnel had any first aid qualifications.

With lack of finance being the most frequent reason for the lack of medical provision, the research found that around one in four clubs had no access to medical personnel whatsoever, or only one person in this role, while two thirds had no access to a defibrillator, and around one in five did not have easy access for emergency services vehicles to reach them.

*

As the game evolved before our eyes, and with rucking and mauling reduced, defences spread more across the field, making the game appear more like rugby league. Coaches quickly came to recognize that they did not need to commit all eight forwards to a breakdown, leaving more to join the defensive line.

One of the IRB's 13 Experimental Law Variations introduced globally in 2008 following trials at Stellenbosch University, geared towards speeding up the game and encouraging attacking play, saw both back lines set up 5 metres back from the hindmost foot of the scrum, when previously they could line up on the hindmost foot of the scrum. In essence this created a 10-metre no-man's-land between the defensive line and the attacking team for both sets of players to run into before contact was taken. It might have looked cleaner for on-screen viewers, but it was another law change which encouraged bigger collisions at higher speeds.

With clear evidence showing concussions were most prevalent in the tackle, including from a two-year study co-authored by Simon Kemp in 2007 titled 'Contact Events in Rugby Union and Their Propensity to Cause Injury', I could see no sense in this.

Players would often talk about the difficulty they would have getting out of bed in the morning following a game. But the stories seemed to be getting worse, and with more and more games being added to the fixture schedule players started saying routinely that the only way for their bodies to recover fully was if they sustained a long-term injury.

I found the new relationship between employer and employee fascinating. Why was professional sport able to operate seemingly outside of the normal parameters of employment law where an employer owed a duty of care to its employees? In the amateur era, players were just turning out for fun, so club accountability was limited. Now, with rugby union clubs and governing bodies being commercial organizations with contracted employees, I could not understand why they were not being held to higher standards when it came to their duty of care. What other job would allow you to be knocked unconscious twice in the space of an hour and expect you to finish your shift?

*

While the players were having a tough time, I was enjoying one of the best years of my life professionally and personally. I left Hayters a few months after the 2007 World Cup to go freelance again and got engaged to my girlfriend Debs shortly after buying our first flat together in Maida Vale, west London.

I was an established rugby and cricket writer, gaining access to all England's rugby Tests and cricket internationals, and with most sports desks' freelance budgets still holding up, just, I was making a decent living doing a job I loved. With Peter Jackson supportive of my work, I'd become a regular matchday reporter for the *Daily Mail*, covering games up and down the country, and occasionally being trusted to look after the whole rugby page on the rare occasion Jackson took a day off and his deputy Chris Foy was covering cricket.

It gave me a huge buzz to see my by-line in the paper, especially opposite Jackson's, while I was also getting regular gigs with the *Evening Standard* and a variety of other newspapers from the *Daily Express* to the *Voice*.

The money was good and with 2007 Heineken Cup champions Wasps based just down the road in Acton and flying high under straight-talking Kiwi coach Warren Gatland and his deputy Shaun Edwards, their established roster of internationals Lawrence Dallaglio, Phil Vickery, Simon Shaw, Josh Lewsey, Paul Sackey, James Haskell, Alex King and Tom Rees afforded plenty of opportunities for high-profile interviews. Danny Cipriani was also now a regular in their starting line-up and it was clear from an early stage that he was courting the celebrity lifestyle. Wasps media sessions were generally open and the appetite from desks for stories about Cipriani was insatiable, even before he'd won a single cap. There was no doubting his talent, and I always found him personable and polite, although that was not always the view of his contemporaries, many of whom resented the media coverage he received before he'd achieved much in the game.

But while I was enjoying life, rugby's injury rates continued to trouble me, especially as I witnessed first hand at Wasps a medical room which routinely resembled a scene from *M*A*S*H*. And while players were being asked to put their bodies on the line almost every day of the week, and while international grounds like Twickenham, where most people experienced professional rugby, were high-tech and well equipped, some clubs' training facilities were unbelievably basic. Way below what you'd expect from a typical second or third division football club, despite rugby's radically higher injury risk profile.

Even understanding what I knew of rugby's culture, having played it all my life, I was still astonished at how much pain these players were prepared to tolerate and how subservient they were. The RPA was toothless when it came to restricting game exposures. The nominal 32-match limit introduced with the Elite Player Squad agreement was not policed at all, while there appeared to be no appetite to reduce contact training from anyone within the game.

No one would entertain a reduction in games based on the widely held view that the only way to increase revenues was by playing more games. The idea that 'less could be more' was not even countenanced. It was dangerously short-sighted. Even without understanding what was beginning to play out in the NFL, with more and more CTE cases being found in ex-players, it was blindingly obvious to me there would be serious consequences for the players. Everyone accepted the long-term risk to knees, shoulders, necks and other joints but what about the possible long-term risk to brains?

*

I was also fascinated by how quickly fans and the media forgot about players once they'd stopped playing. I was complicit in this but the speed with which rugby players – and sports stars more generally – lost relevance once injured or retired was sobering. Only a tiny handful went on to build successful careers in the media after they retired; it was evident only the smartest were making provisions for life after rugby, with few apparently giving much consideration to the fact that one serious injury could end their career and ability to earn money overnight.

The RPA unquestionably did some excellent work in this area, and continue to do so, but it was a hard sell for young players to think about life further down the track when they were living in the moment and desperate for the next contract.

I wrote a few stories that were supportive of the RPA, once interviewing James Simpson-Daniel, a brilliant young player whose career was blighted by injury, highlighting the need to think about life after rugby. But the RPA were not news. A few of the diehard journalists attended their press conferences, notably the *Rugby Paper*'s Neale Harvey, but with little interest from the sports desks in 'sob' stories, why would the other journalists bother attending when they didn't want to miss the main line from England?

With a changing room culture which ensured anyone who spoke out could be labelled a troublemaker – the worst accusation in a tight unit of blood brothers that a successful rugby team had to be – I began to understand there was an *omertà* in the game around injuries, while concussions were simply something players would laugh about, in public at least.

It was entirely understandable current players couldn't put their head above the parapet for risk of losing a contract or being ostracized by a coach. Certainly, the younger players wouldn't dare speak out against the system at that stage, or they ran the risk of having their contracts torn up. 'Banter' was the great saviour, and hanging around Wasps and lots of other rugby training grounds, it was clear to me they felt, on many occasions, like extensions of boys-only private schools where mickey taking and the slightest sign of weakness could be preyed upon and brutally exposed.

'Concussions were seen as funny,' Moody would later tell me in an interview for the *Mail on Sunday*. 'We'd stand around in training and just laugh when guys got knocked out. It was all part of the culture. We didn't know any better.'

To make matters worse, the early data from the RFU's audit contradicted what we were seeing in front of our eyes. The results of the first audit of the 2002/03 season found 42 concussions reported across 139 matches (one every 3.3 matches), while an average of 5.6 concussions occurred for every 1,000 hours of rugby played. According to the data, this had dropped to just 20 recorded concussions across 135 matches (one every 6.75 matches) during the 2005/06 season.

If these figures were to be believed, it meant a solitary concussion was occurring roughly every seven matches. It just did not feel right.

*

Privately, we all acknowledged there was a developing problem. But, for a variety of reasons, few in the media were willing to air private concerns in public. I recall one conversation I had with a friend and national newspaper correspondent around that time when I told him

I thought we should write more about the unfolding injury crisis. He told me: 'Sam, why would I shit on my own doorstep?'

That is a common view for any industry journalist, be it in sport or, say, automotives, where those who challenge the status quo are seen as undermining commercial interests.

In the course of researching this book a good friend who remains a high-profile television pundit gave me their view on professional rugby.

'It's fucked,' they told me. 'The model is completely broken. It just doesn't work.'

I don't for a second believe they will ever air this view in public. Like players, their mortgage depends on it.

As well as anti-inflammatories and other painkillers, the temptation to take performance-enhancing drugs to speed recovery was obvious, although not something I ever encountered directly. Whispers about certain players abounded but I had no direct proof, other than the occasional positive test returned and publicized by the RFU.

'Even without steroids there is no doubt that, thanks to the extra training that professionalism allows, rugby players are getting bigger and stronger,' John Daniell wrote in his 2007 book *Confessions of a Rugby Mercenary*. He continued:

> This has had an unexpected impact on injury statistics. At any given time, of the 600 or so professional rugby players in France about 100 are out with injuries. On the surface, this is no worse than under the old amateur regime, but what has changed is the severity of the injuries.
>
> While the full–time medical and physical trainers employed by the clubs have greatly reduced the number of pulled muscles and other minor injuries, players are now suffering from more serious problems. As speed and strength increase, the amount of energy released in collisions between players also increases,

and although muscle helps stabilize the shock to some extent, the rest of the body – particularly the knee and shoulder joints – is no better equipped than before.

Consequently there is a rise in the number of serious injuries involving ruptured ligaments. It's like an arms race, where the improvement in performance thanks to new technology means you feel stronger and safer – but so does the other guy, and the end result is that you do more damage to each other. There doesn't seem to be any easy solution: no one is about to sign peace agreements.

While I had no doubt the players were conflicted by short-term contracts, often only 12 months in duration, which left them vulnerable to the whims of directors of rugby in charge of clubs' playing budgets, and could terminate with very little recourse, I was also uncomfortable with the literal cheerleading I witnessed from some of the teams' medical backroom staff on the side of the pitch during matches.

The sight of doctors and physios, dressed up in club colours, jumping up and down when 'their' team scored was widely accepted but I always found it odd. I understood why they did it. They wanted to look and feel part of the team and be 'one of the lads', but I felt it undermined any notion that they could act strictly impartially, as you would wish them to. To me, the players needed protecting from the employer, whether that be club or national team, but as long as the doctors were employed directly by the club or national governing body, they were always going to be tempted to act to protect their own position within the organization and not necessarily put the players' interests first at all times. Some will accuse me of naïvety for this, perhaps fairly, but is it too much to ask for doctors, bound by the Hippocratic oath to 'first, do no harm', to act without prejudice?

*

Of his recovery from a severe ankle injury in 2014, Stephen Ferris would later write in his autobiography:

> Mark Anscombe is my fifth coach at Ulster. Everyone calls
> him Cowboy. During my recovery, he always came to me on
> a Monday and asked, 'How are you feeling? How's that ankle
> feeling? You'll be good to go this week?'
>   'Hopefully, Mark. Hopefully.'
>   Then the medical staff would say, 'Stevie's not training
> today.' Mark would turn to me. 'Are you not training today?'
>   'Nah, I'm not, Mark. I don't think so.'
>   Even though the medical staff had told him, he was hoping
> I would say yes, so he could get me out for a couple of sessions.
> That happened a lot.

This was typical of the stories I heard from the start of my time covering rugby union.

Practices which would have been completely out of the question in normal life had become culturally normal in professional rugby union. It was also clear that the medics and the vast army of watercarriers on the touchline were in contact with directors of rugby up in the stands. When a player was injured, they could be seen relaying information to coaches, often sitting among the press benches in the stands, who would then make the final call on whether the player would continue. It was becoming increasingly obvious to me that rugby union's doctors were too close in every sense to their employers.

I struggled with the idea that coaches, clearly conflicted, were able to influence a medically trained physician on the field who had recommended a player be removed from play. Questioning the ethical motivation of doctors was strictly off limits without proof, however, and rightly so. But I'd taken more than a passing interest in the *Sunday Times* sports writers Paul Kimmage and David Walsh's pursuit of cyclist Lance Armstrong and strong insinuations that he was a dope cheat over the previous few years. Having done a fair bit of reading into cycling and its culture, my instinct, combined with the work of the redoubtable pair, told me they were right. And I was fascinated by the conflict of interests seemingly unique to professional sport, where a corrupt doctor had the ability to improve a participant's performance by providing chemical assistance while at the same time inflicting the twin wrongs of risking the individual's medium- and long-term health while completely subverting the level playing field all sports should be played on. The idea a doctor could bury their ethical principles in order to further the interests of a commercial organization fascinated and appalled me in equal measure.

Harlequins were another London club where I spent a lot of my time. The Stoop wasn't far from where I lived and I covered many of their games between 2005 and 2009 when former England player Dean Richards was director of rugby. He was as intimidating off the field as he was on it. At times he could be charming in press conferences, which were held in an oppressive, windowless room underneath the main stand, but when he wasn't in the mood, like a lot of top coaches, he could make our lives extremely difficult. There was an air of menace around Richards, a former traffic cop from Leicester, which I struggled to put my finger on in the early days. I think he knew his reputation went before him and many of the press, me included, were in awe of him.

I'd been a fan for years as a youngster, often rolling my socks down when I played to impersonate Richards, and even had a Nike advert framed on my bedroom wall which showed a muddied and frowning Richards alongside his similarly tough-looking team-mates Micky Skinner, Jeff Probyn, Paul Ackford and Wade Dooley in their full England kit, wearing Nike boots, staring down the camera above the caption 'And for the opposition, we do an excellent line in running shoes'.

When it came to the press, Richards was deeply suspicious. He hated being asked about the England job, as most of the directors of Rugby did, partly out of a sense of loyalty to the incumbent, and partly because it was a Catch-22. If he said 'yes' he wanted it, that was the headline, and vice versa. From that perspective I understood where he was coming from.

I got on with him OK but we clashed in May 2008 after Richards had seen his new club Harlequins narrowly lose 31–28 on the final day of the regular season to his former club Leicester at Welford Road. I could understand Richards being pretty hacked off, as his side had just missed out on a place in the play-offs, but I was taken aback by what happened next. A week before, Quins announced the signing of former All Black fly half Nick Evans, who'd won 16 caps between 2004 and 2007 but, apparently tired of playing second fiddle to Dan Carter, and with a lucrative contract on the table, he'd decided to make the move to England. At 27, Evans was younger than a lot of the imports coming into the Premiership at the time and most of us thought it was an inspired signing.

As a lowkey press conference was winding down, I asked Richards what I thought was a completely innocuous question about Quins' latest acquisition.

'Dean, can you tell a little of your thinking behind the signing of Nick Evans?' It was hardly Paxman but I immediately sensed his hackles were up.

'I'll answer questions about today's match and that's it,' he growled.

Undeterred, I continued.

'Dean, Nick Evans is a fantastic, high-profile signing. I'm just interested to know what you think a player of that calibre will bring to the squad?'

Richards was having none of it and, clearly irritated, snapped back.

'Look. I said I'll answer questions about the game and nothing else. Do I make myself clear?'

But while he was irritated, so was I. He was stopping me from doing my job. Quins had signed a player. Richards was responsible for the deal, and it was not unreasonable to enquire why it had happened. I had no other agenda. So I pressed on.

'OK, Dean. What would Nick Evans have brought to today's game if he'd been playing?'

By now, Richards was livid.

'Oh you are a smart-arse, aren't you?' he said, moving menacingly towards me.

I realized there was a distinct possibility he was going to hit me and I weighed up my options in my mind. Turn around and run out of the room or stand my ground and show I wasn't intimidated. For right or wrong, I stood my ground, working on the basis that if he punched me, I'd have a decent story to tell once I came around.

Sensing things were getting out of hand, Terry Cooper, a seasoned reporter who went back years with Richards, sidled across and attempted to calm things down, putting a fatherly arm around Richards's hulking frame and whispering a few words in his ear.

I don't know what Coops said, probably 'he's not worth it' or words to that effect, but it had the desired effect and the situation was quickly diffused.

I probably had been a bit cheeky but only if you accept that directors of rugby should be able to run press conferences in the same way they run a training session: my way or the highway. I didn't accept that. And Richards evidently didn't appreciate not being in control.

I next saw him at the Premiership launch the following August when he walked straight over to me and, without apologizing, gave me a big hug. I'd earned his respect by standing up to him. It was odd. Either way, I learned a lot about him in that short exchange.

*

On 11 September 2008, Daniel James, a 23-year-old former rugby player who had broken his neck when a scrum collapsed on his neck during a training session 15 months earlier, flew to Switzerland with his distraught parents to terminate his life. In doing so, the former England Under 16 schoolboy hooker became the youngest English person to pay for his life to be terminated at the Dignitas clinic.

Having attempted suicide three times already, twice by overdose and once by stabbing himself, Daniel, who a string of psychiatrists had found to be rational and with full mental capacity to make decisions, was so determined to end his life he told his parents, Mark and Julie James, if they did not assist him to do so, he would move out of the family home and starve himself to death. He said his body had become a 'prison' and he was 'not prepared to live a second class life'.

Even so, his parents who accompanied him to Dignitas and a family friend who paid £12,165 to charter a plane to fly the family to Switzerland were subjected to a lengthy and distressing police investigation as accessories to a crime under the Suicide Act 1961. After returning to the UK, devastated by the death of their beloved son, Mark and Julie were arrested and interrogated by police.

It is a profoundly troubling story and I recount it here so Daniel is not forgotten and to highlight yet another catastrophic injury which occurred around this time and which unquestionably affected my attitude to rugby. Even though the RFU's own research in 2008 described rugby union as 'a full contact sport with a relatively high overall risk of injury and a small specific risk of fatal and catastrophic spinal injury', I increasingly struggled to accept that such extreme injuries were tolerable at all in sport. Our appetite for difficult stories is also finite, but that does not stop me believing Daniel should have his story told.

*

As a sports writer on a national newspaper, you try to convince yourself you are somehow separate from whatever editorial line is printed at the front and it is remarkable how few sports writers share the hard-line right-sided political leanings of papers they work for. I was, and still am, far more inclined to side with a *Guardian* leader column than a *Telegraph* one. So unsurprisingly, I had serious misgivings about accepting the freelance contract to write about rugby and cricket when it was offered by the *News of the World* in the spring of 2009.

But ultimately, and truthfully, the salary and profile the paper brought with a circulation of more than 2.5 million readers was too good to turn down and I accepted a freelance contract.

I still have mixed feelings about the two years I worked there before it shut down following the exposure of industrialized phone hacking by its news reporters. The contract, which still allowed me to work for other newspapers, and came with a hefty travel and expenses allowance, was worth more than five times what I'd started on at PA five years earlier. With a wedding to plan and mortgage to pay, I took the pragmatic decision.

The same week I took the *News of the World* job, Peter Jackson reported the cases of two players in their twenties, Leicester flanker Ben Herring and Bath flanker Michael Lipman. The article reinforced my view that the concussion data being presented was seriously underestimating the scale of the problem and was lulling the entire sport into a false sense of security.

Jackson wrote in the *Daily Mail* on 8 April 2009:

> Another Premiership player has been smashed into premature retirement after being warned of permanent brain damage from one more blow to the head.
>
> Instead of fighting for a place in Leicester's back row against Sale on Saturday, Ben Herring accepted the grim

medical prognosis and quit on the spot on Thursday at the age
of 29.

'The surgeon said, 'You can't replace your brain and you'd
be risking far too much if you go on playing',' said Herring.

'My wife and I have a new-born baby so there wasn't much
of a decision to make.'

While Herring's plight was the main focus, Jackson, who would retire
from the correspondent's job a few months after writing this article,
also reported on Bath and England flanker Michael Lipman's head and
neck problems, commenting: 'Herring and Lipman are just two of an
increasing number of players to suffer from head injuries caused by the
sport's often reckless propensity for collisions on an ever-escalating scale.
Herring's case history supports the theory that, as the game has quickened
and space becomes harder to find, head injuries have increased.'

Herring, a tenacious openside flanker known for his ability 'over
the ball' or 'jackalling', added: 'I've had four big knocks to the head
in the last year. The loss of consciousness from the last one wasn't
as bad as the previous ones, but after the vomiting and dizziness my
eyes were so bad I couldn't watch TV or look at a computer screen.
I had to wear dark glasses.'

Typically, Jackson was also the first to directly challenge the RFU
and Premiership Rugby's self-serving narrative that the professional
game was not getting more dangerous.

The same day the *Mail* ran Herring's story, Jackson received a call
from a senior figure within the RFU's communications department
informing him that the RFU's most senior medical figure had requested
a meeting with him at Twickenham.

'I readily agreed to meet with Simon Kemp,' Jackson told me. 'I
travelled to Twickenham the next day expecting official confirmation
of concussion as an issue within rugby. Instead the party line left me
with the impression "nothing to see here, move along". I pointed out

that if Herring was the only case surely that was one too many. That they were so quick to play it down made me feel suspicious. Perhaps that's the problem with listening to people from within the sport.'

Jackson, as ever, had his finger on rugby's pulse. His line about Lipman 'considering how much more punishment' he could afford to take conjured an image in my mind of a journeyman boxer considering 'one last fight'.

Herring's testimony, along with Lipman's, hardened in my mind the idea that the inherent bravery and loyalty, ingrained in the DNA of 99.9 per cent of professional rugby players, was being exploited for commercial gain. While still attempting to market itself as somehow on a higher moral plane than other sports, 'a game for hooligans played by gentlemen' no less, rugby union's conflicted powerbrokers were, to my mind, losing moral authority.

The day after Jackson reported on Herring and Lipman, Dean Richards was involved in an incident which confirmed some of my suspicions. Bloodgate.

Rumours began to emerge on the Saturday night after Harlequins' 6–5 home Heineken Cup quarter final defeat to Leinster that a major storm was brewing.

Quins had replaced injured regular goalkicker Nick Evans with Chris Malone on 47 minutes, only for the replacement to miss a conversion which would have given Quins the lead, before he himself was replaced by winger Tom Williams on 69 minutes.

With Evans watching helplessly on the touchline, and rugby's replacement laws not permitting a player who had already been replaced to return to the field for any reason other than as a blood replacement – introduced a decade earlier to prevent blood-borne viral transmission – makeshift kicker Mike Brown missed another penalty which would have put the home team in front.

Richards, fast running out of time and options, could be seen prowling up and down the touchline.

With minutes left on the clock, Quins then had the most extraordinary stroke of 'luck' as Williams went down injured for a second time in short succession. Just moments before he'd been attended to by physio Steph Brennan who, as instructed by Richards, handed the player a fake blood capsule, which, it transpired, had been purchased from a Clapham joke shop a few days earlier, and told him to 'do the right thing'. Williams bit into the capsule.

A year later, at a hearing of the Health Professions Council, where Brennan was struck off for his role in the scandal, the physio said:

> In retrospect I should have said no, but in the heat of the moment I did not have that clarity of judgement. I followed orders and wish I hadn't. Yes I went on to the pitch with the intention of deceiving the referee. I wish I'd stood up to Dean Richards. I regret it every day.
>
> I was told this is what I had to do. It was a split-second decision made during a match that had massive pressure on it. Giving a blood capsule to Tom Williams had nothing to do with physiotherapy, it was the stupid act of cheating.

With 'blood' pouring from Williams's mouth, Richards had created the moment he needed to get his first-choice kicker back into the fray. Evans, his star man, was back.

It was, of course, far too convenient to be true and with no one near Williams when he'd suddenly started bleeding, Stuart Barnes in the Sky commentary box was not the only person in the ground to smell a giant-sized rodent.

'Who punched Tom Williams in the mouth? Tom Williams?' Barnes asked.

To make matters worse, as Williams left the field, and for reasons only known to him, he decided to wink in the direction of team-mate Jim Evans, as if to acknowledge his part in the deception, sparking a furious protest from Leinster's coaching staff on the touchline, whose own doctor, the late Professor Arthur Tanner, would later tell a tribunal he 'instantly' knew the blood gushing from Williams's mouth was fake. Tanner also described sports doctors' working conditions as a 'dysfunctional environment'.

Panicking, and knowing Leinster's suspicions were aroused, Williams ran down the tunnel and into the home changing room with Quins doctor Wendy Chapman. Once inside, between them, they decided the only course of action was to cut the inside of Williams's mouth with a stitch cutter to demonstrate he really had been injured. It only served to compound the original sin and dug an even deeper hole for all concerned.

In the post-match interviews Richards decided dishonesty was the best policy.

'Hand on heart was Tom Williams bleeding when he came off?' Sky Sports reporter Graham Simmons asked.

'He came off with a cut in his mouth. The issue is whether he was injured and you have a right if someone has a cut to bring them off, which is what we decided to do,' Richards said with a straight face.

'So your conscience is clear on that one?'

'Yeah, very much so.'

Only the most die-hard Quins fans believed him.

European Rugby Cup (ERC) launched an immediate inquiry which three months later saw Williams plead guilty to swallowing the fake blood capsule and banned for 12 months while Chapman was suspended from practising medicine. In his testimony Williams, who it would later transpire had signed an agreement with Quins guaranteeing future employment in return for carrying the can, refused to implicate Richards or Brennan.

Quins were fined £213,000 but, reputationally at least, Williams was set to be the fall guy.

At the hearing, Richards denied he had ever been involved in fabricating blood injuries, with Quins lawyer Oliver Glasgow telling the panel that 'the idea Dean Richards could stoop so low is so unlikely as to be laughable'.

Within weeks Richards resigned after Williams, shocked by the severity of the ban and on advice of the RPA, blew the whistle on the attempted cover-up. In doing so he accused Richards and Brennan of being the principal culprits in the plot to cheat the substitution system.

With so much new evidence emerging, ERC appealed their own initially lenient sentences, and at the second bite of the poisoned cherry found Richards to be the 'directing mind' with 'central control' over the entire affair, banning him for three years. Brennan received a two-year ban and never practised again, while Williams's ban was reduced to four months.

'His [Richards] was the dominant personality and influence on affairs,' said the judgment. 'He knew or ought to have known that players such as Mr Williams would likely obey his directions whether that meant cheating or not.'

The 'only aspect' the former police officer had not been directly involved in, the tribunal found, was in the cutting of Williams's lip by Chapman. However, he had 'created the situation where intense pressure was brought to bear'.

Williams told the appeal hearing he was injured in a match in Richards's first season in charge, ending the game on crutches. 'In my mid-season appraisal, he criticized my going down injured during play and ordered me to attend a camp with the Harlequins rugby league side to toughen me up. There was no discussion or seeking of my views.' Richards denied this, insisting Williams had willingly attended the camp to improve his skills.

After receiving the longest ban in the history of professional rugby, Richards said: 'I am sorry I got caught but at the same time I know now, as I did at the time I resigned, that I did the wrong thing. I've done something wrong and I've got to pay the price for it. At the time, you have the mistaken belief you are doing the right thing for the club and the players to win the game.'

Richards, for his part, clearly felt he was being singled out for what had become an industry-wide practice. 'I did cheat, I knew it was wrong but I thought it was an accepted practice in rugby,' he said. 'I should have been stronger and not done it. Hopefully, there will be a better system for dealing with this.

'To a point, the people who say that I have damaged the game are right, but it is ironic the reason we went down the route in the first place was that I didn't want to cut people.'

The clear implication was that there were others in rugby prepared to cut players before resorting to blood capsules.

Richards doubled down on that statement the following month when, in his first exclusive interview since receiving the ban, he told me he had 'received phone calls from every other director of rugby in the Premiership saying "we had to clear out our cupboards"'. We will never know for sure if that was true but the idea an overbearing coach could create a toxic environment where players and medical staff were conflicted came as no surprise, even if Richards's capacity for bare-faced lying and coercion did.

Leinster's highly experienced team doctor Tanner, who described Richards's touchline manner as 'arrogant' and 'condescending', shed further light on the coach–medic relationship in rugby. 'We are all human. A doctor is a doctor and that should override everything, but the atmosphere surrounding that match was something that I had not experienced before,' he told the tribunal in Manchester. 'There are massive pressures from coaches and players to do things that are not in their best interests. But, at all times, you have to remember they are patients first, not players.'

For her part, Wendy Chapman was subsequently found guilty of serious professional misconduct by a General Medical Council panel, narrowly avoiding being struck off because chairman Brian

Alderman noted she had been seriously depressed at the time and had subsequently undergone cancer surgery. She was allowed to practise again despite the panel finding that her actions were 'not in the best interests of the patient'. I felt very sorry for her. I'd had a tiny window into Richards's world the previous season and knew at first hand just how intimidating he could be.

'It proved a watershed moment for rugby union,' matchday referee Nigel Owens would later say.

> It raised awareness and let people know that our sport can be affected by cheating as much as any other.
>
> We can't take the moral high ground as things do go on in our sport that are unacceptable. We don't really know whether Bloodgate would have happened in the amateur era. Professionalism involves considerable sums of money and the stakes are raised. People have mortgages to pay and win bonuses to claim, jobs are on the line.
>
> Since the advent of pay for play in union in 1995 an element of win at all costs has crept in. But this was to the extreme.

In my view the RPA came out of the whole affair in considerable credit having done exactly what a trade union is meant to do: look after its members. With so many conflicting interests, players need to know they have someone in their corner.

As if the physical risk of injury of playing wasn't bad enough, the psychological risk posed by coaches was also now clear and present. While professional rugby projects an image of moral virtue, you only need to scratch the surface to unearth the sport's darker side.

*

I boarded the plane to South Africa in June 2009, landing in Johannesburg with a sense of trepidation and excitement. Trepidation, because I knew the *News of the World*'s demands would be extremely high. Excitement because, eight years after Matt and I had enjoyed the time of our lives as fans in Australia, I was about to cover rugby's greatest show: a British & Lions tour.

Predictably, the build-up was dominated by injuries and concerns over player welfare. Rugby's absurd fixture calendar meant that what had previously been a 10-week tour was crammed into six. And the games were set to be more physically demanding than ever. One match stood out, even by modern professional rugby's standards, for its astonishing physical brutality and the toll it took on the players.

What would become known as the 'Battle of Pretoria' was, for those of us who witnessed it, a defining game in professional rugby's short history. To my mind, it was the game where it started to get ridiculous.

27 June 2009 was a perfect winter's day on the high veldt in Pretoria. Most of the travelling press were staying in Johannesburg, where the Lions had spent the week training, an hour's drive from the South African capital along the busy M1 De Villiers Graaff motorway. As always on the day of a big match, there was a nervous energy among us as we boarded the plush media coach.

Big games mean big names and in rugby terms they don't get much bigger than the Lions playing the world champions. As a result, most newspapers had flown out their chief sports correspondent. With the three-match series on the line after the Lions had lost an engrossing first Test 26–21 in Durban seven days previously, the *News of the World* sent out their chief correspondent Andy Dunn to cover the game, alongside me.

We got off the coach and the carnival atmosphere was immediately apparent with smoke filling the air from the meat being cooked on the braais in the car parks around the Loftus Versfeld stadium, invariably by impossibly big men wearing Springbok shirts. As usual, we had some of the best seats in the house.

It took roughly 21 seconds for the tone to be set for one of the bloodiest games in the history of rugby union as Springbok flanker Schalk Burger used the first breakdown as an opportunity to intentionally stick his fingers into the right eyeball of Lions winger Luke Fitzgerald. French referee Christophe Berdos chose only to show Burger a yellow card and with that single feeble act of officiating the tone was set.

None of us who witnessed the game first hand will ever forget the sheer brutality of it as player after bloodied player was taken from the field in various forms of distress.

That Morné Steyn kicked a 55-metre penalty with the last play to secure an insurmountable 2–0 series lead is lost somewhat in the memory of a grotesquely physical game that saw two Lions players – Adam Jones (dislocated shoulder) and Gethin Jenkins (compression fracture of the cheekbone) – rushed to hospital.

Eight days later, Lions team doctor James Robson held what I still consider the most important press conference in professional rugby union's history.

'These have been the most physical three Tests I have been involved in,' Robson told us at the end of a tour which saw no fewer than ten Lions return home injured.

> As a spectator, the games have delivered but I still have anxieties about the number of matches players are subjected to in the northern hemisphere. I hope at some point welfare will become a bigger part of player-management. There is a lot of talk and rhetoric but for the players' sake I hope more action is taken.
>
> We are reaching a level where players have gotten too big for their skill levels. They have become too muscle-bound and too bulky and I think you may see changes in their physical nature in order to speed up the game and introduce a higher level of skill.

You have to look at the midweek games and the length of the tour. Personally I would like a slightly longer tour with less frequent games. I don't want to lessen Lions tours but perhaps it should be eight games over eight weeks.

I had goosebumps on the back of my neck listening to Robson in a downstairs function room of a smart hotel in the Jo'burg suburb of Sandton. He was saying what so many of us felt: professional rugby was too dangerous. But coming from a man of his standing and respect among his peers, it meant so much more than if it came from a member of the media. I honestly thought that that press conference would force rugby to change tack and seek ways to depower the game. Again, this was profoundly naïve.

*

While the Springboks, through Burger, had set the tone, the Lions were far from innocent bystanders.

Simon Shaw and Brian O'Driscoll could both easily have been red-carded for high tackles which would have seen them handed hefty bans today.

O'Driscoll was later left reeling immediately from a collision with Danie Rossouw which left both men demonstrating clear evidence of brain injury. Both played on.

Just a few other incidents in an astonishingly violent game included Lions hooker Matthew Rees almost garrotting Springbok replacement lock Andries Bekker in the 47th minute, Andrew Sheridan punching the same player in the testicles 14 minutes later, and Jamie Heaslip launching a shoulder to Bryan Habana's head when he scored a try in the 62nd minute. If you don't believe me, watch the match on YouTube. It's there for all to see.

Each one of those incidents would have been a red card under today's interpretations of the laws. In those days, some didn't even warrant a penalty.

'The 2009 Lions tour was the second I'd covered,' Dunn would later tell me.

I'd had a taste of it in 2001 when Nathan Grey ended Richard Hill's tour with an elbow direct to the head in the second Test. I was ghosting Phil Vickery's column on that series and I remember going to interview him after one Test and he was just so beaten up and knackered. Coming from a footballing background, I'd never seen anything like it.

What struck me in the build-up to the 2009 series in South Africa was that all the talk was about the 1974 Lions tour and Willie John McBride's famous '99 call'. It was effectively glorifying violence and the authorities and unions were prepared to be lenient because it was what was expected of a Lions tour. It became a self-fulfilling prophecy because the 2009 tour was just brutal.

Dunn was referring to McBride's introduction of a tour rule where if a fight started on the field between two players and '99' was called, it was 'one in, all in', in a collective action of self-preservation and solidarity.

With all of us reeling from what we'd just witnessed, and Dunn writing the main match report, I was at liberty to head off to find a story. And I did, when I spotted, sitting on his own, Luke Fitzgerald, the man who, only a couple of hours earlier, had risked being blinded on the pitch by an act that, if it happened on the street, would carry a hefty prison sentence. I asked him what had happened.

I just felt a hand coming for my eyes. I was lucky enough that I had my hands free and was able to stop him from doing any damage. Luckily enough the eye is fine. We're going to leave the decision up to the citing officer. If the referee didn't see it then fair enough. But he was given a yellow card for what is being claimed [that there had been a gouging incident]. That makes it a strange decision.

I guess part of it was because it was at the start of the game and he didn't want to spoil it as a spectacle. But you'd want to feel that the referee would deal with something like that quite severely.

At the end of the day this is a fella's career and that's a very sensitive area that he is accused of messing around with. We'll have to see what happens at the hearing.

It's surprising that people do take the risk because there are so many cameras these days that they are messing around with their own livelihoods as well as another guy's.

To me, the 2009 tour was the manifestation of 14 years of unfettered and unchecked professionalism where marketing brutality for commercial gain without any acknowledgement of the potential consequences for the players became normalized while high tackles, big hits and recklessness were often celebrated. And the media, me included, was complicit.

Keeping contacts 'onside' is a constant concern for journalists, especially in sport where the demand to break stories is high but the numbers of those truly in the know are relatively low. It's a small pool and the last thing you want to do is alienate a key contact by running a story they don't want in the public domain. But this also acts as a barrier to the truth being told because, often, journalists will choose not to report legitimate stories for fear of alienating a contact. It's no coincidence that the end of a coach's reign is always met with a slew of new stories. Once you don't need them you can write what you want. How else did Eddie Jones suppress his tyrannic approach to coaching England for so long before his overdue sacking in December 2022?

The day after the Pretoria Test, with five Lions in or recently in hospital, Springbok coach Peter de Villiers chose to up the ante.

'What we must understand is that rugby is a contact sport and so is dancing,' he told us at a press conference.

> But in this game there will be collisions. There are no collisions in ballet. And the guy who wins the collisions hardest is the guy we will always select. If we are going to make it soft because we won a series and people don't like it then I can't do anything about it.

> So make a decision. There were so many incidents in that game that we could go and say we want to cite this guy for maliciously jumping into another guy's face with his shoulder. Why don't we do it? The reason we don't do it is because this game will always be a game to us.

> If that's not the case, why don't we all go to the nearest ballet shop, get some nice tutus and get some great dancing going on? No eye gouging, no tackling, no nothing. Then enjoy. I know Schalk Burger is an honourable man and he would never, ever commit an act such as eye gouging.

The thrust of what de Villiers said encapsulated the sense rugby was becoming 'less manly', softer and sanitized through the scrutiny of the media. The emergence of citing commissioners, responsible for assessing incidences of foul play in a post-match review, and close-up cameras was, in some eyes, causing the sport to lose its very soul. I thought this was complete and utter horse shit.

As a youngster, I'd lapped up rugby folklore like the legendary '99 call' on the 1974 tour to South Africa. One of my favourite videos was the highlights package of that tour, basically a collection of the greatest fights with some decent rugby thrown in. One memorable scene showed Lions full back JPR Williams, who happened to be a practising doctor, running 30 metres to join a mid-pitch brawl with a look of pure relish.

Another scene showed an interview with legendary Scotland lock Gordon Brown telling the story of him punching South African lock

Johan de Bruyn at a lineout, in retaliation for an earlier punch of course, only to look on in horror as he realized he'd knocked his opponent's glass eye clean out of his head. Fortunately, de Bruyn was otherwise unscathed and both teams were gracious enough to stop fighting in order to search for his eye in the mud. For decades, fighting had sold rugby.

But while some harked back to those days, it was evident to me that rugby could no longer have it both ways. If it wanted to survive commercially, it had to reach new audiences outside of the old amateur bubble where culturally it was OK to laugh at a man having his eyeball punched out. On the other hand, the more professional it got, the harder the hits and the more severe the injuries.

And if it wanted to survive, flourish even, its lifeblood was new players. And for new players, you need parental buy-in. To me, as someone who'd spent his entire life immersed in rugby, the second Test in Pretoria made seriously uncomfortable viewing. Things were getting out of hand.

And far more important than the commercial viability and reputation of the sport was the health of the players. Whereas Gordon Brown was considered a giant of a man in his day at 6ft 5in and weighing close to 17 stone, Bakkies Botha stood fully 6ft 7in tall and weighed more than 19 stone. His opposite man at Loftus Versfeld was 6ft 9in, 20 stone Simon Shaw.

The press conference comments made by James Robson, widely recognized as a 'player's doctor', should have set immediate alarm bells ringing. Especially as everyone present, all rugby lovers and experienced campaigners, agreed with him. But if anything, things were about to get even worse.

5

Nothing to see here

By 2009 I was deeply uneasy about rugby's trajectory. Bloodgate had exposed that a high-profile coach, a former hero of mine, was a cheat, while the Lions tour had been brutal enough to watch, let alone to play. Hearing De Villiers's comments following the second Test also made me question just how the influence of a coach with a reckless attitude to player welfare could directly influence on the field in the way his players behaved.

It was clear how influential coaches and directors of rugby were within organizations, often responsible for everything from player recruitment to media and communications. Many a time a request to interview a player was put in via the normal channels of a press officer, only for it to come back that the director of rugby wouldn't approve the interview. It seemed nonsensical to me that a coach could have control over the comms strategy of an organization which, almost always, desperately needed media coverage in order to attract sponsors, sell tickets or simply allow the player to raise their own profile and, by extension, that of the professional sport they were playing.

Coaches' primary concern, understandably, was winning games. Anything else was a distraction. For most, the press fitted into this category. There was little scrutiny of international cultures, with players unwilling to speak out against bad practice and the media unwilling to call out abuse of match officials and players, even when we witnessed it first hand. On occasion this was for fear of physical intimidation – witness Richards exuding menace simply for asking a question he didn't like – but more often because coaches could be the source of privileged information while also controlling access to players.

But following Bloodgate it was clear for everyone to see that, under the wrong set of circumstances, when a director of rugby gained influence and believed they were untouchable, as Richards had at Quins, serious cultural problems could emerge, with players especially, but also medical and backroom staff, compromised.

It was thus in the spirit of seeking to protect players that I went to the RPA and offered their chief executive Damian Hopley the opportunity to share his thoughts on the situation just a few days after the publication of Tom Williams's evidence to the appeal panel where he outlined the untoward pressure being exerted on him from above.

It was the first time I'd met Hopley and he was affable and engaged and certainly didn't hold back when talking about the protections needed for vulnerable players.

'I wrote an open letter to the players the day after Tom came to see us,' Hopley told me.

> I told them if they are put in this position they have to come
> to the Players' Association to talk about it and whistle-blow. If
> you are put in those difficult positions there has to be a route to
> unpicking that. The events of the last few months have sent out
> a very clear message that you can't take liberties with players.

> You can't put players in this compromised position and
> if you do there will be a process that will be followed and
> the RPA will fight tooth and nail for them. Clearly Tom was
> complicit and played a major part in Bloodgate. But rather like
> in a military operation where the orders come down from on

high, it takes an incredibly strong person to turn round to his General and say: 'Sorry, I'm not going to do that.'

Dean's ban is severe but it sends a very clear message that this kind of behaviour won't be tolerated. Administrators, coaches and players now know it is entirely unacceptable to treat an employee in this way. If people doubted why the RPA existed there is no doubt now.

I was encouraged by Hopley's position. He appeared to be taking the opportunity to draw a line in the sand and it was clear he meant business. I also thought, in this instance, the military reference was entirely reasonable. To me, Richards, and no doubt other directors of rugby as well, were acting like dictators and, under intense pressure for results, were abusing their powerful position. Having dealt first hand with a large number of directors by that stage in my career, I was in no doubt similar abuses of power could happen again. So too, by my understanding from our interview, was Hopley.

I filed a story with a strong but I felt entirely warranted introductory line: 'Players' chief Damian Hopley today calls on Premiership stars to blow the whistle on bullying bosses who force them to cheat.'

With a strong 'newsy' exclusive interview secured, with an angle few could argue with considering the astonishing events of the past few weeks, I went to bed on the Saturday night, satisfied with my week's work and with a strong belief the article would be beneficial to players. Of all those, I believed, who would be happiest with the story and promotion of their organization it would be the RPA and their chief executive Hopley, who had spoken so strongly on the subject of protecting players; the very thing he'd set his organization up to achieve more than a decade earlier.

The next morning, my phone rang at 8am. It was Hopley calling from his holiday home in France.

'You've stitched me up,' he said.

'What?' I replied, completely lost.

'You've stitched me up,' he repeated. Since joining the paper earlier that year I'd been the first to get onto the desk to complain when they overspun a headline or rewrote something I'd written, but on this occasion I believed the intro, which Hopley also strongly objected to, was entirely representative of what he'd said to me.

I apologized profusely, although I had no idea what I was apologizing for, but Hopley was having none of it. I'd stitched him up and that was that. He hung up and we did not speak again for another three years. To this day, I genuinely have no idea what he was so annoyed about, but the incident unsettled me and alerted me to the fact Hopley wasn't always as straightforward as he appeared.

The fallout from Bloodgate would have profound implications for rugby but so too, I believed, should the events in South Africa that summer.

While Bloodgate had provided clear evidence of the corruption which could occur under the wrong set of circumstances, so too had the Lions tour highlighted the mounting risks facing top players. The truth was, with this generation of players the first to spend their entire careers as professionals, no one could honestly say what the consequences would be.

Phil Vickery, by now a Wasps player after signing from his home club Gloucester, and whose neck and shoulders had been twisted, battered and crunched even more than most Lions players in South Africa, under pressure from Tendai 'The Beast' Mtawarira, had surgery on his spinal cord in October 2009, a few months after returning home. Surgeon Peter Hamlyn was required to make a 12cm incision at the front of Vickery's neck before moving his voice box and larynx to one side, removing the worn down vertebrae, and replacing it with a brand new one made of titanium. Most people undergoing such an operation would avoid any sort of contact or collision involving their neck, head or spine for the rest of their lives. Vickery, who had previously spoken of being unable to lift his newborn baby out of the cot, would be back playing professional rugby again later that season. I interviewed him at Acton as he was working through the final stages of his gruelling rehabilitation regime when the popular 18 stone World Cup winner went into graphic detail about the surgery. The headline accompanying the interview read: 'Vickery: I had my throat cut for England'.

The headline may have been tabloid gold but beneath it there was a darker message. I found it increasingly unconscionable how badly beaten up these guys were becoming and it actually concerned me that, as modern medicine progressed and surgical techniques advanced, players' careers may actually be extended, not shortened. That was certainly the case with Vickery, who in any other generation would have been forced to retire some years earlier. You could argue his neck would not have been in the same condition in other generations, but that would be a moot point.

The RFU's data for 2008/09, which showed the number of matchday injuries to be remarkably stable at 100 per 1,000 playing hours and concussion rates actually lower than in the first season with 38 recorded in 135 matches (one every 3.55 matches), was still not reflecting what we were seeing with our own eyes.

However, by removing the figures from the first audit in 2002/03, which appeared anomalous, it was possible to see a noticeable upward trend in the frequency of both matchday injuries and concussions. Critically, although this was rarely highlighted in the reports, the severity of matchday injuries was also tracking upwards with six injuries requiring more than 84 days' – or 12 weeks' – absence in 2008/09 as opposed to just three in 2002/03. Training ground injuries were also significantly on the rise, up from 159 in 2002/03 to 318 in 2007/08. Despite a slight reduction in 2008/09, training ground injuries, including concussions, would continue to climb over the coming years.

Indications of a serious looming problem were starting to present in the data.

Perhaps as a combination of Bloodgate and the shocking scenes we'd witnessed in South Africa that summer, players felt emboldened to speak out, not least the impressively articulate Simon Shaw.

In an interview with the *Mirror*'s rugby correspondent Alex Spink, Shaw said he believed professional rugby was in danger of producing a generation of 'gym monkeys' prioritizing power above skill and brute strength over finesse. One of nine players in head coach Martin Johnson's Elite Player Squad for the upcoming autumn internationals sidelined through injury, Shaw pinpointed the ever more crammed fixture schedule, allied to overtraining, as causes for concern:

> There is an argument people are spending too much time in the gym and they are creating more of an athlete than a rugby player.
>
> If you take your body to a peak physical state then it is also more liable for tears and strains. There is a limit to how far you can stretch your body.
>
> We shouldn't be trying to create gym monkeys with technique, we should be trying to create rugby players.
>
> The expectation is on the players to be fit for an entire season. Whether they are playing or not is almost irrelevant.
>
> But it is asking a lot to be training every week for an entire season and then perhaps a summer tour and then a pre-season tour, and then it's back into the season again.

Helpfully, the paper had a chart highlighting the schedule of one of England's top stars.

July 1: Return to clubs after four-week break following summer tour with national side/Lions

July: Pre-season training begins with clubs. Intensive fitness work building strength and stamina

Early August: Three-day intensive England fitness assessment

Early September: Guinness Premiership begins

October: Two Heineken Cup games plus Premiership

November: Three/four autumn internationals versus the southern hemisphere's best

December: Return to club action in the Heineken Cup and Guinness Premiership

January: Premiership – possible short mid-season break

February/March: Six Nations. Five internationals against the best of the northern hemisphere

April: Premiership play-offs. Heineken Cup semi-finals

May: Premiership final. Heineken Cup final

Late May/June: Lions tour (nine matches). Or two-match national tour to southern hemisphere

Late June–early July: Four weeks' rest before pre-season

*

That November, and with Johnson's squad decimated through injury, no doubt in some significant part due to the residual effects of the Lions tour, Rob Andrew, the RFU's elite rugby director, joined the growing chorus of concerned voices. In an interview with Rob Kitson in the *Guardian*, Andrew said:

There has been a rise over the last season from 20–25% [of players unavailable] up to around 30% and through this autumn we were operating at both 40% of the seniors and Saxons squads being unavailable. That is unsustainable as far as the game is concerned. We don't have figures yet as to whether the breakdown laws are contributing to the injuries, but there is an anecdotal view that the increased collisions are

contributing to a greater risk of injury. It's important the IRB
have a look at both areas pretty quickly. There is a bigger issue
which the game has to address if the upward curve of injuries
is heading where it appears to be going. I think the game has to
look at it very seriously for the longer term. We can't continue
with the current rate of injury.

In January 2010, Simon Kemp gave an interview with *Rugby
World* signposting his belief that a 'head bin' should be introduced
to allow medics more time to evaluate players away from the field.

Rugby's substitution laws had been relaxed to allow tactical
substitutions in the professional era with three first permitted in 1996
and up to eight changes permitted by 2009. A 'blood bin' had been
introduced around 2001 as in many other sports, allowing a player
to leave the pitch temporarily to have a wound treated to avoid the
transmission of blood-borne diseases, notably HIV/Aids and hepatitis.
But at this stage, despite mounting evidence of a brain injury pandemic
playing out before our eyes, if not being recorded in the official data,
no provision was being made to allow players with potentially serious
head injuries to be removed from the field for assessment.

'If you take the injured player to the side line, your team plays
on with 14 men – not an option anyone takes – so you make an
assessment in the short break in play,' said Kemp. 'Making such
a decision in the middle of the pitch in less than two minutes is
an almost impossible challenge. In the less clear-cut cases, because
replacements are permanent, doctors tend to allow players to stay
on and see how things unfold.'

In reality, you did not need to be a doctor to realize players like
Moody, Volley or Dallaglio, to name just a few, had suffered brain
injuries and should have been immediately removed, in line with
IRB regulations at that time that any player with a 'suspicion of
concussion' should be removed immediately and not returned to play.

The problem was that the genie had escaped the bottle and rugby's concussion issue was now so significant, any attempt to address it would only highlight how serious the problem really was.

It's important to stress that Kemp was by no means alone in allowing concussed players back on the field. In fact, it had become standard practice to 'watch and wait' when a player had suffered a head injury.

It was clear by now the old 'three-week stand-down' had gone out of the window and medics, led by Kemp, were arguing for more time to assess players away from the glare of the pitch and shorter return to play protocols.

*

On the field there was no sign of any let-up in the injury toll. At the 2010 Six Nations, James Robson, the Scotland team doctor, was again on hand to save one of his players' lives when winger Thom Evans collided with Wales full back Lee Byrne during Evans' side's dramatic defeat at Cardiff's Millennium Stadium. Evans would later describe the impact, which severely damaged two vertebrae and required emergency surgery, as 'like being hit by a sniper's bullet'.

Mercifully, Robson identified the immediate risk and ensured Evans was kept motionless on the field for 10 minutes before being moved onto a spinal board and away for emergency surgery.

'I owe my life to James Robson,' Evans would later say.

That summer I covered England's two-Test tour to Australia. It was a quick in and out affair, with a few days in Perth for the first Test followed by 10 days in Sydney for the second Test, with a short bus ride up the coast to Newcastle for a midweek game against the Barbarians. With Lewis Moody, Martin Johnson's former team-mate, now installed as captain, England were soundly beaten in Perth.

But in the second, an outstanding back-row performance by Moody, Nick Easter and Tom Croft, with notable contributions from

Ben Youngs, aged 20, and Courtney Lawes, aged 21, saw England claim only their third ever victory on Australian shores.

The fact Moody played on yet again after being knocked senseless has largely been lost in time. But, in the course of researching this book, I was reminded of the moment when Quade Cooper's knee smashed into the side of the England captain's head and Moody was sent careering across the field.

Moody would later say:

All I could hear was Floody [Toby Flood] shouting at me. Everything was in slow motion and my legs weren't really working.

I was heading in one way but my body was going in the other direction. It was a really weird feeling. It was a little bit like an outer body experience. It was so surreal. You hear the voices in slow motion just desperately trying to get you back into the line and that's what drives you.

You know you have to get up and help your team-mates even if it's just a case of standing there and showing the opposition there was another man there in defence. Not that I'd have been much use because I would have just fallen over if they had run at me. It's just part of playing this game, our bodies get tested to their limits.

Moody's testimony reminded me of Tom Williams. Not because there was any allegation of cheating in this instance, but because of the absolute acceptance that it was your duty to be in the defensive line, no matter how badly beaten up you were.

But the RFU's figures continued to tell us there wasn't a problem. According to their data, the number of reported concussions in 2009/10 was just 31 in 135 matches (one every 4.35 matches), compared to 42 in 139 matches (one every 3.3 matches) in 2002/03. Meanwhile, the severity of these concussions was also apparently coming down, with players on average sidelined for 56 days per

1,000 playing hours through concussion in 2002/03, almost halving to just 27 days' absence per 1,000 hours by 2009/10.

So, despite players being bigger, stronger, faster, and ball-in-play time increasing steadily through these years with far more contacts happening at higher velocities, we were being told there were fewer concussions and, on the rare occasions they occurred, they were half as serious as before. It was, palpably, nonsense.

*

Moody's head-related issues continued. As time progressed, far less force was required to render him woozy or cause tunnel vision. Upon returning from Australia to join Bath, after Leicester declined to offer him a new contract, the 32-year-old suffered another head injury against Gloucester in early October 2010. He suffered permanent damage to his eye when he collided with Charlie Sharples's knee while attempting to charge down a kick. Initial concerns about a fractured eye socket were unfounded, but Moody, in journalistic speak, 'faced a race against time' to be fit to face New Zealand.

Later that month, Moody's fellow World Cup winner Phil Vickery finally accepted his race had been run, retiring on medical grounds aged 34, a year after undergoing major spinal surgery. Vickery confided to reporters he was concerned that if he carried on he could end up seeing out his days confined to a wheelchair.

For Moody, he had his fitness to prove following his latest head injury. Playing against Harlequins a week before facing the All Blacks, he may have needed 10 stitches in yet another head wound but this was not deemed significant enough to prevent him playing for England the following weekend.

After the game Moody, attempting to make light of his ongoing vision problems, made a cricketing reference to 'getting his eye in' while admitting: 'I was a bit nervous I wouldn't be able to pick the ball up as quickly but even in the dwindling light it was fine. It's still blurry but when the game gets going your brain ignores it. I was just really happy to get out there and get 70-odd minutes. In an ideal world I'd have played last week as well but you have to listen to the specialists.'

While Moody was publicly putting on a brave face, privately he was struggling with concussions, which were becoming more and more frequent. But with little to no information provided to players in those days, and no apparent cause for concern in the RFU's own injury data, why should he have been worried? Players were routinely being allowed to return to the field, even as further evidence was emerging in the United States linking repeated head injuries with long-term neurological damage.

Two weeks before the start of the 2010/11 Premiership season Boston University's Center for the Study of Traumatic Encephalopathy (CSTE) had published their latest research which provided 'the first pathological evidence that repetitive head trauma experienced in collision sports might be associated with motor neuron disease'.

The research was led by Professor Ann McKee and supported by former professional wrestler turned concussion campaigner Chris Nowinski, who established the Concussion Legacy Foundation as a not-for-profit organization around this time, along with another world-renowned brain injury expert and Boston researcher Professor Robert Cantu, having experienced debilitating symptoms following a professional sporting career beset by concussion.

Nowinski's unenviable but heroic job was to encourage families of dead athletes to donate their loved ones' brains for research. McKee and her team examined the brains and spinal cords of 12 deceased athletes, three of whom, former professional footballers Wally Hilgenberg and Eric Scoggins, as well as an unidentified military veteran and professional boxer, developed motor neurone disease (MND) late in their lives.

The study, funded in part by an unrestricted gift from the NFL to the CSTE, found that when they died 'all 12 athletes showed neuropathological evidence of chronic traumatic encephalopathy... In the three athletes with motor neuron disease, abnormal tau protein deposits were not only found throughout the brain, but also in the spinal cord.'

The researchers also discovered '10 of 12 CTE victims had a second abnormal protein, TDP-43, in their brains. Of those 10, only three had TDP-43 in the brain and the spinal cord, and those were the three athletes diagnosed with motor neuron disease.'

But despite these alarming findings, professional rugby carried on largely oblivious. And with no reason given for them to do otherwise players did what players do: they got up, dusted themselves down and played on.

A week after receiving 10 stitches in a head wound, four weeks after being knocked out against Gloucester, three months since playing on after being knocked out against Australia and three years after being knocked out twice in the same game and playing on against Tonga, England's captain declared himself ready, willing and able to face New Zealand at Twickenham the following week. And the doctors signed him off.

With the Ashes being played down under, it was back to Australia on cricket duty that winter for me but being on the other side of the world would not stop me, watching England playing rugby and I decamped to a bar in downtown Adelaide with my old friend and fellow rugby lover Dean Wilson to watch Johnson's men take on the Springboks in the third Test of the autumn.

Yet again, rugby's desperately substandard head injury protocols were horribly exposed as winger Chris Ashton, who a week earlier had scored one of the all-time great England tries at Twickenham in his side's win over Australia, one of the few times in my journalistic career I felt compelled to let out a yelp of excitement as he careered towards the line, was allowed to play on after he was clearly knocked unconscious attempting to tackle Springbok lock Victor Matfield, and took more than a minute to regain consciousness.

'He's nearly asleep,' referee George Clancy told the England medics attending the winger on the pitch. 'He's slurring his words. Make a responsible decision now.'

Instead, they made the irresponsible decision to keep the player on. Speak to many ex-players from this time, and believe me I have, and they will tell you 'the knowledge wasn't there in those days'.

Former England, Saracens and Bath prop David Flatman told a discussion panel on Tortoise Media in 2022:

> We were worried about our necks, our backs, our knees, our shoulders, our eye sockets, our jaws, our noses, our ears, we were not worried about our brains. That isn't because we were glib or arrogant, or dismissive, or we ignored it. We were literally ignorant. We didn't know that was a problem, it was never spoken about.
>
> The doctors worked seven days a week to take care of us. Maybe there was information that everybody knew that they kept from us? That feels unlikely, but I don't know, so I won't declare either way. But I think the attitude has changed towards it completely, because players are now… well, they're better informed. They know a lot about it.

The IRB regulations stated at this time that players with 'suspected concussion' should be removed from the field but more often than not they played on. At least the Ashton farce led to some questions, which continued in the days that followed.

Twelve days later, having been passed fit to play again for Northampton, Ashton was quizzed about the incident at a Saints media day at Franklin's Gardens.

'At the time you don't really think whether it is the right thing to carry on, you just want to play – but coming off would probably have been the right decision for me and for the team, more importantly,' said Ashton. 'I have watched it and I do appear to be all right but I didn't play how I normally play. I didn't get involved in the game as much as I normally like to, so I definitely wasn't with it.

'The medical staff kept checking every five minutes and I kept saying I was all right, so I kept up a good act,' he explained. 'I was very convincing. The ref wanted me to go off and I can't remember anything about the game, so obviously I wasn't fine. All I remember is coming off and sitting on the bench. I think I remember the bus journey, but then again we did the same bus journey every week so I might not.'

Northampton forwards coach Dorian 'Nobby' West had no objection to the way the incident was handled.

'Rugby is rugby. I've been in that position myself and you just want to stay on and play,' he said. 'Chris wanted to stay on the pitch and the only thing you can do in that situation is monitor a player.'

With impeccable timing, and perhaps seeking to ward off growing concern around the mismanagement of head injuries, the *Guardian* reported on 9 December that the IRB was set to harden its stance on head injuries. They could hardly have softened it.

Paul Rees's article reported:

The International Rugby Board is set to change the regulations next year to ensure that players who suffer serious head injuries, such as Chris Ashton, who insisted on carrying on after being knocked out during England's Test against South Africa last month, are permanently replaced.

The IRB set up a concussion working party after its first medical conference last year and it is due to report in the next few weeks. There is agreement among the medical teams of the major unions that concussion is a growing cause for concern and that it is in the interests of players to be cautious even

when, like Ashton, they plead to stay on. Players would also
be closely monitored during their recovery to ensure there is
a graduated return to play. Under a proposed change in the
regulations that will be put to the IRB's council next May, any
player who suffers a head injury that gives cause for concern
will have to be taken off and replaced permanently...

Referees are likely to be given the authority to order a
player with suspected concussion to be replaced but the desire
is for team doctors to take a stand. All World Cup matches next
year will have an independent doctor who will assess whether
it is safe for someone who has suffered a blow to the head to
continue.

To me, it was beginning to appear more like smoke and mirrors.
What other regulations did the sport need when it was already clearly
stated within the IRB's own guidelines that if a player was suspected
of having a concussion, they should be removed from the field of play
immediately and permanently? Was Ashton not suspected of having
a concussion? And why was the decision about whether they played
on being left with the player?

While players playing on through concussion was nothing new, it
was clear to me that it was now happening, to coin a phrase, on an
'industrial scale'. It wasn't that players were occasionally not taken off
through concussion, now they were almost never taken off. Witness
Moody and Ashton, where two of the highest-profile England players
could be knocked completely unconscious in live televised games
but permitted to carry on in defiance of the regulations without any
repercussion for those charged with looking after them. Of course,
players wanted to carry on playing. International rugby players, male
and female, are imbued with a warrior spirit. To put the onus on
them to make a decision, when potentially suffering from the effects
of a brain injury, was simply absurd.

It was evident to me and other observers, including Jackson, that as the game grew faster and more physical and collisions occurred more frequently and with more intensity, doctors were, for myriad reasons, becoming far less conservative in the way they managed brain injuries. It was evident they were taking far more risks with players' brains. And that was just in matches. Away from the cameras and media scrutiny, I could only imagine what was going on in training.

With coaches holding huge power within club or national set-ups, as exposed in graphic detail by the Bloodgate scandal and anecdotally, medical professionals were being placed in the invidious position of being damned if they did remove a player and damned if they didn't. In my potentially naïve eyes, though, their duty of care lay entirely with the players, not their employers. Doctors like Scotland's James Robson showed it was possible to survive, just, within the system without betraying the Hippocratic oath to first and foremost 'do no harm'.

But while there was no doubt in my mind, and among a growing band of other rugby lovers who believed the sport had become dangerously weighted in favour of brute force and power, there remained a number of challenges to reporting this in the sports pages. The biggest obstacle was that no one wanted to hear it.

Meanwhile, the RFU and Premiership Rugby continued to deny professional rugby was getting more dangerous. Worse still, the line given to the media following the publication of the 2009/10 season professional injury audit in February 2011 was that rugby was actually getting safer. The press release containing the report, distributed just minutes before it was published and therefore providing next to no time to critically assess it, carried a photograph of Simon Kemp at Twickenham in 2008 attending the stricken Mike Tindall, his liver lacerated and lung perforated. It was an odd picture to accompany a press release which, somewhat triumphantly, told us the 2009/10 season had seen a 20 per cent reduction in the likelihood of sustaining a match injury while there had also been an overall reduction in the severity of injury from 23 days to 22 days (average time sidelined) and as a result a reduction in the total number of days absent of 26 per cent. The following year (2010/11), both injury severity and frequency rose again, but this slight drop in 2009/10, defying all logic and anecdotal evidence following the most physically demanding Lions tour ever witnessed, was seized upon.

A headline in *Rugby World*, still edited at this time by Paul Morgan, read: 'Rugby is getting safer in England's top flight'.

I was appalled by what appeared to be a lack of journalistic rigour and willingness to swallow the 'party line'. Here was a one-off drop in severity which certainly didn't represent a downward trend being presented by the RFU and Premiership Rugby as something far more significant than it actually was. Surely Morgan could see what the rest of us could see? A few months later, Morgan accepted the lucrative position as Premiership Rugby's director of communications, a post he remained in until March 2023.

In the big picture, I thought it irresponsible to make some of the claims in the press release, especially considering the previous year's report had shown a 20.5 per cent increase in injury severity; a more important measure of the injury picture which went largely unreported. In my view, to suggest rugby was getting safer off the back of a one-off decline in the frequency of injuries seemed improbable at best.

By now, Kemp had assumed a new title: RFU Head of Sports Medicine and Chair of the England Rugby Premiership Injury and Training Audit Steering Group, which produced the report. He said in the press release: 'The data… shows a welcome reduction in the likelihood of match injuries and in that regard is much closer to the results of previous years. There was a reduction in the severity of injuries across all categories and a marked reduction in the recurrence of match injuries. That suggests a more complete and effective rehabilitation of all injuries by club and England medics.'

Just 31 concussions were reported, suggesting just one was occurring every 4.35 games. This simply did not tally with what we were witnessing or hearing in the professional game on a weekly basis. By now I was convinced the figures in the report were seriously underplaying both the extent of the problem and the risk posed by playing at the top level.

But the status quo remained. Even England head coach Martin Johnson was convinced, according to the RFU press release:

> I am encouraged by the results of the latest injury audit and the reduction in both the likelihood and severity of injury. Investment in the injury audit has been crucial, providing the game in England with a robust, clinical programme of research that allows the kind of accurate assessment of the injury risk involved in training for and playing elite rugby union that no other country can replicate.

Phil Winstanley, rugby director at Premiership Rugby, added:

> The reduction in injury rates shown in the latest audit is encouraging, however the value is in the ongoing analysis of data and the changes that can inform. The injury audit is the main part of what is a much wider programme of medical initiatives taking place in England designed to promote the safest playing and training environment in world rugby and an example of what can be achieved when clubs, players and the union work together.

The report paved the way for rugby union, at a professional level, to carry on as normal. Whatever normal was.

6

Death of a schoolboy

On 31 January 2011, Benjamin Robinson's life support machine was turned off. Two days earlier the 14-year-old schoolboy sustained three separate head injuries in a game between two schools in Northern Ireland.

A happy-go-lucky boy with everything to live for, Benjamin was a strong-running centre from a rugby-loving family who lived to play sport. On three separate occasions, in a game between Carrickfergus Grammar and Dalriada, he was allowed to play on, having been examined following blows to the head.

Benjamin's mother, Karen, had earlier been told to calm down by the referee after she voiced grave concerns about her son's continued participation in the game.

When he collapsed, seconds from the final whistle, Karen rushed onto the field.

'Benjamin, Mama's here,' she said as she attempted to keep her little boy warm. But it was too late. Despite her best efforts, her young son's brain injuries were too severe.

'I was hit with the very cold, hard, realization that the son I love and adore, my only son, my youngest, had gone,' Karen would later tell the *Guardian*'s Andy Bull.

The doctors who treated Benjamin at the hospital were shocked by the severity of the injuries to his brain, which had swollen to such an extent it pushed into the base of his spinal cord. Had it not been for the rugby kit he was admitted in, they would reasonably have assumed Benjamin had been involved in a road traffic accident.

Two days after the game, and showing no outward signs of life, doctors injected cold water into Benjamin's ears with a syringe, a test used to determine brainstem death known as the caloric reflex test. There was no response.

His father, Peter, himself a former rugby player, had flown over from Edinburgh the moment he had heard of his son's plight and was at his bedside when they turned off his life support machine.

'It's really hard to know that if just one person had recognized the signs of concussion he could still be alive today,' Peter said.

You would imagine the incident would have been reported on by those of us whose job it was to cover rugby union. But it wasn't. Not enough, anyway. In fact, Benjamin Robinson's death was hardly reported outside his local area. The first I heard of it was when the coroner found Benjamin had died from second impact syndrome, the condition Dr Paul McCrory had in 2001 dedicated part of a paper towards effectively denying the existence of. The coroner also found Benjamin had 'passed all the tests'.

It would be another three years before I even began to understand the suffering his family had endured, when I met Peter for the first time. Peter, a tireless campaigner and one of rugby's true heroes who now lives in Edinburgh, has vowed to keep his son's name alive with his 'If In Doubt, Sit Them Out' campaign. Along with the likes of Dr James Robson and Professor Willie Stewart from Glasgow University, Peter has been a hugely influential figure in Scottish sport, securing a more unified approach to concussion management than has so far been achieved in England or Wales including a joined-up approach to head injury management in all sports in Scotland.

The thinking behind the message of the 'If In Doubt, Sit Them Out' campaign focused on erring on the side of caution, whereas

World Rugby's preferred 'Recognise and Remove' slogan implies the need to actually diagnose a concussion. Meanwhile, the RFU's decision to name their principal concussion education tool 'Headcase' was considered clumsy by brain injury charities. Their failure to acknowledge the potential risk of fatality associated with concussion also meant the message failed to cut through. 'If In Doubt, Sit Them Out' is simple, concise and to the point.

'Rugby is just a game,' Peter told me. 'No one should die playing a game. It is not war, whatever some people would have you believe. If there is any suspicion a player has suffered a brain injury, they should leave the field immediately.'

If In Doubt, Sit Them Out key messages

- A concussion is a brain injury.

- All concussions are serious.

- Most concussions occur without loss of consciousness.

- Anyone with any symptoms following a head injury must be removed from playing or training and must not take part in any physical activity until all concussion symptoms have cleared.

- Specifically, there must be no return to play on the day of any suspected concussion.

- Return to education or work takes priority over return to play.

- If in doubt, sit them out to help prevent further injury or even death.

- Head injury can be fatal.

- Most concussions recover with time and a staged return to normal life and sport.

At the time of writing, Labour MP Chris Bryant continues to push hard for a UK wide national strategy on acquired brain injury but, to date, and to my knowledge, Scotland's government-backed protocols remain far superior to anything available in England. Crucially, they recognize that concussion can be fatal, something English sports authorities have been reticent to state in their literature.

*

Five years before Benjamin Robinson died, 13-year-old Seattle high school American football player Zackery Lystedt had suffered a brain injury attempting to make a tackle. Like Benjamin, Zackery played on. After the game, as he was walking away from the field, Zack collapsed and was airlifted to a specialist hospital, where he spent the next 93 days.

'He had a bleed on the right and left side of the brain that was compressing his brain, and that required them not only to take off the bone on each side of his brain and leave it out, but actually take out the blood clot,' Richard Ellenbogen MD, Zack's neurosurgeon, told ESPN.

As Zack embarked on a lifetime of rehabilitation, his parents campaigned for new legislation which, they hoped, would spare other families going through what they'd suffered. In May 2009, Washington State Governor Christine Gregoire signed the Zackery Lystedt legislation into law. The new law essentially prohibited young athletes suspected of sustaining a concussion from returning to play without the approval of a licensed healthcare provider. The law aimed to mitigate the consequences of concussion through education and medical intervention. Similar laws have been adopted in all 50 US states.

To this day, no such law exists in the UK.

Far from implementing new directives which would have made returning to play following concussion more difficult around this time, it can reasonably be argued rugby union chose to do precisely the opposite. On 2 June 2011, the IRB announced an end to rugby's mandatory three-week concussion stand-down, introduced in 1977 in response to decades of research demonstrating the 'cumulative effect of concussion' in athletes. Instead a 'graduated return to play' (GRTP) programme at elite level enabled players, if symptom free, to play again within six days of incurring a diagnosed concussion.

It was a hugely significant moment for rugby union brought about and enabled by, I and many others would argue, the reports of the Concussion in Sport Group, of which Paul McCrory and Michael Turner were among the lead signatories, and who consistently downplayed the longer-term risks and asserted the need for more individually tailored return to play programmes instead of a blanket 21-day stand-down.

McCrory alone published no fewer than 164 articles while editor of the highly influential *British Journal of Sports Medicine* between 2001 and 2008, consistently raising doubts over previously accepted science linking repetitive head injuries with poor longer-term neurological outcomes while also calling into question conditions such as second impact syndrome. In doing so, he facilitated a sporting culture which treated concussion as no more than a short-term inconvenience.

Rather than treat concussion as a uniquely serious injury, professional rugby players, coaches, fans and media were by now taking the diametrically opposite position.

'I will not apologize for having laughed at and brushed off concussion because we didn't know it was serious,' former Bath and England prop David Flatman later told me. 'We just thought "happy days we haven't broken our arm so we can play on". It wasn't toughness or machismo, it was ignorance. Plain and simple. We did not know.' Why would they know? No-one was telling them otherwise.

Many viewed the newly drawn-up six-day GRTP window as extraordinarily convenient as it allowed top players precisely enough time to prove their fitness for the following weekend. The myriad commercial and competitively driven reasons for this move were obvious.

It may be hard to believe now, but, at the time, there was next to no interest paid to this seismically important development from rugby's media, me included.

Rather, there was a sense of inevitability about this push towards ever shorter return to play times as it was completely in keeping with the overall picture in which players were treated as dispensable commodities and where television and marketing executives were placing more pressure on top players to be available for more matches. Commercially, having the stars available week in, week out was hugely appealing and that pressure did not just come from the TV companies but also from players and coaches. Doctors and physios were the ones who could facilitate it happening.

The six-day Graduated Return to Play programme differentiated for the first time the brains of professional players and amateurs and, crucially, potentially removed neurologists or brain experts from the process of 'signing off' a player before they returned to play following a diagnosed concussion. When all the evidence was pointing to the need for more conservative concussion management, professional rugby moved decisively in the opposite direction.

*

The *News of the World* closed in July 2011 amid damaging allegations that news reporters had illegally hacked voicemail messages to gain stories. The allegations, most of which proved accurate, sickened me and in many ways I was relieved when the decision came to close the paper. Fortunately, I'd maintained excellent relationships with the other sports desks, and as I'd already booked a non-refundable trip to the World Cup in New Zealand, I offered my services around to other News Iternational titles, with *The Times* offering me paid work.

Before departure, several of us were invited to a sponsors' dinner at Twickenham, laid on as a farewell for the team by O2. I was seated next to James Haskell and thought little of the fact he arrived almost an hour late. As a journalist you get used to waiting around for players.

When he did eventually arrive, James and I got on well over dinner, as we did most of the time, but relationships between journalists and players were about to get seriously strained when, barely a week into the tournament, photos emerged of Mike Tindall, married in July that year to the Queen's granddaughter Zara Phillips, appearing rather too familiar with an unknown woman in a bar in Queenstown.

In a surreal twist, pictures also emerged of England players attending the 'Mad Midget Weekender' party at the Altitude nightclub which, apparently, involved manhandling dwarfs on the dance floor.

With tabloid news reporters descending on New Zealand faster than Tindall could say 'I'm a celebrity get me out of here', the tournament became a PR disaster off the field while fortunes were hardly better on it, England losing to France in a drab quarter final display.

I felt sorry for Martin Johnson. He'd trusted his players and they let him down badly. Moody also deserved better, and at their final press conference together in Auckland before they headed home it was sad to see two good, trusting men crushed by events on and off the field.

Back on the field, Wales captain Sam Warburton was sent off in the first half of the semi-final against France for a tip tackle, another dangerous new development of the professional era which saw the defender upend the attacker by driving upwards from their midriff, lifting their opponent's legs above the horizontal and often driving them down into the ground head, neck or shoulder first.

Initially, commentators Michael Owen and Nick Mullins believed Warburton had been handed a yellow card for flipping France winger

Vincent Clerc's legs 'beyond the horizontal' and allowing his head and neck to thud into the turf.

'I think that's very, very harsh to get a yellow card for that,' Owen said. 'You're playing rugby. It's a pretty ferocious game. It's very hard to bring someone down...'

But referee Alain Rolland, following the IRB directive to the letter, had actually shown Warburton a straight red.

'Hang on,' said an audibly shocked Mullins. 'Is that a red card rather than a yellow card? For this? It's a red card. Sam Warburton has been sent off. In a World Cup semi-final. One of the most controversial decisions in the history of the World Cup.'

Mullins was far from alone in being shocked. Outraged even. But Rolland's call had sent the strongest message, and players and coaches reacted by changing their approach to tackling. This type of tackle simply hadn't existed before professionalism and while there was no malice intended from Warburton, or indeed most of the players who deployed it, what mattered was the outcome. The tackler was responsible for the way the ball carrier landed and recklessness was being clamped down on. Within a year, the tip tackle had almost completely disappeared from rugby and spines, necks and brains were safer for it. But while that incident showed tip tackles were now being properly policed, concussion management, when it happened, was as poor as ever, and four years after Moody's double knockout, France fly half Morgan Parra was knocked out in the final, only to go off and come back on again. It barely got a line in anyone's match reports.

Moody's international retirement a few weeks later came as no surprise; nor did Johnson's sacking shortly afterwards. It was a poignant way for two great warriors to end their associations with England. Johnson's sacking was unusual in that it came following the leaking of a highly sensitive tour report for which the RPA had gathered evidence via confidential questionnaires circulated to players. Although the leak was widely believed to have come from within the

RFU, it damaged the RPA's standing with players, with one telling me it caused an 'irrevocable breakdown in trust'.

Things got deeply unpleasant with players portrayed as money hungry and lazy, while Johnson's coaching team was shredded. Relationships, reputations and mental health suffered across English rugby as a result.

There were stories being leaked left, right and centre, and when one Premiership coach told me the players had been late for the pre-departure dinner because they were threatening to strike over image rights and distribution of sponsorship, I filed the story for the *Mail on Sunday*, where I'd struck up an excellent relationship on the road with their rugby correspondent Ian Stafford.

The story was on the money in every sense. It convinced sports editor Malcolm Vallerius of my credentials and he offered me a rugby and cricket reporting role on the paper.

Early in 2012, I became even more convinced that the RFU and Premiership Rugby were misrepresenting the data generated from their annual injury audit. Despite a reported 16.25 per cent rise in the frequency of matchday injuries, essentially offsetting the drop from the year before, which had been presented as 'rugby is getting safer', an increase from 80 injuries per 1,000 playing hours in 2009/10 to 93 in 2010/11 was presented as 'within normal levels'. Meanwhile, the undeniable fact players were now bigger, faster and stronger was described by Kemp as 'perception'.

'People like playing and watching rugby union because it is a collision sport. We try and make it as safe as you can while keeping it recognizable as rugby. Despite the perception players are bigger, faster and stronger there isn't any evidence that the injury rate has increased in professional rugby since 2002,' Kemp said in an interview with the Press Association. What he failed to say was there was lots of evidence the injury rate had increased dramatically before 2002, while many observed that the severity of injuries, if not the frequency, was getting worse.

He contined, 'although the studies before 2002 were not as comprehensive, there is some evidence that there was an increase in injury risk between 1995 and 2001, but the risk has now stabilized. We do see differences in risk from season to season, as you would expect, but they are those that reflect differences that have arisen as a result of normal statistical variation.'

Thanks to some heavy top spin, the headlines shifted subtly from 'Rugby is safer than ever' to 'Rugby is no more dangerous than before'.

Kemp, with the support of the RFU's PR department and a complicit media, was using individual statistics to bolster the 'rugby is safe' narrative, such as the 20 per cent drop in injury frequency the previous year, while inferring that the appalling toll we'd witnessed on the Lions tour the previous summer should not be taken out of context. All the while, reported concussion, still inexplicably below the rate first reported in 2002, barely got a mention.

'At the last IRB meeting we looked at all the good quality data since the turn of the millennium. There simply isn't a year-on-year rise of injury risk,' Kemp said. 'The value of studying the whole league is that it smooths out the club-by-club variations. To infer rugby is more dangerous from looking at the injuries sustained by a single club or team at one point in time is invalid.

'This study gives strong enough information to be able to draw sensible conclusions.'

Crucially, the rise in one-off potentially career-ending injuries had doubled from three (2002/03) to six (2008/09) and would continue to track upwards over the coming years. By 2014/15, the risk of sustaining a one-off career-threatening injury was 200 per cent higher than in 2002/03, with nine occurring in the season. By 2017/18, this figure had risen to 300 per cent higher, with 12 injuries requiring more than 12 weeks out. But in 2012, those of us calling out rugby's dangerous evolution were told to keep calm and carry on. Clearly, we weren't drawing sensible conclusions.

It was next to impossible to challenge the findings when it came to the data. The RFU's medical department gathered it from club and national physios and medical teams, which was then effectively processed in-house through their close commercial relationship with Bath University. The bridge between the two organizations was made by Professor Keith Stokes, Professor of Applied Physiology at University of Bath and Medical Research Lead at the RFU.

Stokes became a senior lecturer at Bath in February 2002, the same year the injury audit was launched, shortly after completing a PhD at Loughborough University.

The University of Bath's website states:

> Professor Keith Stokes has established strong partnerships with stakeholders in Rugby Union and other sports to investigate injury risk in sport and to develop and evaluate strategies to reduce injury risk. He also has a strong interest in the prevention of frailty in older adults.
>
> He has published over 150 articles in journals such as the *British Journal of Sports Medicine, Sports Medicine, American Journal of Sports Medicine, International Journal of Sports Physiology and Performance*, and the *Journal of Applied Physiology*.
>
> Keith has attracted over £5 million in external funding from agencies such the Rugby Football Union, The RFU Injured Players Foundation, World Rugby, United Kingdom Sports Council and BBSRC.
>
> He is editor for the *International Journal of Sports Medicine*, is on the editorial board of *PLoS ONE*, and is on the Advisory Board (Biological Sciences) of the *Journal of Sports Sciences*.
>
> He is a Fellow of the British Association of Sport and Exercise Sciences and a Fellow of the Higher Education

Academy. In 2013, Keith received a University Knowledge Exchange Award in partnership with the Rugby Football Union.

Stokes was still in this role at the time this book went to print. But the audit process was hopelessly opaque and inaccessible. All I could be sure of was that the concussion figures reported were wholly inaccurate and the sport's injury profile was being completely misrepresented as a result. I knew the sport was getting more dangerous because I witnessed it and its participants told me, but for the time being, rugby union seemed determined to hold the line.

*

That summer provided a welcome break from life on the road. I'd covered close to 200 Premiership and European matches and over 70 internationals in seven years and that was before all the cricket Tests and one-day internationals.

Much as I loved travelling around the grounds and clubs with my friends in the rugby pack – we affectionately referred to each other as 'the Jacks' – I welcomed the opportunity to draw breath when Malcolm offered me a role on the desk at the *Mail on Sunday*.

I'd do two or three shifts a week in the office, sub-editing copy, answering the phone and helping Malcolm and his deputy Mike Richards filter out the best stories. This also gave me a chance to gain a little more understanding of what was going on in the States.

The previous year I'd read that retired NFL player Dave Duerson had committed suicide by shooting himself through the heart. The 50-year-old, a key figure in the Chicago Bears' 1985 Super Bowl winning squad, had planned his death meticulously. Having suffered mood swings, searing headaches and struggling with simple spelling tasks following his retirement, the previously affable and mild-mannered Duerson chose to kill himself. Among several notes he left behind, setting out financial and other arrangements, one read: 'Please, see my brain is given to the NFL brain bank.'

In the spring of 2012, another NFL star, Junior Seau, also killed himself by taking a shotgun to his chest. A few months later, I read a report in the *LA Times* stating that 'Junior Seau had brain disease when he committed suicide'. Slowly, the penny was beginning to drop. Meanwhile, details emerged of the legal case involving around 4,000 former NFL stars and 2,000 families of former players claiming negligence against the NFL in its handling of head injuries.

And the reason they were bringing the case? Because the league had failed to inform them of the long-term risks associated with repeated brain injuries and many of them were suffering serious neurological conditions in their retirement. A couple of quotes in the *LA Times* article really stood out to me.

Former NFL linebacker Gary Plummer, a team-mate of Seau in San Diego, said:

> Your entire life, that is probably your most revered characteristic as a player – your toughness, your ability to handle pain, your ability to overcome adversity… You've got to be mentally tough, you've got to overcome. Just block out this pain. It's taught from coaches from the time you're in Pop Warner [equivalent of mini rugby]. I've done it myself as a coach, coaching my kids through high school.
>
> Junior was obviously very good at it. He'd play through ridiculous pain that some people wouldn't even get out of bed with to go to an office job. Sometimes you play a game with those.

I was also interested in a comparison made by a director from the UCLA Brain Injury Research Center, Dr David Hovda, comparing the mindset of gridiron stars to the military: 'Athletes are like military personnel in that they don't tell the truth. They want to go back to play, or they want to go back and be with their unit, so they're less likely to be straightforward with a physician or trainer or coach.'

The article struck a chord and I asked myself: 'If this is happening in NFL, why not professional rugby?'

*

Stuart Lancaster took over as interim England head coach from Johnson at the end of 2011. I immediately liked him. With no public profile to speak of, and a refreshing absence of ego, Lancaster knew he had to work with the media and not against us. He was open, collegiate and unfailingly polite with everyone he dealt with. He also had a deep knowledge of England's future stars and, given some slack, I believed he could be just the sort of progressive, open-minded leader English rugby desperately needed after so foolishly forcing Woodward to walk away seven years earlier.

There was also change at the top of the *Mail on Sunday*. New editor Geordie Greig was appointed in March 2012 and he didn't waste much time before sacking Malcolm who, despite some eccentric tendencies, I'd enjoyed working for and was sorry to see go. The industry rumour mill immediately cranked into action and all sorts of names, all of them men, were suggested as potential successors. But I'd wager not one person in sports journalism saw the appointment of Alison Kervin coming.

I'd known of Alison's work through the rugby books she'd ghost-written and, growing up sports-obsessed, I recognized her byline from the sports pages of *The Times*, *Rugby World* and other outlets. But I'd never met her face to face.

As soon as I did, I immediately liked her. As the first female sports editor on Fleet Street there was a lot of scepticism around her appointment and I was shocked at how scathing some of the comments were from other reporters. But, having chatted with her,

I was more than willing to give her the benefit of the doubt. She seemed personable and decent.

With next to no experience inside the office, Alison had little choice but to trust her writers. While a few other editors I'd worked for took a controlling, top-down approach, treating reporters either as schoolchildren or incompetent, or both, Alison showed great faith in her reporters from an early stage.

Right from the beginning she seemed keen to back what I was doing and, as she had a far broader interest in and knowledge of rugby than any other sports editor I'd worked for, I saw no reason why I couldn't work effectively with her. I also liked her deputy Mike Richards, a detail-driven, quietly spoken Oxford graduate with an impressive intellect and extraordinary sports knowledge. Roger Lacey, the chief sub-editor, was grumpy and seemed to dislike all the reporters but, having spent time in the office with him, we had built up a good rapport and mutual respect. Above all, Lacey was bloody good at his job.

Cara Sloman, the desk secretary, made the desk tick and provided the role of mother hen to the often high-maintenance group of mainly male reporters. Cara is also a highly effective journalist in her own right and one of the kindest people I know.

I soon made my concerns about rugby's direction of travel clear to Alison. I told her of the dangers I saw on the horizon, commercially and in terms of player welfare. I told her the injury picture was far worse than it was being portrayed.

Peter Jackson had taught me that money-related stories always generated interest, even if the numbers in rugby didn't come close to matching those of football, but injury stories rarely got quite the same level of traction. Sure, it was important to report on them as they impacted on selection and by extension a team's chances of winning or losing, but they were not 'sexy'. Much of sport's success around the globe is built on the fantasies of fans, many of whom imagine the participants on the field are in some way superhuman.

That is certainly what sports marketing, advertising and PR, costing countless millions, would have most people believe.

While all this was going on, the Pitchside Suspected Concussion Assessment (PSCA) was being trialled at the IRB Junior World Championship in South Africa and the following year it would be rolled out across the professional game.

According to the IRB's website at the time, a PSCA could be requested by a team doctor or match referee if they 'suspect that a player may have a suspected concussion' with a temporary replacement taking the field. Crucially, and in a clear response to Bloodgate, the temporary replacements were 'not allowed to take kicks at goal'.

The rules stipulated that the PSCA would incorporate a series of questions relating to cognition known as the 'Maddock questions' and 'must be completed within five minutes'.

Similar to the abolition of the 21-day mandatory stand-down, the drive for a 'head bin' first flagged by Simon Kemp two years previously drew little media attention. But some in the sport were taking it very seriously indeed.

Dr Barry O'Driscoll is an Irishman with a Mancunian accent who, like his brother John, cousin Frank and Frank's son Brian – yes, that one – played rugby union for Ireland. O'Driscoll followed his Army doctor father into medicine, and played full back for Lancashire before being spotted by Ireland's selectors following a brilliant performance against Ulster on a stinking night at Ravenhill.

In 1968, he was called up for the Five Nations Championship but before the days of tactical substitutions spent the entire campaign on the bench. 'In those days you had four subs: a scrum-half, hooker, utility forward and utility back,' O'Driscoll said. 'But for four years, none of the backs were injured.' He eventually made his debut in 1971 and went on to win four caps for Ireland, while also having the rare honour of beating the All Blacks while playing for North West Counties the following year.

O'Driscoll retired aged 31 and proceeded to land a series of influential roles within sports medicine, becoming Irish Exiles' medical rep at the Irish Rugby Football Union (IRFU); chairman of the IRFU Medical Committee; Anti-Doping Commissioner at the IRB; and World Cup Commissioner in Australia (2003), France (2007) and New Zealand (2011).

Like me, he had watched the game change radically during that time and found himself frequently out of step with other senior doctors at the IRB.

Unbeknownst to almost anyone outside the IRB's small medical advisory board upon which he sat in an advisory role, O'Driscoll had clashed repeatedly with head of medicine Martin Raftery in the lead-up to the introduction of the PSCA in 2012. He had also previously raised concerns with his own doctors' union over what he perceived to be Kemp's attempts to remove a neurological expert from the process of assessing whether or not a player was deemed to have a concussion.

On 2 June 2012, O'Driscoll wrote to IRB chairman Bernard Lapasset, copying Raftery and acting CEO Robert Brophy, describing the proposed pitchside assessment as 'ill thought out research on teenagers using a minimal and virtually meaningless protocol', adding: 'We in rugby are about to use these teenagers as guinea pigs. We will be playing Russian roulette with their brains. If anything goes wrong either when one of them RTP [returns to play] after five minutes or at some stage in the future, the IRB may be held vicariously liable and rightly so.'

He went on: 'We have in rugby done much by endorsing Zurich [i.e. the Consensus Statement of the CISG] and producing our fine guidelines. We will do more good work in the future but do not destroy it by this research project, which is dangerous and does not even start to stand up to analysis.' O'Driscoll also highlighted the mounting NFL legal situation, the risk posed by sub-concussive impacts and the fact rugby had a higher concussion rate than American football, with NFL stars playing a maximum of 17 regular games in a short season, as opposed to more than 30 across nine months in professional rugby union.

The letter prompted a furious response from Raftery who accused O'Driscoll of being 'offensive' to those who had devised the protocol while insisting NFL and rugby union could not be compared as 'attacks to the head were only outlawed in 2010!!' whereas 'attacks to the head in rugby have been illegal since William Webb Ellis picked up the ball.' Raftery also bullishly stated that 'multiple studies from the US confirm that players are continuing to use their heads as offensive and defensive weapons in NFL and this action is still the major cause of concussion at all levels of their game'.

Raftery also referenced Paul McCrory a number of times, citing 'McCrory's latest article in the Medical Journal of Australia 2012 [which highlights] that in the US, the media and the lawyers are driving the debate and science is not supporting this non medical "push"!'

The first many of us heard of O'Driscoll's concerns came in March 2013, when Tom English conducted a bombshell interview with him in the *Scotsman*. O'Driscoll told English:

> Rugby is trivializing concussion. They are sending these guys back on to the field into the most brutal arena… There is no test you can do in five minutes which shows a player is not concussed… We have all seen players who have appeared fine five minutes after suffering a concussive injury then vomiting later in the night…
>
> If a boxer cannot defend himself after ten seconds he has to have a brain scan before he comes back. And we're not talking ten seconds for a rugby player, we're talking maybe a minute that these guys are not sure what is going on. They don't have to have a brain scan, they have to have five minutes where they

have to stand up straight without falling over four times, they have a basic memory test – 'What's the score? Who are you playing against? Which half did it happen in? And do you have any symptoms?'

These questions should serve as a landmark for when you examine them six hours later to see if they're getting worse or if they're bleeding into their brain. That's why you ask them, not to see if they can go back on. They are already concussed at that point. You don't need to ask questions to find that out. If six hours later their responses are worse than they were earlier you say 'Wait a minute, this shouldn't be the case, is this guy going to bleed?' That's why you ask the questions and so it has always been. But we're going in the other direction now. We're going from being stood down for three weeks to one week to five minutes with players who are showing exactly the same symptoms. The five-minute rule came out of the blue. I couldn't be a part of it so I resigned from the IRB. It saddened me, but I couldn't have my name attached to that decision.

In response, the article quoted the IRB's Raftery as stating 'evidence supporting the theory that collision sports have a negative effect on cognitive function has been questioned by many scientists.' It just so happened most of those scientists had close ties to sport.

A few years later I witnessed O'Driscoll walk into an RPA end-of-season awards dinner held in Battersea, south London, where he was greeted as a long-lost brother by current and former players alike. Like Robson, O'Driscoll was, and is, a 'player's doctor'.

In the article, English also wrote about a visit to Murrayfield for a Six Nations game between Scotland and Wales made by three men: Chris Nowinski, former wrestler and founder of the Concussion Legacy Foundation; a neuropathologist from Glasgow University, Professor Willie Stewart; and American documentary maker Steve

James, who was making a film about concussion in sport called *Head Games: The Global Concussion Crisis*, set to be released in the UK the following year. Coincidentally, on the same day, Ireland captain Brian O'Driscoll, Barry's relation, was allowed to carry on playing against France while clearly suffering the effects of concussion.

'I couldn't believe the physicality of that Scotland versus Wales game,' Nowinski told English. 'Then I watched the Ireland versus France game on television where there were two very obvious concussions and only one player was removed. The other was allowed to continue in such a state that if it happened in the States there would be an outcry. It's exploitation for a concussed player to be allowed back on the field. It's like you giving a drunk the keys to his car because he tells you he's fine.'

Nowinski himself had experienced terrible mood swings, headaches and other post-concussive symptoms after retiring from professional wrestling and had first had chronic traumatic encephalopathy explained to him by Professor Robert Cantu.

Cantu worked alongside Professor Ann McKee at Boston University School of Medicine – also known as the Boston brain bank – and explained that CTE was a degenerative disease caused by repeated head trauma, leading to all the symptoms Nowinski was experiencing. He also explained that – in the worst cases – CTE led to early onset dementia.

At that time, the Boston Group had examined around 100 brains of deceased former athletes, including former San Diego linebacker Junior Seau, who had shot himself the previous year. Evidence of CTE was found in the overwhelming majority of brains examined, and this formed the central part of the class action legal case being brought against the NFL by thousands of former American footballers and families of former players, alleging the league had underplayed the risks of head injuries in their sport while owning, controlling and misrepresenting research into the long-term effects. By controlling the narrative, the NFL had controlled the information flow.

'It was a big battle with the NFL,' Nowinski said. 'We had years of trying to convince them that concussion and CTE was something they needed to take seriously.

'The idea that rugby wouldn't have it [CTE] is silly. Rugby's physicality is extraordinary. Also, the five-minute rule doesn't make sense to me. It's ludicrous. It's simply a matter of time before CTE is found in a rugby player.'

Professor Stewart, himself a former amateur rugby player, spoke of his frustration at some major unions' refusal to recognize CTE and the long-term risks of repeated brain trauma.

He said:

> America has moved on but in the UK and internationally there is talk about concussion but there is also denial about it. James Robson of the Scottish Rugby Union is different in that he is fully on top of the situation, but elsewhere there seems to be an attitude that this is not a problem for the game and that worries me. There is nothing different about an American brain compared to a British or Irish brain.

O'Driscoll shared Stewart's concerns, relating some of the conversations he'd had with senior doctors in rugby including Raftery and Kemp:

> The IRB said to me when I wrote to them about the lessons of American football, they said it's a different game, that you can't compare, they wear helmets, they have (or used to have) head on head collisions, but concussion is concussion is concussion. To say that we cannot take any of the facts that they've discovered in America because it's a different game is head in the sand.

I have no reason to doubt that we are going to get cases of CTE in rugby... it is our responsibility to learn from what is happening in America and act on that. We have to presume that it can happen in rugby or else we might have a very big debt to pay years from now.

That last point drove home the urgency of O'Driscoll's message and resonated with me as someone who had long held reservations about rugby's increasing tolerance – that shifting baseline – of serious injuries, especially concussion. Finally, here were informed experts challenging what, since the advent of professionalism, had become rugby's new normal.

We were witnessing a generation of professional rugby players being exposed to hitherto unimaginable forces, more collisions and risk than any players had been for more than a century of the game's codified existence. Surely we would prefer to sit down in 20 years, having been too risk averse, but with a generation of players with all their faculties intact? The alternative was unthinkable.

*

I'd read Paul Kimmage's book *Engage: The Fall and Rise of Matt Hampson* late in 2012, in which he brilliantly recounted Matt's life story. The *Telegraph* would describe it as a 'hellish, inspiring and often hilarious account' which left me in tears on a several occasions. Like Andy Bull's coverage of Ben Robinson's death, Kimmage's sensitivity, empathy and compassion shone through in his writing and portrayed Hampson as both utterly vulnerable and heroically brave. It was among the most honest and challenging books I have ever read but also convinced me great sports writing needn't be soft shelled. In fact, the opposite was true. The further under the skin you got of a subject the more information you could give your reader.

As soon as Alison Kervin was appointed, I suggested I interview Hampson. She thought it was a good idea and I contacted him to see if he was keen. Thankfully, he was. It proved among the most uplifting experiences of my life, meeting a young man, his body broken by rugby, who held no bitterness or resentment towards the sport whatsoever. His resilience and love for life moved me profoundly.

I rang the desk afterwards and spoke to Alison about the interview. She gave me almost no direction in terms of what to write or an angle to take but simply said: 'I'm really looking forward to reading it.' It may sound silly, but this gave me enormous confidence. Even though I was now an established sports writer, I still feared my words being spiked or rewritten at the whim of a sub-editor. Alison backed her reporters.

Despite Hampson's lack of public profile or the hook of a news line, my interview was given a page lead in the sports pages. It was unashamedly emotional and pulled on the reader's heart strings, and I sensed there was a noticeable shift in editorial direction which would be more human-focused across the paper. More empathetic.

Having spoken to several players in recent years who'd suffered serious neck injuries, most recently Phil Vickery, spending time with Hampson was a sobering reminder that the risks of catastrophic injury in rugby, while played down by the authorities and pigeon-holed as 'freak accidents', were a clear and present danger for its participants.

With the Premiership getting to the business end of the season, Tom Croft, who I'd witnessed break his neck in a game between Leicester and Harlequins the previous season, was named in the Lions tour squad to go to Australia that summer. His return from career threatening surgery was a remarkable story and, for a different angle, I rang the 27-year-old's surgeon, Peter Hamlyn, the man who had operated on so many rugby players before him, including Vickery.

'If you have an injury to that level, you are most likely to be paralysed, but there's certainly a risk to your life, too,' Hamlyn told me. 'Tom needed to be operated on through the back of the neck to decompress all the nerves and then through the front to reconstruct his injury.'

Hamlyn also told me rugby 'has a problem' with acute neck injuries such as the ones suffered by Croft and Hampson. But the surgeon, who had worked across a large number of sports, also spoke in glowing terms about the RFU's data collection programme, which he believed, if used appropriately, would provide the same benefits for rugby safety as Formula One's data programme had provided following the deaths of Ayrton Senna and Roland Ratzenberger, and act as a catalyst for change in the laws. He pointed to the work already done around the scrummage engagement as evidence of this potential.

On 12 May 2013, Rowan Stringer, a 17-year-old Canadian rugby player, died from what a coroner found to be second impact syndrome, having ignored symptoms of a previous concussion, only to suffer another heavy blow to her head when she was tackled hard to the ground. In the days before the game which would eventually kill her, Rowan had experienced headaches, fatigue and bags under her eyes, confiding in friends that she thought she was experiencing the symptoms of concussion but 'nothing would stop me unless I'm dead.' A few days later, she was.

Twelve days after doctors turned off Rowan's life support machine, Leicester Tigers fly half Toby Flood was knocked out in a typically forceful tackle by Northampton Saints lock Courtney Lawes early on in the Aviva Premiership's showpiece final at Twickenham.

Covering a desk shift in the office, I'd been sharing my concerns with Alison and Mike about how rugby was dealing with concussion when we looked up to watch one of the television monitors and saw Flood lying prone on the floor, surrounded by doctors. Having been poleaxed by Lawes, Flood was demonstrating all the signs of being concussed and, under the IRB's own directives, should have been removed from the field. But, as had become customary in rugby, he wasn't.

With Tigers director of rugby Richard Cockerill in close conversation with his medical staff over walkie-talkie, no doubt voicing his will for his key playmaker to stay on, Flood played on until another Lawes hit downed him again. Finally, several minutes after the collision, he was removed from the action.

But there was no outrage. No strong opinion pieces condemning the mismanagement of a brain injury. Just a collective shrug of the shoulders. This was rugby, after all. Nothing to see here, move along.

7

The campaign begins

I was delighted when Alison asked me to cover the Lions Test series in Australia for the *Mail on Sunday* in the summer of 2013. We'd secured the services of Wales and Lions scrum half Mike Phillips as a guest columnist for the trip and after a few initial conversations I sensed I'd find him easy to work with. With sponsors HSBC to satisfy, Phillips played in the Lions' opening game in Hong Kong in 80 degree heat and close to 100 per cent humidity. Phillips had an excellent game but, in doing so, also ruptured knee ligaments.

It was abundantly clear for the rest of the tour that he was struggling, but he kept soldiering on, despite inevitably damaging the knee further in doing so. In one conversation, he told me the Lions' management team, with his permission, had chosen not to scan his knee because they knew they would have to rule him out of the tour if they did. Such was the lure of playing another Test series for the Lions, Phillips was willing to risk his entire career. His comments once again made me consider the conflicted relationship between players and medics. It was becoming something of a theme now.

By the end of a typically gruelling tour both teams were on their knees with Australia's reserves so stretched they sent out an SOS call to former captain George Smith, who was almost four years into his retirement from the international game after 110 Tests.

With the series perfectly poised at 1–1 and just three points separating the two sides in the first two Tests, another nail-bitingly tight affair was anticipated when the game kicked off at 8pm.

But the Lions played on a different plane that night, physically, tactically and emotionally, running out comfortable 41–16 winners to put to bed their agonizing defeat at the same ground more than a decade earlier.

Inevitably, some detail would be missed in the limiting and pressurized environment of live reporting on a match which saw the final whistle blow close to 10pm, with the press conference and other formalities wrapping up closer to midnight.

But the fact that almost no one in the British media, including me, even referenced the appalling sight of Smith, having become one of the first international players to undergo a Pitchside Suspected Concussion Assessment, returning to the field after a thunderous clash of heads with Lions hooker Richard Hibbard less than five minutes in is indicative of where concussion sat on the news agenda around this time. In simple terms, it wasn't on it.

Even then, with all the concerns I had about mounting concussion and injury rates, and a little knowledge of the US picture, I was unsure how to present the story. Having been repeatedly told by rugby's most powerful medics and administrators that there wasn't a problem, who were we to say differently?

Rugby, just like the NFL before it, was in a state of collective denial. In the weeks before, having witnessed Wallaby centre Christian Leali'ifano being knocked out in the first game and playing again the following week, and following the Premiership final incident when Flood had played on after being banjaxed by Lawes, I'd tweeted several times about my concerns over rugby's increasingly flippant attitude to brain injuries. The deafening silence was noticeable.

As a result, and to my eternal shame, I declined to comment on the Smith incident in my match report or any of the accompanying news stories I sent through to the sports desk.

'Just keep filing,' deputy editor Mike Richards told me over the phone. 'We'll find room for it all somewhere.' Even then, I didn't touch the Smith story. I just couldn't see them publishing it. I was far from alone in taking that view. For the UK press, George Smith was not 'the line'.

I focused instead on Warren Gatland – the Lions' tough-talking New Zealand head coach – being vindicated in his controversial selection of 10 Welshmen in his starting line-up and, in doing so, dropping Ireland and Lions legend Brian O'Driscoll.

I wrote: 'This makeshift team, playing a brand of power-based rugby the Wallabies could not come close to matching, produced one of the great Lions performances. It will go down as a selectorial masterstroke.'

But as I wrapped up my match report, something nagged and I looked up from my desk in the middle of the vast media room. In the far corner, I saw Smith, standing alone after conducting a media huddle with the assorted Aussie press.

'It obviously affected me,' he said when asked by an Australian journalist about the sickening clash of heads with Hibbard. 'You saw me snake dancing off the field. I passed the [concussion] tests that were required within those five minutes and I got out there.'

As he wandered off, clearly still dazed and unsteady from the earlier incident, I asked him if he was OK.

'I guess so, mate,' he replied, unconvincingly. I watched as he tottered off out of the room. It made almost as uncomfortable viewing as the incident itself.

But for me, it was not for now. With the clock approaching midnight, my work had only just begun. I had a column with Phillips to ghost-write and a ton of 'colour pieces' to decorate the back and inside pages being prepared back in Kensington in recognition of the Lions' series triumph.

With the media centre located on the other side of the enormous stadium to the players' changing rooms, I jumped in an official golf-cart with man-of-the-match Leigh Halfpenny and a couple of Lions backroom staff.

One of the undoubted perks of being a sports reporter is being granted access to places fans can only dream of going.

This would be one such moment. As I stepped off the golf-cart behind Halfpenny and walked past the coach parked under the stadium, I was handed a beer by the grinning Phillips, whose company I had thoroughly enjoyed throughout the tour.

'Hang on a minute, mate, I'm just going to have my photo taken with James Bond.'

In the space of 10 minutes I'd gone from pondering the possible long-term neurological damage caused by rugby to gate-crashing a party with James Bond.

The actor Daniel Craig had been watching the action in the stands before being invited into the party with the team. As I waited for Phillips, I called the desk again.

'James Bond is in the Lions dressing room,' I told Mike. 'I'll try and get some pics.'

I filed my last word just after 4am back at the team hotel near Sydney Harbour Bridge and four hours later was in a taxi to the airport for the long flight home accompanied by several hundred elated Lions fans.

My memories of the tour were manifold. But above all what lingered was the image of Smith shambling back into the action moments after somehow passing the test designed to stop precisely this happening. How could they be getting this so wrong?

Although I had neither the scientific knowledge nor understanding of the data to support my position at that stage, a combination of instinct and experience told me the concussion problem ran far deeper than the authorities were letting on, and almost as soon as we touched down at Heathrow I set to work. I was far from alone in believing rugby had a player welfare crisis. Across the board, there were grave concerns about the extreme physical demands, length of season, lack of recovery time and relentless schedule for the top players. Anyone who didn't see it was choosing to bury their head in the sand. But seeing it and reporting on it were not the same things.

In 2013, it was clear professional rugby's status quo was unsustainable but most felt powerless to effect change. A combination of uncertain financial waters, confused science, misleading data presentation and fears over 'shitting on your own doorstep' had a chilling effect on the reporting of rugby's concussion crisis.

But for me, the uncomfortable truth was becoming undeniable. From speaking to players at the start of their careers, over the next decade we'd witness many of their facial features alter, flatten almost, as the impacts took their toll. Mike Tindall, mockingly nicknamed Lord Shitnose by his team-mates for his dual association with royalty and multiple nasal fractures, estimated he broke his nose at least eight times during his professional career. Despite a game-wide clampdown on fighting and punching, more and more players began to resemble boxers in their facial appearance. Their heads, and by extension their brains, were taking punishment on a scale never previously witnessed.

*

Clearly concussion was an issue taking up a lot of the rugby authorities' time, if not yet media attention. Although that was beginning to change.

I saw some value in the idea doctors should be provided with a means by which to make a judgement on a player away from the field of play. As the IRB stated on their website:

A particular challenge faced by the healthcare practitioner working in rugby union, and other sports, where there is no

temporary interchange for the assessment of injured players
(other than those with bleeding wounds) is the difficulty in
creating an appropriate environment for the on-field of play
initial clinical assessment. As a consequence, there has been a
tendency for concussed players to remain on the field of play.

But my concern was that, knowing how poorly resourced the sport
was lower down, any attempts to 'copy' this process in the amateur
game could be potentially catastrophic. I also could not understand
why any player-welfare-driven initiative should have a strict five-
minute time limit placed on it. Surely that would put doctors under
undue pressure?

There was an obvious risk the PSCA could be abused to allow
players who'd suffered clear concussion signs – including loss of
consciousness (which occurs in less than 10 per cent of cases), ataxia
(loss of balance), vomiting or tonic posturing (fencing with the arms),
or convulsions – time to recover their senses and return to the field.

Barry O'Driscoll argued that the merest suspicion of brain damage
should be enough for a player to be permanently removed from the
field. I agreed with him.

Ethically, the PSCA trials were also open to question, with
O'Driscoll himself having raised serious concerns as to the morality
of trialling it the previous year at the IRB Junior World Championship.

With the trial also set to be rolled out in the English Premiership
that season, it was unclear if players had signed anything remotely
resembling a consent form to participate in an experiment which,
ultimately, could cause more problems than it solved.

Without commenting upon, or knowing, the motivation of the
medics involved, the George Smith case seemed, on the surface at
least, to perfectly illustrate people's concerns. Here was a player,
showing several clear indicators of a brain injury, perhaps most
notably dragging his left leg behind him and nursing his left arm

which appeared in spasm as he was helped from the field, returning to play within five minutes.

A few days after the third Lions Test, Peter FitzSimons, a former Wallaby lock turned journalist and campaigner, wrote a coruscating article in the *Sydney Morning Herald* headlined 'Sideline Concussion Test a Disgrace'. Pulling no punches, FitzSimons described the Smith incident as a 'disgrace' while taking aim at the new concussion tests, demanding 'if Smith was not suffering concussion on Saturday night, what the hell was it – freaking FLU!?'

FitzSimons quoted neurological physio Phillip Sweeney, who had written to him following the incident:

> When Smith was dragged to his feet and helped off his left leg was all over the place. He was clearly shaking his left hand and trying to tell his attendants that he was troubled by this. The left leg kept collapsing as he walked. Now, it's clear that the right side of the brain governs the left side of the body... The man had clearly suffered no injury to the left leg, nor hand/arm. This was... a neurological injury. It's a classic example of a head injury during sport, and for the great man to come back on the pitch amounts to negligence.

FitzSimons went on to ask:

> In what other field of employment would an employee who had just suffered major brain trauma be allowed/encouraged to get back to it five minutes later? If you or I had been engaged in a work practice that, through misadventure, made our brains bleed, just how legally liable would our employer be in having us get back to it a few minutes later – doing exactly the same thing, except this time we would not be so alert? And just what would have happened to Smith if he had received exactly the same knock, on exactly the same spot of his head? And how

many junior rugby clubs around Australia, and around the world watching this epic clash, taking their cue from what happens in the big leagues, would have got the message that concussion is no big deal? See, even when you are knocked motherless, you can get back out there! You will be considered 'tough'!

I repeat: I accept the medical professional involved, who gave Smith the PSCA test, acted with integrity. He or she is not the problem. This newly instituted test is...

This rule is a disgrace and runs entirely contrary to the medically informed tide of the 21st century, when it comes to the way to treat concussion. Yes, the imperatives of big business sport wants the stars out there, come what may, most particularly in enormously important matches like the third and deciding Lions Test. But simple decency, basic sanity and – make no mistake – legal liability, says when a sportsperson is concussed, when THEIR BODY IS GOING INTO SPASM, they need to sit it out.

It was the article I wished I'd filed from the media centre at Stadium Australia a few days earlier.

Every word revealed the depth of FitzSimons's anger at what he saw as an abdication of duty by the sport's governing bodies and clubs who paid the players. And while he stopped short of accusing the doctors of negligence, no doubt for legal reasons, I was growing increasingly concerned about the clearly conflicted position many sports doctors found themselves in when trying to assess a player and make the right medical call, while also trying to 'please' or at least placate a coach. All the while, it was increasingly clear players needed protecting from themselves. A fundamental reason they had achieved so much success in their chosen sport was due to their willingness to take risks with their body.

In August 2013, I found a video, hidden away deep on the RFU's website, promoting their 'Headcase' concussion awareness campaign.

'Do I think it [concussion] is a problem within our game long term? No. Not at the moment,' Simon Kemp said in the video.

> I do think, though, that we are moving towards much more of a zero tolerance towards leaving players with successive concussion on the field. And certainly the minimum threshold to make a diagnosis at the development or age-group game I think needs to be very low.
>
> If you have any suspicions as a coach or a parent or fellow player or referee, if a player has been concussed then I think we are all obligated to get that player to leave the field.

Kemp's public refusal to commit to concussion being a long-term problem put a speed bump in the way of reforming rugby's culture and protecting players. If the most senior medic at the most commercially powerful union played down the long-term risks associated with head injuries, the ripple effect through the sport would be huge.

Up to this point, I'd trodden a careful line between raising serious concerns about professional rugby's mounting injury risk while not wanting to turn people away from the sport, upturn the applecart or 'shit on my own doorstep'. I'd also not previously had enough authority to start reporting on such a complex and challenging subject with any degree of confidence. Reporting what happened on or around the playing field was very much the reporter's role, while interviews, press conferences and the occasional radio or television appearance were our bread and butter. Challenging a sport's very culture would be an altogether more difficult proposition. At the time, I had no idea just how difficult.

*

That summer, with Alison in charge and willing to back me in the office and on the road, I felt in a stronger position. With seven Six Nations campaigns, back-to-back World Cups, two Lions tours and more than 200 Premiership matches now also under my belt, not to mention thousands of press conferences and interviews, I had built up a bank of experience and felt confident enough to hold my own in a variety of scenarios. Crucially, I had also demonstrated how deeply I cared about the game.

I still had enormous admiration for the players, perhaps more than ever, but I'd grown deeply untrusting of the 'suits' obsessed with driving growth while steadfastly refusing to acknowledge the collateral damage. With the governance of the sport terminally conflicted and seemingly every governing body or league in direct competition with each other – Six Nations, International Rugby Board, Rugby Football Union, Welsh Rugby Union, British and Irish Lions – it was impossible to say who owned or ran the sport and by extension who controlled the players. As a result, the players were pulled in every direction with no one accountable for the consequential damage.

Each administrative body was commercially self-serving. Take the autumn international, for example, where the international window had historically seen one or two Tests played, with clubs choosing to play friendlies or not at all to give the internationals room to breathe. This was stretched to three Tests in November almost as soon as professionalism was introduced, and by the mid-2000s four back-to-back Tests had become the norm.

Meanwhile, the end of the English domestic season crept from April into May and, following a Lions tour or World Cup, June.

So while the games were getting more physically demanding, seasons were actually getting longer and return to play times shorter. It was a toxic combination for player welfare.

As my knowledge about the damage being caused grew and all the while I continued to witness brain-damaged players return to the field, the more I resented the PR spin about rugby being 'safer than ever' and the lack of urgency in addressing the problem. Player welfare was patently and evidently not the authorities' 'number one priority'.

Deep down, I feared it may already be too late for many.

The *Mail on Sunday* was my platform, and I decided to use it in defiance of the governing bodies who were no longer serving the best interests of a sport I was, in truth, beginning to fall out of love with.

Dan Schofield was a young agency reporter who'd impressed me whenever I'd worked with him. He was studious and quite serious, for a rugby journalist at least, but also thorough, methodical and occasionally painfully direct. All good traits in a journalist. I'd been happy to put a bit of match reporting work his way in the previous few months and Dan, aware of my growing concerns over player welfare, rang me early in July to ask for a meeting.

We met near Oxford Circus and Dan proceeded to fill me in on the latest research being carried out at Boston University, the *Head Games* book Chris Nowinski had written outlining his experience of suffering repeated concussions while wrestling, and the pending multi-million-dollar lawsuit being pursued by the former NFL stars with long-term neurodegenerative issues linked to repetitive head injuries. Dan also agreed that Barry O'Driscoll's resignation as medical advisor to the IRB should have set alarm bells ringing throughout rugby, and the George Smith case that summer had been symptomatic of the sport's increasingly worrying management of head injuries.

Having been reading up on the medical research since returning from Australia, it was also interesting that Dan saw the Concussion in Sport Group as shadowy, opaque and potentially dangerously conflicted.

Led by Paul McCrory at the time, the group, a small cohort of fewer than 40 experts organized and funded by international sports federations including FIFA, the International Olympic Committee and the IRB, met approximately every four years to establish a consensus on the scientific understanding of concussion in sport. This group may have been small in size but it was massive in terms of influence and power.

At the time, to my knowledge, not a single person in the UK media had written, discussed or scrutinized this group but it was obvious to both Dan and me that they were worthy of further attention, especially as rugby's senior doctors were increasingly referencing them and relying on their statements. Reading their statements up to this point (2002, 2004, 2008, 2012), it was clear the CISG's position when it came to the long-term risks associated with repetitive head injuries was very much 'watch and wait' while also warning of the risks to participation which could be caused by 'fears' from 'media pressure'.

The group's first statement in 2002, made 74 years after Harrison Martland's discovery of dementia pugilistica (aka punch-drunk syndrome), had made no reference to the possible long-term effects of concussion other than to say more research was needed.

By the group's fourth meeting in 2012 in Zurich their position had moved to:

> Clinicians need to be mindful of the potential for long-term problems in the management of all athletes. However, it was agreed that chronic traumatic encephalopathy (CTE) represents a distinct tauopathy with an unknown incidence in athletic populations. It was further agreed that a cause and effect relationship has not yet been demonstrated between CTE and concussions or exposure to contact sports. At present, the interpretation of causation in the modern CTE case studies should proceed cautiously. It was also recognized that it is important to address the fears of parents and athletes from media pressure related to the possibility of CTE.

On a warm summer's day in central London, Dan and I agreed the subject was worthy of more digging, although I remained concerned that the *Mail on Sunday* would struggle to see the value in reporting on a complex issue which could, when broken down, directly link participating in contact sports with a heightened risk of developing dementia.

With several weeks before a new Premiership season began, I piled into background reading, poring over research papers including the 2007 'Epidemiology of Rugby Injuries' which Simon Kemp co-authored and the 2001 paper 'Concussion in Rugby: The Hidden Epidemic' from University of North Carolina researchers. I also examined the concussion consensus statements released by the CISG and sought to understand their position and who was part of the group.

I read Nowinski's *Head Games*, upon which Steve James's film was based, as well as *League of Denial* by ESPN's award-winning journalists Mark Fainaru-Wada and Steve Fainaru, charting the NFL's concerted attempts to play down head injury risks and hide potentially life-changing research from players. I studied as many injury audits as I could lay my hands on and tried to recall as many of the incidents and conversations I'd been party to around the subject in rugby as possible.

I spoke to friends playing professionally and tried to understand how concussion affected their day-to-day lives. The more I dug, the more apparent the parallels between the NFL experience and professional rugby union became.

To convince the *Mail on Sunday* to run such an emotive and powerful story, I needed every base covered and I began feeding the information through to the deputy sports editor Mike Richards. Richards had an extraordinary capacity to retain information, and gradually, between us, and with no little input from Dan, we began to frame what an article could look like.

To me, if there was a long-term issue relating to head injuries in the NFL, there would inevitably be one in rugby too. The assumption had always been that the NFL operated in a different stratosphere to rugby

union in terms of its sheer ferocity, physicality and brutality. Players
wore helmets, pads and other protection, and films such as Oliver
Stone's *Any Given Sunday* betrayed an image of a sport prepared
to sacrifice young men at the altar of winning. And winning meant
money. Surely rugby union, the previously amateur game played with
Corinthian Spirit and built on the shoulders of Muscular Christians,
would not be so louche as to place profit, or the blind pursuit of it,
over its people? Two years later I'd attend the UK premiere of another
film, *Concussion* in which Will Smith plays Dr Bennet Omalu, which
showed how the NFL had done precisely that.

Previously, I'd shared precisely the same misgivings about
comparing professional rugby to American football. But in recent
years, as I'd witnessed rugby's evolution, it was obvious to me the
sports were becoming comparably physical. Visually, the sports were
also merging, with opposing lines of attackers and defenders now
forming across the field in rugby union as defensive coaching became
more sophisticated. In some ways, with rugby players now obliged to
hit multiple rucks and mauls while also carrying and defending and
sometimes playing more than 40 matches in seasons with less and less
time between them, it could reasonably be argued that professional
rugby union was now the most physically demanding sport on the
planet. To suggest there would be no consequences to this heightened
physicality defied logic and the evidence in front of our eyes.

*

Following O'Driscoll's resignation, there came another 'red flag'
moment when former Scotland player Rory Lamont spoke to the
Scotsman's David Ferguson in July 2013 about his concerns over
concussion in rugby.

In the article headlined 'Rugby players are "cheating" concussion
protocols', the 30-year-old revealed he'd undergone 16 surgeries
during his career, an average of almost two every season he'd played

professionally, while also suffering a litany of concussions. Lamont was also heavily critical of the handling of George Smith's case:

> Everyone saw George wobbling his way off the field, clearly concussed, and then come back on. I have suffered clean knockouts, real sleeping-on-the-floor episodes in a game, so I know the protocols inside out, the symptoms and recovery periods, and there is no way a player should be allowed to stay on the pitch after a head knock. It's insanity. People might get annoyed with me saying this, but we are seeing reckless disregard for players' welfare right now.

On the subject of the CogSport tests, upon which the new six-day Graduated Return to Play protocols were so heavily reliant, Lamont's comments were damning.

> Players regularly pass the tests. In many cases that is because they cheat. Players all talk about it. A test is done at the start of the season as a baseline test, and players who suffer from concussion have to return to that level to be passed fit to play.
> But some players will deliberately do stuff in the baseline test so that their results are low, making it easier to pass after concussion. And I've seen players carrying concussion into games. They'd come off a fairly straightforward tackle, but be sitting on the ground, staring into space... I've experienced that. I didn't hide it, but you are often ostracized by coaches who assume you are being dishonest or shirking by saying you can't train or play, so with that pressure boys do play when they have head trauma.

At this time, Lamont was one of the few players with knowledge of the picture emerging in America and brave enough to air his concerns publicly, saying: '[The US] are further ahead of pro rugby and are beginning to see the effects, and it doesn't look good. I know that with the concussions I've had, for example, there is a high risk of me developing neurological issues associated with the early stages of "Parkinson's Disease". But what's done is done. All I can do now is look after my body as best I can.'

The article also highlighted the resistance SRU medic James Robson had encountered from other unions when attempting to introduce more conservative concussion protocols, while Lamont emphasized the conflicting pressures on players to play when not fully ready. He added:

> I'd like a return to a minimum three weeks out after concussion, because that would take away the pressure from coaches and medics to try to get a player back too early.
>
> But, for me, the route to change lies with the players. The message is pretty clear: if you take the pitch with concussion you will not perform to the levels you can, will let team-mates down, and will run the risk of causing yourself serious long-term damage.
>
> Once you start losing your mind there's no coming back from it. You can be an alcoholic and have cirrhosis of the liver and get a new liver and come off the booze, but there's no coming back from brain damage.

I immediately flagged the interview to Mike and Alison and insisted there was now more than enough evidence to run a hard-hitting feature pulling together the various strands of rugby's growing concussion story. Smith, Flood, O'Driscoll resigning, Lamont, a looming law case, NFL stars with early onset dementia, CTE denial all rolled into one story which, I believed through what I'd witnessed myself, was a significant problem for rugby. But even I would be shocked to discover how big that problem actually was.

A few things struck me about the injury audit data. Firstly, there wasn't any from before 2002, meaning that in the very period when players' physicality was changing faster, hits were getting harder and higher and the game was getting rapidly faster, it was incredibly challenging to compare the amateur era with the professional era through these figures. Certainly, any definitive claim the game was 'safer than ever' was at best misleading and at worst extremely dangerous for those hoping to be able to make an informed choice about whether to pursue a career in the sport or allow their children to participate.

I was also struck by how many injuries were occurring in training. In 2002/03 – the year England won the World Cup – there were 159 injuries in training, accounting for just 18 per cent of total injuries. These were the Wild West days when, so we were told, training was still brutal and with far too much contact.

But by 2007/08, by which time players' training loads should have been routinely monitored and limited, this figure had almost doubled to 318 training ground injuries, accounting for 33 per cent of total injuries.

By 2013/14, the number had continued to rise to 414 training ground injuries with the number of days absent per 1,000 hours now at 73 days, as opposed to just 56 days when the audit begun. In essence, training injuries were getting more frequent and more severe.

The narrative that training was being more carefully managed and scientifically conducted continued during the decade and by 2019/20, the last audit published before this book, there were a record 551 training ground injuries – almost four times higher than the first year of the audit.

As injuries in training got more frequent, so too did concussions. And while the data was not showing it yet, there was no doubt to anyone observing or playing the game that injuries were getting more severe. Soon that picture would become abundantly clear.

As part of my self-schooling in brain injury I decided to speak with the real experts who'd dedicated their entire career to the issue. And it was eye-opening the first time I picked up the phone to Professor Willie Stewart, the neuropathologist at Glasgow University whose name I'd first spotted in Tom English's article back in March. Stewart not only impressed me as one of the world's foremost authorities on head trauma, but he also struck me as being highly knowledgeable about rugby and its evolution as a sport. Professor Stewart shared my concern that the professional game was in danger of reaching a tipping point where it became prohibitively dangerous as a mass participation sport. The big hits may have been superficially attractive to marketing execs and aloof, highly paid medics who rarely dealt face to face with players, but the true cost was only just beginning to be understood.

Stewart was at that time the only neuropathologist in the UK with the knowledge, experience and equipment to diagnose CTE. While he said the jury was still out on precisely how, when or to what degree head injuries caused CTE – with all the associated presentations including depression, suicide, mood swings, memory loss and sleep disorders – it was now clear from extensive studies into the brains of deceased military veterans, victims of domestic abuse and retired sports stars that CTE was common in them all. Alcohol, drug abuse, stress and other factors were present in many of the cases. But one factor and one factor alone was present in them all: repetitive head injuries. He told me:

> CTE is a form of dementia we've known about for almost a century. It was first recognized in boxers who demonstrated a unique form of dementia which was the punch-drunk syndrome. What we're now recognizing is that it can happen with exposure to virtually any head injury.
>
> If you and I are having a conversation about knee injuries in sport and somebody within sport said there was no evidence of causality that damaging your knee leads to arthritis in years to come, that would be ridiculous. Because of course it does.

Your brain is an awful lot more complex and fragile than your knee. Why on earth would your brain be any more protected than your knee? It doesn't bear scrutiny. Knees heal. Brains don't.

The following year, Professor Daniel Perl, head of the CTE brain bank for the US Department of Defense, said in an article on ESPN by Steve Fainaru and Mark Fainaru-Wada: 'CTE is only seen in the setting of repeated head trauma. At the end of the day, this is produced by head trauma. I'm sorry, that's what all the research says.'

With O'Driscoll's resignation, allied to the Smith case and Lamont's comments hinting at a culture of secrecy and flawed medical practice in rugby, the conversation around the issue was beginning to change.

Players like Lewis Moody, former Ireland hooker Bernard Jackman and Lamont all came forward and voiced their concerns. Between Dan and myself, we spoke to them all, with some of their stories stopping me in my tracks.

With an article such as the one we were writing, calling into question whether rugby was sustainable on this current trajectory and challenging some of the medical and safety practices in place, it was only reasonable and fair to go directly to the sport's two biggest governing bodies: the IRB and the RFU.

Both the RFU's head of medicine Simon Kemp and the IRB's Martin Raftery stated their support for the CISG position that no causal link between CTE and concussion had been proven and both men were quoted in the article. I even returned to the RFU's senior press officer Dave Barton to make absolutely certain his organization wanted to repeat this line. They did.

I sent my first take at the article to the desk on the morning of Thursday, 29 August 2013 to give the sub-editors and picture graphics team, not to mention the newspaper's legal department, plenty of time to fit everything together on the page.

That evening, I went out for dinner with Debs and our friends Ben and Mimi and I explained the article I'd filed and the ramifications it could have for rugby and contact sport more broadly. I knew it would cause waves, but didn't for a second imagine it would be more than a one-off article adding more weight to the argument that concussion in rugby was a serious issue which needed urgently addressing.

It was a warm evening and we were sitting outside a Mexican restaurant just along from Camden Market when my phone went. It was Dan.

'Have you seen the news in America?' he asked, one step ahead of me as usual.

I hadn't.

'The NFL lawsuit has been settled. They've agreed to pay $765 million in compensation to retired athletes with CTE.'

A story on the NFL's own website confirmed Dan was right:

> The NFL has reached a tentative $765 million settlement over concussion-related brain injuries among its 18,000 retired players, agreeing to compensate victims, pay for medical exams and underwrite research…
>
> More than 4,500 former athletes – some suffering from dementia, depression or Alzheimer's that they blamed on blows to the head – had sued the league, accusing it of concealing the dangers of concussions and rushing injured players back onto the field while glorifying and profiting from the kind of bone-jarring hits that make for spectacular highlight-reel footage.
>
> The NFL long has denied any wrongdoing and insisted that safety always has been a top priority. But the NFL said Thursday that Commissioner Roger Goodell told pro football's lawyers to 'do the right thing for the game and the men who played it.'

Two thoughts ran through my mind. Firstly, it was a staggering amount of money. The second was that our feature piece was as good as spiked.

The reason I assumed our story would be spiked, the newspaper equivalent of being left on the cutting room floor, was that there were still two days before the Sunday papers went to print. Surely the other papers would pick up on such a massive development, even if it was playing out across the Atlantic in a sport which remained relatively niche in the UK. In sporting terms, this was an absolutely seismic moment. To me, it was as clear as night followed day that if this was a problem for one sport where head injuries repeatedly occurred it was a problem for all contact sports, not least rugby where the true extent of the problem had, in my view, been hidden for years and was getting shadily worse.

Although the news broke on Thursday evening, I assumed all the UK's leading national papers would cover the story the next day. To my astonishment, only one did, *The Times* running a short paragraph in their News in Brief section that simply stated the facts. Either I had completely misread the global significance of this story or every single news and sports editor on Fleet Street had. It turned out to be the latter.

With our rivals unwilling to touch the story, I headed into the office on Saturday to work the feature, alongside Alison, Mike and Roger.

Alison, eager to make her mark a few months into the job, was clearly excited. She had excellent sources within the RFU from years working on the rugby beat, and had heard the organization was nervous about the concussion story running.

We chose to use the image of Smith 'snake dancing' from the field. It was a picture that has since become iconic. But no sooner had we laid it out on the page, one of the sub-editors shouted out: 'Have a look on the wire [paid news feed]. Flood's been knocked out again.'

Toby Flood, playing in a pre-season 'friendly' against Ulster, had been caught with a stiff arm by opposition second row Dan Touhy and immediately knocked unconscious. A state in which he remained for about another 12 minutes. In only his second game back since being allowed to play on against Northampton at Twickenham, the Leicester and England No.10 had been felled again.

Grim as the image was, Flood lying prostrate, unconscious and face down in the mud provided the perfect up-to-date illustration for our story.

Rugby's ticking timebomb! Fears grow as evidence links brain damage and dementia to increasing number of serious head injuries suffered by top players
By Sam Peters and Daniel Schofield
31 August 2013

The sight of Toby Flood lying unconscious on the Welford Road turf surrounded by anxious medics on Saturday provided another unwanted reminder of the dangers rugby players face on a match-by-match basis.

The 28-year-old Leicester and England fly-half, whose last competitive game saw him knocked unconscious during the Aviva Premiership final at Twickenham in May, required 12 minutes of on-field treatment yesterday before he was taken from the pitch on a stretcher and rushed to Leicester Royal Infirmary, his neck in a brace and still requiring oxygen.

Ulster lock Dan Tuohy received a yellow card for his actions, and could yet face further sanction after his forearm appeared to make contact with Toby Flood's head. Mercifully for Flood, early indications last night appeared to show no more serious short-term damage than a nasty gash above his left eye and a sore head.

But the consequences for his long-term mental health are less clear.

With the new Aviva Premiership season about to get under way this week, urgent calls have been made for more to be done to protect players from the frightening consequences of head injuries.

Concussion is the most common injury suffered at the top level of English rugby, with statistics showing one player concussed in every five Premiership matches. But there are growing concerns that concussed players are being allowed to stay on the field or being returned to play after only a perfunctory examination.

Despite a clear link being established between repeated concussion and early onset dementia, depression and other neurological diseases, rugby's governing bodies have been accused of 'playing Russian roulette' with players' long-term health by not implementing more stringent safety procedures.

The man making that claim is Dr Barry O'Driscoll, a former Ireland international who resigned as the IRB's chief medical officer last year in protest at the introduction of the controversial Pitchside Suspected Concussion Assessment (PSCA), a protocol which aims to establish whether a player has been concussed during a game.

O'Driscoll, whose nephew [sic] is Ireland rugby great Brian O'Driscoll, said: 'It is going to take a tragedy for the reality to hit home.'

He believes the protocol's controversial insistence on the assessment being completed within five minutes of a player leaving the field is 'completely discredited'. He added: 'There's absolutely no justification for the five-minute rule. It is a completely unjustified experiment, and it is playing Russian roulette with rugby players' health.

'We have to protect the players from themselves because they will pay for it later in life. Hips and knees can be replaced, but we only have one brain. If players show signs and symptoms of concussion they should not go back on the field for another seven days. It is not difficult to implement. It is what every other professional sport insists on but rugby thinks it is a law unto itself.'

O'Driscoll's son Gary, who is Arsenal's chief medical director, shares his father's concern and refused to consider being part of the Lions medical team for a third time for this summer because of his worries over the handling of concussion. 'I pulled out because I did not feel comfortable with it,' he said. 'I have big concerns about the way the IRB are going about it.'

Earlier this month Dr Willie Stewart discovered the first evidence of Chronic Traumatic Encephalopathy (CTE) in a former rugby player. Since then a further 10 potential cases have been presented to the Glasgow neuropathologist.

'If we liken this to a marathon, then the gun has only just gone off,' said Dr Stewart. 'It would be foolish to think rugby is immune to brain damage.' The IRB insist they are doing everything they can to mitigate risks to players – and strongly refute Barry O'Driscoll's position – but fears remain that there could be a ticking timebomb of mental-health issues for a sport in which collisions are all too common.

The RFU's head of sports medicine, Dr Simon Kemp, said yesterday that the union were committed to delivering best practice in the handling of concussion cases. But he also said: 'We understand that there is no proven causal relationship between head injuries sustained while playing rugby union and the reported cases of CTE and early onset dementia.'

The now notorious George Smith affair in Australia, which saw the Wallaby flanker allowed to return to the field just moments after leaving it barely able to stand up following a sickening clash of heads with Richard Hibbard in the third Test against the Lions, followed closely on from the disquiet over the incident which saw Flood remain on the field for several minutes during the Premiership final despite being knocked unconscious in a tackle by Courtney Lawes.

Senior figures at the International Rugby Board, the game's rulers, privately admit to being 'devastated' at the decision by Australia's team doctors to allow Smith back on to the field when he was clearly concussed. The incident drew widespread criticism and an added focus on the IRB's concussion protocols.

Former Scotland winger Rory Lamont, who retired last year through injury, said: 'The current IRB concussion protocol is simply dangerous. I don't know what research the IRB used for this trial but it is seriously flawed. Everyone saw Smith wobbling his way off the field, clearly concussed, and then come back on. There is no way a player should be allowed on the pitch after a head knock. It's insanity. We are seeing reckless disregard for players' welfare right now.'

Lamont also claims some players intentionally underperform in pre-season cognitive tests – taken to establish 'baseline' data against which further tests can be compared – in order to pass them later in the season if they go on to sustain a brain injury which impacts their mental agility.

The outcry over Smith's reintroduction in Sydney led to calls for the five-minute rule to be scrapped. But the IRB insist the global experiment has been 'highly successful' while promising to review the findings of the past year.

'The IRB are interested in protecting players,' said Dr Martin Raftery, who succeeded O'Driscoll as the IRB's chief medical officer. 'We are trying to move forward in a scientific, logical fashion. The inference that the IRB have made up this PSCA rule without thinking about it is ridiculous. We spent months and months developing it and looked at all the research available and were advised by independent experts. We have the support of player associations on this.'

Pioneering research on American Footballers published last year by Boston University in the United States demonstrated a clear link between successive concussions and degenerative brain diseases later in life. There is mounting evidence to suggest professional rugby players are being exposed to similar risks. The findings in the US led to more than 4,500 former players suing the National Football League. Last week the NFL agreed to pay out almost £500 million in compensation to former players, deceased players' families, as well as funding further research into concussion-related illnesses.

The Boston research revealed that degenerative brain disease (CTE) had been found in 30 former NFL players, who, before they died, had shown symptoms similar to those found in boxers suffering from 'punch-drunk syndrome'. Former American Footballer and Harvard graduate Chris Nowinski – co-founder of the Sports Legacy Unit – was at the forefront of this research along with his colleague, Dr Robert Cantu.

'There is evidence of a concussion problem in rugby similar to that in the NFL,' said Nowinski, who suffered multiple concussions during his own playing career. 'It is not just an American Football problem, this has been found in boxers and ice hockey players. When you engage in something that involves repeated brain trauma with force, it opens the door to serious problems.

'At some point that damage turns into a disease. The damaged proteins have the ability to spread to other healthy proteins and damage them as well. It is like a crack in a windshield that keeps spreading by itself.'

Within rugby, there is serious concern over the pressure allegedly exerted on team doctors by coaching staff to pass players fit when they should be removed from the field. 'It takes a strong or experienced medic to turn around to a director of rugby or head coach and say 'This player is coming off',' said recently retired Scotland captain Rory Lawson. 'I've no doubt that less experienced medics feel intimidated by their seniors.'

While Test matches governed by the IRB will see independent doctors on hand in the changing room capable of overruling team medics, this season's Aviva Premiership will have no such provision.

'In the five-minute test, the medic asks the player four or five questions when they are back in the dressing room,' said Barry O'Driscoll. 'They then have to stand for 20 seconds with one foot in front of the other without falling over. If they are able to do that, then they will ask them, 'How do you feel?' That's ludicrous because at the top level these guys are real warriors – they are never going to say, 'Can I stay off?' I suggested to the IRB five years ago that when you have a concussive incident the independent match doctor should go on. They have these at every game and they can overrule a team doctor. He is completely independent and he is the guy who should go on the field. If he says, 'This is concussion', then the player comes off. The pressure comes off the team doctor and you get an objective, clinical view.'

There is also evidence that players are attempting to deceive medics into believing they are fit to play on. David Barnes, rugby manager at the Rugby Players Association, has invited Nowinski to address the union's board next month and is anxious to educate players about the risks of playing on with concussion.

'We have come a long way in how concussion is managed but it remains a big area of concern,' said Barnes. 'I've dealt with a number of players who have had to retire with head injuries and it is alarming when you speak to those guys and realise what they are going through.'

Earlier this year, the family of former NSW Waratahs coach Barry Taylor, who had died after developing dementia at the age of 57, donated his brain to Boston University for research purposes. Taylor suffered multiple concussions during a lengthy playing career but, according to his wife, 'just played through them'.

Dr Willie Stewart said: 'Just as we discourage people from playing on with a damaged knee, so we should strongly discourage people playing on with a damaged brain.'

Toby Flood's injury yesterday demonstrated all too clearly the dangers rugby players at all levels face in today's highly competitive arena.

In the course of researching this book I have gone back over the numbers and can reveal that with 135 matches played in 2012/13 and 54 recorded concussions, the picture even then was actually far worse than I was reporting at the time, with an average of one concussion per 2.5 matches, not every five matches as I stated in the report. This compared to just 20 reported concussions in 2005/06, at an average of one every 6.75 games.

That rate would get considerably worse over the course of the next decade. I should not have been surprised by the leadership Lewis Moody showed on this issue and his testimony for that first article we ran gave credibility to a feature which set the cat among the pigeons at Twickenham. 'I've never seen the RFU Council so rattled,' one well-placed source told Alison at the time.

The captain: Lewis Moody
*Former England captain, nicknamed Mad Dog for his
combative style. Retired from rugby in 2012*

I have been out cold five times, but towards the end of my career I was getting other forms of concussion far more frequently. It got to the stage that whenever I had a blow to the head I had the feeling for a minute or so that the game was going in slow motion. I had a couple of really bad ones for England against Australia in 2010, when I was stumbling around the pitch for several minutes, and against Tonga in 2007. I got knocked out twice in that game and that was the only time I had really severe migraines afterwards. The big problem is when it happens in a big match and the club and player want to play on. I have played on in games when I have been knocked out cold. The doctor will come on and ask a series of questions such as 'say the months of the year backwards' and crucially they will say 'are you OK?' As a player you will do whatever you can to stay on. Concussion is viewed as a minor injury you can run off in a couple of minutes. We need to change that mindset.

The player: Bernard Jackman
Former Ireland and Leinster hooker who retired in 2010 after being concussed 20 times in the last three years of his career

When you're playing, there's a feeling of invincibility. You're so focused on your goals and your team goals. Concussion can't get in the way of that. It was an honour to play for my country and for Leinster and I have some fantastic memories, so I feel the toll on my body was worth it. But what if in a few years' time I am diagnosed with dementia or another brain disease. Will it have been worth it then? I now suffer not only from pain like a migraine, but from longer-term problems like mood swings. There's a culture in rugby where concussion isn't taken as seriously as it should be by the players. Other players often joke and laugh about it. You enter a strange place called 'self-denial'. You accept that this is a normal part of your working life. The headaches, the sickness which follows, you know you have to get on with it, so you pop tablets more frequently than you know you should. I've heard more about head injuries in the last 12 months than ever before. I've read that the effects of concussions are cumulative, how one concussion leaves you more vulnerable for a second concussion and so on. I'm the living evidence of this.

The doctor: Willie Stewart
Neuropathologist at Glasgow's Southern General Hospital

I have seen the same pathology in a former rugby player in his fifties as that described in American footballers and boxers. It used to be called Dementia Pugilistica but it's now known as chronic traumatic encephalopathy. It came as no surprise to see a former rugby player with this pathology. No game which involves repetitive head injury can be immune to this. The big questions now are: How many people will be affected? How many times does someone need to be hit? Are there other factors like genetics that might increase the risk? The size and athleticism of players now is considerably advanced from the Seventies and the frequency and severity of contact has increased. We might assume that players would be at greater risk today but that would only be an assumption. I expect there will be more cases out there. Whether there are many more, I couldn't say. In the past two weeks I have been notified of 10 people who died of dementia after playing rugby or are currently living with early onset dementia. That doesn't prove anything – there are many reasons why people get dementia – but at least in a couple of those cases the families who got in touch have always believed their father had dementia because of playing rugby. I have seen the George Smith incident and I don't think anybody within the game would support people coming back on to the pitch with concussion. That was an aberration and I don't think we should assume it will happen every week. I'm sure it's not what the rugby authorities want to happen. We're currently setting up a study looking at living people who have been exposed to head injuries and monitoring them over a number of years to try to test if there is any neurological impairment. From that we hope to be able to add information in terms of how many times someone needs to be hit, how hard, and the frequency required to trigger dementia.

8

Pulling the pin

By the time I filed 'Rugby's ticking timebomb', I'd spent the summer investigating concussion in rugby. And that was off the back of more than a decade covering rugby and more than 30 years living and breathing it. If anyone was going to have a reasonable grip on the scale of the problem, it was me. As it turned out, I hadn't even the remotest clue.

Within days of publishing the first article, I began to receive calls, texts, tipoffs and messages from people within the game, several of them current players, who had a concussion story to report or knew someone else who had. The sense of relief from some at being able to tell their story was palpable. I'd anticipated a response, but nothing like this. At times, I had so many leads to follow up, I didn't know where to start. Very quickly it became clear that by highlighting concussion in rugby, I'd opened Pandora's Box.

The day after the first story ran, a friend suggested I give former Wasps scrum half Nic Berry a call. I remembered that the press release reporting his retirement the previous summer had mentioned he'd suffered from concussion but otherwise it had been functional and lacking detail. Before arriving at Wasps in 2010, Berry had been a high-calibre performer who'd played for Queensland Reds and Racing Metro but injuries, and by that I mean concussion, meant he'd never really made his mark at

Adams Park. Relatively unknown in the UK, his retirement went largely unnoticed by the media.

After checking with Nic it was OK for me to give him a call, our mutual friend passed me his contact details. At this time, it really wasn't the done thing in English rugby to lay bare your problems, while the idea of seeking a wife or girlfriend's view on dealing with their partner's injuries was, to my knowledge, almost unheard of. Especially on an emotive subject such as brain injury.

When it came to concussion in rugby, players and their families had up to this point been both unseen and unheard. In English rugby particularly, there seemed to be a 'code of honour' around the issue which stopped players speaking out. That silence felt dangerous.

I spoke to Nic on the phone. At first, understandably, he was nervous. He'd barely heard of me and was still trying to come to terms with what was happening to him. He was still experiencing symptoms and was unsure what the future held for him or his young wife, Mel. It was a tough time for them and I needed to tread carefully and sensitively. Nic was at pains to state he had no grudge against anybody at Wasps, who he said had treated him extremely well. He also held no grudge against rugby.

What concerned him was the uncertainty this had created for him and his young family, and, of course, the potential repercussions down the line. No one could give him answers about that, not even the consultant who'd finally told him it was time to call it a day: Peter Hamlyn.

In what was to become a common theme, Nic explained initially how it took a lot for him to be knocked unconscious but in recent times it was taking less and less to 'spark him out'. He admitted he was fearful for the future.

Several times he mentioned Mel and the fact she had to live this nightmare with him. I asked if Mel would be prepared to speak on the record. Nic said 'yes' and the following evening I caught the bus to their small flat just off the Fulham Palace Road.

En route, I picked up a copy of *The Times* and wasn't entirely surprised to read Simon Kemp, in what appeared to be a direct response to the 'ticking timebomb' article, being quoted in a story by Alex Lowe. The headline read: 'No concussion fears, says Dr Simon Kemp'.

> Dr Simon Kemp, the RFU's head of sports medicine, does not expect the sport to be the subject of an NFL-style class-action lawsuit over concussion. American football's governing body agreed a $765 million (about £491 million) settlement last week over concussion-related injuries suffered by 4,500 retired players.
>
> Rugby's handling of suspected concussion has been revised after an incident in the second Lions international when George Smith, the Wallaby flanker, returned to the field soon after being helped off after a clash of heads. Medics are now urged to act on suspicion. Even if a player passes the cognitive tests, he can be removed if the doctor suspects concussion.
>
> Dr Kemp says that there is no proven link between rugby and the early onset of dementia. 'I don't see a silent epidemic of retired players with significant cognitive impairment,' he said.

This begged the question: had the RFU or any other major sporting body bothered to look?

Undeterred, I arrived at the Berrys' flat with *The Times* tucked away in my rucksack. Nic and Mel were so welcoming. They were at pains again to say they did not wish to denigrate the sport but they had a truth to tell and they told it with a frankness and honesty that made the hairs on the back of my neck stand on end. I remember thinking as they unburdened themselves of more than two years of hidden suffering: 'This feels like real journalism.'

Mel, in some ways, held it together better than Nic. Although her concern for her husband was clear, it was also clear how hard this had been for her, watching the man she loved suffer in silence in front of her eyes. They spoke of Nic being knocked out in a tackle during the curtain raiser to the Premiership season against Harlequins held at Twickenham the previous year when, following countless concussions in the previous few months, Nic's comeback game had lasted just a few minutes before he'd been knocked out cold attempting to tackle Nick Easter. Shamefully, I admitted I'd covered the game but hadn't even noticed the incident. At the time, he was just another bloke who'd been knocked out. Not a single person in the press box that day had the remotest clue they'd witnessed the end of a young man's career.

Mel told me that by the end of Nic's career she didn't even care who had won the game, all she cared about was whether he was still conscious by the final whistle. It took a while for the comment to sink in.

The interview was even more powerful than I'd expected. Without throwing a single stone at rugby, they had articulated what had happened and why they were fearful for the future. It was extremely moving to sit there and listen to their testimony. I felt protective of Nic and chose not to file one of the lines he told me: 'Everyone at the club was incredibly supportive but only a small handful had a clue what I was really going through. Guys would come in the morning and ask me how I was. I'd say I was fine but I really wasn't. How do you tell your team-mates that you'd cried yourself to sleep that night?'

I filed the next morning and headed into the office again. It's not where a reporter wants to be, but the senior editors were keen for me to be on hand, such was the importance of the story and the lack of knowledge at the time over this complex issue.

Concussion: The invisible killer. Former Wasps player Nic Berry talks about the worries that forced him to quit
By Sam Peters
7 September 2013

By the end of Nic Berry's career the only thing his wife, Mel, thought about when she watched him play was whether he would finish the game conscious.

She had long since stopped caring about anything as trivial as the result.

'The longer things went on the longer it would take Nic to recover from the head knocks,' said Mel.

'There was an immediate concern for Nic's health and, with two young kids, we started thinking seriously about his future.

'Every time he ran on the field I was anxious, just hoping he'd get through the game without being knocked out. The result or his performance didn't matter as long as he was still conscious at the end.'

The end – in a professional rugby-playing sense at least – came on the opening day of last year's Aviva Premiership season, when London Wasps took on Harlequins in front of a 60,000-plus crowd at Twickenham.

Berry was on as a second-half replacement after spending the off-season without taking any contact in a desperate bid to allow his brain to recover from nine concussions the previous year.

But when Nick Easter made a trademark burst through the middle, he felled the Quins No 8 in typically fearless fashion.

Berry did not get up.

Mel, watching on television at the couple's flat in west London with their young son, Will, was distraught.

'I'll never forget that moment,' she said. 'I was almost

inconsolable. It was so upsetting. I needed to be there with him
but I couldn't. Our son was sick at the time and I was with him.

'All sorts of things went through my mind. Should he have
been playing? Was he fit for this game? How unlucky could he
be? My heart broke for him.

'When Nic got back, his career was not at the forefront of
our minds. It was just about getting through the night, making
sure he was OK. I was just so happy that he was home and
I was able to take care of him and monitor the symptoms. It
took several days, maybe four or five, before he came back to
something like his normal self. He was confused for about two
or three days, not sure what to do or what would happen.

'It was about three days later that I felt it was the right
time to sit down with him and tell him how I felt. I had to say:
'Enough is enough, you can't keep going on like this'.'

Two weeks later, Professor Peter Hamlyn, one of the
world's leading neurologists who the previous season had told
Nic that he was risking his long-term health by continuing
to play, took the decision out of the 28-year-old's hands by
refusing to sign him off as medically fit.

'It wasn't until I retired that I realised how much stress it
was putting them all under,' said Berry.

'Especially Mel, she was there before and after every game.
She saw the full effects of everything. It was rough. It was a
hammer blow when they said I couldn't play again. But then
you look back and think: 'That went on for a long time'.

'Players will always want to continue, but I don't believe
they know about the long-term consequences. Unfortunately,
the neurologists can't really tell you that. They can't say what
you're going to be like in 15 years. I really hope I haven't done
any permanent damage that will come back to bite me later
on.'

The last meeting with Professor Hamlyn was the end of
a long road for Mel and Nic, who had pleaded for 'one more
chance' to prove his fitness more times than he should have
done.

'It got to the point where it just took so little to spark me
out that it was scary,' he said.

'I had an incident during a training session when all I did
was bump into a bloke and I was completely out of it, in pieces.

'I wandered off the field and one of the management team
– Kev Harman – scooped me up, put me in the car and sent me
home.

'I went back a couple of days later and asked for a video of
the session. I asked one of the coaches: 'Who hit me or was it a
tackle?' and they said: 'Mate, you need to have a look at this.'
When I saw how innocuous the contact was, I knew it was
getting serious. That was the one that scared me most. It took
me a long time to recover.'

On other occasions, Berry would suffer anxiety, mood
swings and depression, sometimes as a direct result of the
neurological damage caused by the concussions, on other
occasions because of a sense that his life was spiralling out of
control.

He would find himself back in the dressing room in floods
of tears, not knowing why or how he had got there.

'It was awful,' he said. 'I'd be panicking all the time. I'd
get home and couldn't remember if I'd done or said something
inappropriate. I had this feeling of being out of control and
completely losing track of my emotions. I'd get up in the
morning and forget where I'd put my keys or wallet the night
before. Then I'd realise they were right in front of my face.

'Everyone at Wasps was incredibly supportive, but I
wouldn't let on how bad things were.

'I learned to cope. It almost became normal. I'd get through a training session, then get home and slump on the couch for a day-and-a-half.'

Neither Nic nor Mel bear any resentment towards a sport which has afforded them a comfortable, if not lavish, lifestyle, and provided him with a weekly adrenaline rush and a sense of camaraderie almost unmatched outside of top-level sport.

They are especially grateful to the compassion and support shown by Wasps, their medical team, and, in particular, director of rugby Dai Young.

They also have a huge debt of gratitude to the Rugby Players Association, who provided professional support before and after Nic took the decision to call time on his career.

Nic has since gained a teaching qualification from Harrow School and secured a job at a top school back in Brisbane, from where he originates.

Mel has her hands full with the recent arrival of their second child, daughter Mila.

But there is a worry for the future.

'The scary thing is the dementia side of it and not knowing how far the damage has actually gone,' said Mel.

'It's something Peter Hamlyn brought up. I remember sitting in that room when he was talking about it and I could feel the tears welling up in my eyes thinking: 'I can't imagine that... it would be absolutely awful."

Nic adds: 'It's sobering not knowing what's going to happen.'

He believes rugby's attitude towards concussion has matured as more research is done into one of the most complex and sensitive of issues.

'For me there has to be a line drawn where they say: 'OK, you've had this many, you're done.' I'd like to think that 20-year-olds now will take concussions much more seriously.'

Nic has since gone on to enjoy an outstanding career as one of the world's leading referees on the international circuit. I haven't spoken to him for some time but it would appear, for the moment at least, the worries about his future brain health have been allayed. But, like Lewis Moody before him, his decision to speak publicly about what he'd been through showed real leadership and courage.

Even as someone who had suspected for some time that rugby's concussion problem was worse than anyone was letting on, I still found the Berrys' testimony shocking. They had opened a window into an unseen world of despair, anxiety and, on occasion, real darkness. This was not a side of rugby – or indeed sport – the marketeers and broadcasters wanted telling. But it was the truth. Laid bare and raw.

The important questions, for me, were how many Nic Berrys were out there and how many players could be affected in this way?

Neither Nic nor Mel had a bad word to say about rugby or the people in it. Perhaps if they had, it would have been easier for those whose purposes it served to sideline them. But this simply was not the case. In fact, while it wasn't hard to find people with stories to tell about concussion, those who also felt bitter towards rugby, around this time anyway, were vanishingly few. Sadly, that picture would change over the coming years.

But, thanks in no small part to Nic and Mel Berry's honesty, and Lewis Moody's, rugby was finally facing up to the reality of concussion.

What was increasingly clear was that concussions didn't just fix themselves. With almost everyone I spoke to, there was a cumulative pattern which saw them get worse over time. The idea, promoted by some, that concussion was akin to a computer rebooting itself with no adverse effects was little more than wishful thinking. Speaking to players like Moody, Berry and Jackman, along with the mounting evidence from the NFL, there was very obviously a cumulative effect. Current and recently retired players were living proof of this.

With so many players coming forward with stories, it became increasingly clear Nic's would not be the last interview we ran. Concussion could be the inconvenient truth which risked being a check and balance on the unfettered growth of the sport. That wasn't my concern. I was more interested in getting to the bottom of how big the problem was, why it had taken this long to emerge and how we could start the process of solving it.

It took courage for Nic to speak up. Like many other players going through the same ordeal, there were concerns that by baring their soul and being truthful about their suffering, they would be portrayed as weak, 'soft' or even lazy. Because you couldn't see a concussion, it was easy to dismiss it or portray those suffering from it as shirkers or, as some medics would describe them in academic literature, 'malingerers'.

*

My phone was red hot in the days afterwards, including a call from one of the RFU's senior comms team, Dave Barton, 'enquiring' about whether there were more articles to come.

It had also piqued the interest of senior editors at the *Mail on Sunday* and Alison was engaged in what was unfolding. Any early doubts she or any others at the paper may have had about the newsworthiness of the concussion story had been allayed by the power and depth of the testimonies we'd heard.

That summer Alison had called all the *Mail on Sunday*'s sports reporters into the office for a meeting and asked us to think about possible campaigns. Delivering these had been part of her brief when she'd taken over. I hadn't thought too much of it at the time but here I was, a few weeks later, wondering what a concussion campaign might look like.

The next few weeks, months even, were a relentless blizzard of stories. I had so many, I literally couldn't write them all. One that did make it into the *Mail on Sunday*, though, was my interview with Gloucester legend Andy Hazell. I visited him in his house just a stone's throw away from Kingsholm where I'd covered dozens of Gloucester matches and watched him play on time after time with what we now knew to be a significant brain injury.

I sat with Hazell for almost two hours in his modest home. Like Moody, Berry, Jackman and Lamont, he again bore witness to the increasingly debilitating cumulative effects he'd experienced, as the concussive symptoms would arrive with more frequency and from increasingly innocuous contacts. He also confirmed Lamont's assertion that the CogSport baseline tests were unfit for purpose.

After a concussion hit the previous season, the warm and affable Hazell described his desperate attempt to extend the 16-year career which had already made him a Cherry and Whites legend for just one more year.

> I had a really good pre-season. I played about 25 minutes against Toulon and everything felt fine and then had a friendly... a friendly... against Plymouth. About 30 minutes in I made a tackle. I can't really remember much but I can remember feeling my face and feeling a cut. It felt like it was a big blow. I don't think I was unconscious but I definitely wasn't right.
>
> I went off and got my face stitched up and did the concussion protocol. I got all the answers right and passed. I jumped off the bed to go back on and my legs were like jelly. I needed a minute to calm down. I waited another five minutes and then said: 'Right, get me back on.'
>
> I played another five minutes up to half time and then came back in and did the concussion protocol again. I passed again. I was coherent and knew what was going on but did feel odd. But I thought I was OK to go back on.

I started the second half. I can't remember much of the game. I can just remember feeling more groggy as the game wore on and with every hit I felt more light headed and light legged. After about 15 minutes the physios came on and grabbed me and took me off. They could see I wasn't myself.

As soon as I came off I sat down and put my jacket on and I was in a different world. Really bad. In hindsight I should have come off before. But it was nothing different to what I'd done time and time again for the past 16 years.

As we spoke in the modest terraced house, it struck me again how much these guys were risking for relatively little reward. Within two weeks of running the first story, I could have been writing 10 stories a day. I had, in journalistic terms, tapped into a vast seam of previously unreported information. And there was much, much more to come.

I was acutely aware there were many in the sport who thought I should back off, journalists included. Dan emailed me shortly after the first article had been published and noted he was 'surprised by the lack of follow ups in other papers'. I started to notice the hushed voices when I walked into the media centre before a game while increasingly every time there was a concussion incident during a match, which was more often than not, my friends and colleagues would turn to me knowingly as if to say 'over to you, Sam'.

Some players also sensed this could be damaging to the sport's reputation. One of my friends, an experienced Premiership player, said to me: 'Mate, they're important stories and hard to read but it's not great PR for the sport, is it?'

I responded: 'Mate, I'm not in PR.'

One of my course tutors at City, Phil Derbyshire, had once told us: 'News is something somebody doesn't want printed; all else is advertising.' It was a quote from legendary American newspaper publisher William Randolph Hearst. I had never forgotten it.

Although I'd grown up a fan, I was now a journalist first and a fan second, and had long since been wary of falling into the trap of becoming a cheerleader for the sport. My only agenda was to follow the story.

I'd never been one to choose the easy path in life, perhaps to the detriment of my blood pressure and relationships with those closest to me. I'd always found the harder people butted up against me, the harder I'd push back. It was in my character, for better or for worse. I just couldn't let this drop. It was potentially a matter of life and death for some of these players.

Alison called me into the office at Northcliffe House on Kensington High Street and I got the lift up to the second floor where the sports desk was located. Roger and Mike were smiling.

'Geordie wants us to run a concussion campaign,' Alison said.

'Fuck,' I said.

Gradually, the penny was dropping. This was not going away. Although at that point I still naïvely thought a few more articles would knock things into shape. Surely rugby would see the error of the NFL's ways and recognize the need for radical change to the fixture schedule, training methods, tackle technique and concussion education to reduce exposures across the sport. If they didn't, it was obvious to me this could only end up in one place: a court of law.

We sat down in Alison's office and set about outlining our list of demands for rugby to change.

CONCUSSION CAMPAIGN

The Mail on Sunday believes rugby's ruling bodies must:

1. Commission independent, scientific research into the incidence of concussion in rugby and the effect of repeated head trauma, including any links to serious neurological conditions.

2. Compel coaches and players at all levels of the game to undergo training in concussion awareness and treatment.

3. Introduce compulsory medical examinations by independent doctors for any player suffering more than one concussion within a three-month period.

4. Oblige all clubs and encourage all rugby-playing schools to display concussion information posters in clubhouses and changing rooms.

5. Enforce penalties for any failure to implement the above.

I called Lewis Moody's agent Mark Spoors. I knew in order for the campaign to fly we needed a high-profile player with the leadership skills, empathy for players and the ability to communicate with a wider room. A player who had given everything in the cause and whose love of rugby could not be questioned. A player with integrity.

SP: 'Spoorsy, how's it going?'

MS: 'Good, pal, you?'

SP: 'Good mate. We're going to go big on the concussion story. Really big. We're going to run a campaign calling for change. Do you think Lewis would donate his brain to medical science?'

MS: 'Do what, mate?'

SP: 'You heard. Would Lewis be prepared to donate his brain to medical science?'

MS: 'What, now?'

SP: 'No, you idiot. When he's dead! We're going to run a campaign around concussion in rugby. We think it's a massive issue. Massive.'

MS: 'Oh, right. OK, I'll ask him.'

A couple of hours later I received a text from Spoors.

'Lewis is up for it.'

We arranged to meet at a hotel in South Kensington the next day and I explained the plan to run the campaign, which was designed to put pressure on rugby's authorities to change the sport's culture of habitually allowing brain-damaged players back on the field – Moody, Ashton, Smith, Flood, Hazell, Berry were just a few we had identified.

If we didn't, we argued, the sport was facing a train crash further down the track with inevitable legal consequences. Lip service was no longer enough. Action was needed.

Lewis listened attentively before explaining he did not want to be part of something which would damage participation in the sport. Having played mini rugby from a young age, like me, he loved the game to its core. But, like me, he saw a direction of travel which, if it continued unchecked, was storing up serious problems for its participants, especially those at the highest level where most was being demanded and extreme risks were being taken.

My argument was that if parents continued to see top stars being evidently concussed but allowed to play on by the top doctors in the sport, they should vote with their feet. Culture is set from the top and their protective instincts would kick in and playing numbers would drop. In fact, there was already anecdotal evidence to suggest that was happening.

Lewis, showing true leadership, agreed to support the campaign.

Moody: We used to treat concussion as a joke…
now I worry about dementia
By Sam Peters
21 September 2013

When Lewis Moody called time on his 16-year career at the sharp end of English rugby, the tributes poured in. People spoke of the 33-year-old, World Cup-winning flanker's bravery, loyalty and willingness to put his body on the line for his team.

His scant disregard for his own safety had become the stuff of legend, earning Moody the nickname Mad Dog.

But as he announced his retirement in March last year, no one, not even the former England captain himself, mentioned the countless concussions he had suffered and the possibility that, in later life, there could be repercussions for his mental health.

At that stage, the link between multiple head traumas and early onset dementia – now referred to as Chronic Traumatic Encephalopathy (CTE) – had been made in American Football, ice hockey and boxing, but not in rugby.

'For me, concussion wasn't a big deal,' Moody told The Mail on Sunday.

'It was something you could just shake off. Nobody ever said concussion could lead to permanent brain damage or even death if it was not dealt with properly.'

Today Moody joins The Mail on Sunday's campaign to get rugby's ruling bodies both to help fund research into the medical consequences of repeated concussion and to accept their responsibility for ensuring everybody in the game is aware of the risks they face.

Moody has no wish to undermine the game he loves. But he does want to protect players from the dangers of repeated concussion and the reluctance of many to take the issue seriously.

'When I was playing if someone got knocked out it was always a laughing matter,' admitted Moody. 'Guys would get asked if they knew what they were doing on the pitch or where they were. Now if players really understand the risks, they will take it more seriously.'

Moody is so concerned by possible links between head injuries and dementia that he wants to donate his brain for medical research. Concussion is now the most common injury sustained by players, and Moody, along with top British neuropathologist Dr Willie Stewart, wants rugby to fund more research, introduce mandatory concussion training for players and coaches, and insist on independent medical examinations for players who are repeatedly concussed.

Nobody in the campaign wants to knock rugby. But the consequences of failing to deal with its most serious injury are too frightening to ignore.

There are signs that rugby's authorities are prepared to do more. A high profile forum will be held at Twickenham on November 7 to discuss the issue, with senior figures from the Rugby Football Union, Premiership Rugby and the Rugby Players' Association attending. While the RFU's website does provide information and advice on concussion, there is no obligation on players, coaches or clubs to undergo any training on the subject. The RFU's own 2011-12 injury audit showed concussion, which is usually defined as impairment of brain function resulting from head trauma, to be the most common injury in the professional game, with 5.1 instances for every 1,000 hours of rugby played. Anecdotal evidence indicates a significant number of concussions are also going unreported.

Another review of rugby union and league showed an even higher figure, 9.05 concussions for every 1,000 hours. That compares with 6.5 instances in ice hockey – traditionally viewed as the most dangerous sport for head trauma – and 3.35 in American Football.

Moody believes players need to be better educated about concussion and better protected when they suffer it. He acknowledges that attitudes have to change. 'It's about making players realise that if their mate is still on the pitch while he's concussed he could actually be damaging the team's prospects, as well as his own health,' he said.

Moody was the first England player, to my knowledge, to publicly support a wider conversation around concussion. It was an act of integrity, risking the schoolboy mockery of those less informed who couldn't see past the macho bullshit which demanded you 'get up and man up' regardless of the state of your brain. He risked a lot by taking that stance and I will always admire him for that.

The fact concussion was treated as a joke, and brain-damaged players the subject of derision, may have come as news to many of us, but for medical historian Stephen Casper, there is a long history of mocking this subject and portraying concussed athletes as 'losers' while glorifying those who could 'soldier on'.

In his paper 'Punch-Drunk Slugnuts: Violence and the Vernacular History of Disease', published in *Isis: A Journal of the History of Science Society* in June 2022, Casper wrote:

> The observation that neurological illnesses follow recurrent hits to the head was tempered by the terms that first called the diseases into scientific existence: 'punch-drunk,' 'slugnutty,' 'slaphappy,' 'goofy,' 'punchy,' and a host of other colloquialisms accompanying class identities. Thus the discovery of disease and its medicalization ran straight into a countervailing belief about losers – losers in boxing, losers in life, losers in general. To medicalize such individuals was to fly in the face of a culture that made them jokes. Yet a subculture began to emerge around

pathological understandings: first in medicine, then in journalism, then in the courts, and finally with patient accounts about illness.

As it became obvious we were not going to stop in this campaign, players, doctors, physios and coaches kept coming forward with stories about how ineffective the protocols were, while the harrowing testimonies kept coming like a tidal wave. In the past, I'd get to Friday worrying about which story I was going to put into Sunday's paper. Now I was getting to Friday worrying about which story I was going to have to leave out. At times, it was almost overwhelming.

I spoke to Jon Patricios, a South African neurologist and advisor to the IRB, who, in an interview printed in the *Mail on Sunday*, confirmed the CogSport test was 'open to manipulation'. He explained:

> Because we don't have a blood test to see if someone is concussed or not there are ways of getting around the system.
>
> The IRB have tried to bring in other parameters to allow better assessment but have players worked the system and doctors manipulated the system? In all honesty, probably yes. But it's not for want of the IRB trying to look after their players. We're trying to find parameters in the absence of an absolute test for diagnosing concussion.
>
> There are difficulties. The pre-injury test may not be 100 per cent accurate. There may be distractions or deliberate attempts by the player to score poorly. There are checks built into the CogSport test so if you really are scoring poorly in a baseline test it will give you an invalid score and you should really repeat that.
>
> There are some checks, but there is no silver bullet.

The RFU began a charm offensive including offering free tickets and matchday hospitality to senior people on the desk – notably Alison – and invites for lunch with RFU president Bill Beaumont in his corporate box at Twickenham. All the offers were, to my knowledge, declined. It may have been pure coincidence that these offers came so soon after we started running stories about brain injuries in rugby. But then again, perhaps not.

Soon, even more players were coming forward and Moody's testimony, supported by the likes of Harlequins captain Will Skinner, who I'd also witnessed play on countless times after suffering head injuries, was as hard-hitting as we'd hoped.

We had so many stories, it was hard to know which one to lead on. With space at a premium, Skinner's and Hazell's stories made just a few lines in the paper, but by speaking to them both at length, I became even more convinced I was on to something huge. And having watched the transformation of rugby's breakdown and the grotesquely dangerous 'jackal' becoming normalized, it came as no surprise that a high percentage of players coming forward were back-row forwards, who specialized in this 'art'.

Joe Worsley, Tom Croft and Tom Rees were just three whose careers had been decimated by neck, shoulder, head and other breakdown- or jackal-related injuries and I'd long been concerned about how dangerously exposed the backs of players' necks and heads were, especially with so little regulation about how they were 'cleared out' by opponents. During my career the number of times I was knocked clean unconscious was probably into double figures,' Skinner said in an interview for the *Mail on Sunday*.

> When I first started it was a case of taking a knock on the head, possibly be knocked unconscious, but then it would be a case of asking the player how they were feeling and if you said you were all right you could carry on.
>
> As a player, very rarely would you say 'I want to come off because I am worried about my head'. It just didn't happen. Rugby has changed a lot in the last 10 years with the size and

impact of collisions and the sports science behind it all. The registering of these concussions means we will probably start to see similar patterns to the NFL.

If you look at the number of injuries that are happening around the breakdown in rugby and the concussions around that particular area of the game it's because of the collisions there. It is a danger. I'd like to see more education, not just for the players, but for rugby as a whole. NFL is one of the richest and most scrutinized sports in the world and it's only just come out there that this is potentially a very big problem.

The medical teams at various clubs are getting more savvy about this, especially at Quins. Clubs are increasingly conscious about looking after players. But even today a lot of the power is down to the player and whether they say they have symptoms. It's very hard for a doctor to assess you properly if you say you are fine and want to carry on playing.

You always have to look into the player's welfare. Yes, we love the game but players have to realize there are another 40 or 50 years on your life after you stop playing. If you want to be running around with your kids when you are 40 or 50 years old there are certain considerations you have to take in to play.

But while many players were coming forward, others were backing off. Many of my fellow rugby journalists were openly sceptical. Over years of travelling around the world, covering the sport we all cared deeply about, I'd built close friendships with a number of the Jacks. Working mainly on the Sunday newspaper beat – which by then had become something of an anomaly as most of us were also contributing to daily papers and online as well – guys like Adam Hathaway, Steve James, Michael Aylwin and Stephen Jones were all close travelling companions, while Dan Schofield, Gavin Mairs, Alex Lowe, Chris Foy, Duncan Bech, Alex Spink, Neil Fissler, Mick Cleary, Owen Slot,

Sarah Mockford, Martin Crowson, Neil Squires, Hugh Godwin and, latterly, Jonny Fordham were just a few of the group I considered friends. I still do. On the broadcast side, Chris Jones of the BBC and BT Sport's Ali Eykyn were guys I enjoyed a beer with. In fact, there was literally no one within the Rugby Union Writers' Club I wouldn't have happily sat down for a drink or bite to eat with.

So it troubled me personally that their response to the stories I was writing was largely silent. Certainly to begin with, other newspapers hardly touched the concussion story.

One of my friends on a national broadsheet told me a senior editor had said to them: 'Concussion is boring. A non-story. Leave it.'

Other contacts, including surgeon Peter Hamlyn, began to back off. I emailed Peter asking if he'd support the campaign but his response made it clear he was lukewarm about talking to me.

He wrote: 'This is a complex issue and a highly charged one. Rather than be interviewed by you again how would it be if I wrote a couple of paragraphs laying out where I feel rugby stands in relation to the other sports and our knowledge of dementia in general?'

I replied: 'I understand this is a complex issue but would be most grateful if you would be prepared to lay out where rugby currently stands in relation to other sports. Could we talk off the record tomorrow?'

He didn't respond. Later that year I would see Hamlyn at an RFU concussion symposium but he kept his distance. For whatever reason, he had been spooked and it was my strong belief he'd been spoken to by the RFU, who had provided the surgeon with a great deal of work over the years. Although I have no evidence to suggest this happened in Hamlyn's case, I have spoken to a number of former players and administrators over the years who have told me Kemp contacted them soon after they'd given interviews about concussion, insisting the problem was not as severe as being claimed while attempting to deter them airing their concerns publicly again.

In the week I'd been convincing the former England captain to donate his brain to medical science, Dan Schofield was also busy.

First, he telephoned Paul McCrory, the man with a direct interest in promoting CogSport, having written the handbook while also featuring in promotional material. In 2002, he had co-authored a paper with Kemp titled 'A Guide to CogSport's Handbook' explaining how it worked when it was first trialled among Premiership clubs and players around that time before being formally integrated into the six-day Graduated Return to Play protocols in 2012.

'It was clear as soon as he picked up the phone McCrory didn't want to speak to me,' Dan said. 'I asked him why the research he had done was superior to the research being done in Boston. How could he be so sure there were no long-term implications to concussions? He was obviously unhappy at being challenged. He told me he didn't do media and hung up.'

Shortly after we'd run the first piece, around the time Kemp confidently told *The Times* he 'did not see a silent epidemic of retired rugby players with significant cognitive impairment', Dan had interviewed him on the record at a pre-season media event at Twickenham.

'His demeanour and attitude were dismissive and it was clear he didn't appreciate my line of questioning,' Dan would later tell me. 'He rolled his eyes whenever I asked a question and sought to play down the issue while constantly referring back to the Zurich Concussion in Sport Group. He seemed to have absolute confidence the whole concussion issue would just disappear.'

In a sport founded by the top public schools and universities, and historically riven by class and social hierarchies, the RFU, where Kemp had become one of the most influential figures, still felt like an old boys' institution.

When pressed on CTE and a possible link with repetitive head injuries, Kemp would constantly fall back on the latest position of the CISG, which had met in Zurich in 2012 for the fourth time, with McCrory again lead author, when it was agreed 'a cause and effect relationship has not as yet been demonstrated between CTE and concussions or exposure to contact sports' while recognizing 'it is important to address the fears of parents/athletes from media pressure related to the possibility of CTE.'

And when it came to restricting the PSCA to five minutes, Kemp also insisted that 'operationally the feedback from the medical practitioners is that five minutes is long enough' to carry out the pitchside assessment.

My suspicion, which Kemp would later confirm was correct, was that one of the factors in limiting the time permitted for the assessment to five minutes was concern over coaches manipulating the ruling to create 'rolling substitutions' which had always been fiercely resisted in rugby union. Yet again, reputational risk was trumping player welfare. The spectre of Bloodgate remained. Dan had also pressed Kemp on the burden of proof needed to accept there could be long-term consequences to repeated blows to the head being sustained by employees of clubs or unions. Kemp turned the question on Dan:

> Without there being any data about risk on CTE, it is very hard to know what is a proportionate response. Do you want us to turn contact rugby into touch rugby? There are very significant health benefits to playing rugby. If there are negative health consequences regarding trauma to the head, you have to factor those into the positive health consequences of regular exercise, effect on heart disease, cancer and self-esteem. So what's your position?

None of us doubted there were benefits to playing rugby. But why on earth should that deter us from trying to understand and articulate the risks as well? To me that was enabling informed choice. I still occasionally enjoy a cigarette, knowing full well it increases my risk of developing cancer, and I also drink alcohol, knowing it could damage my liver and cause heart disease. But the point is I know because the companies making these products are legally obliged to tell the consumer. Why should professional sport be any different?

I was hugely impressed with Dan's work. Still only in his mid-twenties, and cutting his teeth in the industry, here he was doing what journalists are meant to do: holding power to account. Kemp was, and is, an influential and authoritative figure willing and able to make an underequipped interviewer squirm. Challenging his position required nerve, bravery and a solid grasp of a complex brief. Dan possessed all these qualities, as a verbatim account of his conversation with Kemp reveals.

> DS: So how long do you wait for definitive proof when the evidence is starting to point in that direction? You go back a couple of decades and cigarette companies were saying that there was no proof of cigarettes causing cancer.
>
> SK: We have been working 10 years setting up a good epidemiological study in the Premiership so I think my call here is that rugby needs to show leadership and clarity. But what we do has to be data driven and the challenge here with the CTE is that rugby has always balanced its response on an understanding of risk.
>
> DS: Would you accept that every time an incident like George Smith happens, and I know that was not a Premiership incident, it will have a big impact on parents watching with young children and undermines the message that it is an improving situation? Surely something needs to happen there, even a disciplining of a doctor responsible for returning a clearly concussed player to the field of play.
>
> SK: I will only talk about the Premiership.
>
> DS: Fine. What about Toby Flood in the Premiership final?

SK: We have a process within Premiership Rugby where we have the ability to have a serious untoward incident inquiry. If something happened which we believe was a serious untoward incident, we have the ability to investigate it. I am not prepared to discuss the details of the Toby Flood case, but my sense is that we are trying to change and optimize behaviours that have been in place for some time among players, coaches and medical staff. You don't do it overnight. Are we moving in the right direction? Absolutely yes and I would suspect that episodes where the assessment is contentious to become less common. There are some subtleties. Concussion is a clinical diagnosis. I would not want to get in a position where there is repeated trial by television.

On Saturday, 5 October 2013, Leicester winger Blaine Scully was knocked unconscious early on against Northampton, underwent a PSCA and was passed fit to continue.

'He was removed from the field with a suspected concussion but answered all the questions correctly and was deemed fit to play,' said Leicester backs coach Paul Burke, apparently oblivious to the fact Scully should not have even undergone a PSCA. Even the 'suspicion of a loss of consciousness' should have led to the player's immediate removal from the field.

*

That same month I came across a PhD researcher at Auckland University of Technology (AUT) in New Zealand, Doug King, whose groundbreaking work in rugby league, using microchipped mouthguards, had shown far greater impact forces involved than had previously been recognized.

King's research also showed that as many as three out of four concussions in rugby went unreported.

King, who began his research after witnessing the death of Leonardo Va'a, a young rugby league player who sustained a head injury in a club game in 1998, described his findings as 'frightening'. But perhaps just as worrying were the efforts deployed by rugby's two most powerful unions, the RFU and New Zealand Rugby Union (NZRU), to undermine King's research and suppress the findings.

'I have been belittled professionally and personally,' King told Dan, and continued:

> It got so bad I had to resign my position as a rugby club medic and walk away from the game. I have been hounded out. The threats made to me have taken such a toll that I have had to consider whether to go on with this.
>
> I received a phone call from the [AUT] communications manager who said a major sporting organization would not look favourably on AUT as their preferred research provider in future negotiations if I talked to the media.

Asked if he was referring to the NZRU, King replied: 'Yes. It was about $500,000 in research for the AUT, so it is big money.'

I picked up the story in the *Mail on Sunday*, writing: 'King is also in possession of an email from a well-placed source shedding light on a bitter exchange between a senior English RFU figure resistant to King's findings and a world-renowned neurologist supportive of his work. In the email, which The Mail on Sunday has seen, King's medical credentials are ridiculed by the RFU man and his research programme dismissed.'

With so much focus on the RFU and the game's wider approach to concussion management, the sport's governing body were adamant their views should be represented and I was 'invited' to Twickenham to interview Kemp along with the RFU's head of community medicine, Mike England. While the communications we received were civil and professional, this felt unmistakably like a summons, just as it had for Peter Jackson four years previously when he first wrote about Ben Herring and Michael Lipman. And why did the 'invitation' come from the RFU's communications department rather than Kemp himself? I had the personal mobile numbers of every England coach, several captains and the majority of directors of rugby, who would all, at that time, pick up the phone if I rang. And vice versa. But for some reason, Kemp felt the need to involve comms experts.

It was early October 2013 when I arrived at Twickenham Stadium, the monolithic home of English rugby I'd got to know inside and out since first watching London Welsh lose to Bath in 1985. Inside the 82,000-seat stadium lies a network of corridors, meeting rooms, hotel facilities, lecture theatres, medical rooms, hospitality suites, bars and other spaces mostly designed to facilitate commercial opportunities for the betterment of the union. On this occasion a hospitality box overlooking the pitch was provided for the head of medicine to speak with me. I wasn't anticipating a warm welcome and nor did I get one.

When I entered the room, Kemp refused to make eye contact or even acknowledge my presence. He was too busy concentrating on his laptop screen and the notes in front of him. England was slightly more forthcoming, although the atmosphere was frostier than Murrayfield in midwinter.

We covered a range of topics, generally conversing reasonably well on questions around the PSCA, which, as I'd suspected, had been constructed with Bloodgate and cheating in mind.

Kemp told me:

In the post-Bloodgate era there are some sensitivities to introducing initiatives which might be open to manipulation. To be blunt here the feeling is that in a five-minute trial there is unlikely to be any competitive advantage to bringing a player on because the feeling is that it will take that player at least five minutes to get up to match speed. I stress we have got no evidence that this trial has been manipulated but we are trying to balance a welfare initiative with something the broader game will accept and feel comfortable with.

But I'm really clear that in my 15 years of being involved with professional rugby I do not have any concerns about the integrity of the healthcare practitioners who work within the professional game.

Four years after Bloodgate had demonstrated with crystal clarity how doctors' ethics could be compromised, this felt, at best, complacent.

While our exchanges remained civil, if distinctly on the prickly side, Kemp's disposition soon became disdainful when we moved on to the elephant in rugby's room: CTE. I made a point in the transcription I sent back to the sports desk of annotating it with comments about his body language.

SP: I'd like to move on to the CTE issue. It's a huge subject but it's something people need to understand where the RFU stand on this. What is the RFU's position on the Boston research?

SK: Frame the question more specifically.

SP: Do you believe there is a link between multiple concussions and chronic traumatic encephalopathy?

SK: So I think the RFU's position would be aligned currently with the Zurich consensus. Which is that there is no proven association between head trauma and CTE. The RFU is watching, monitoring and evaluating the research as it emerges but it would appear likely that different research will be needed to answer this question. The subtlety here is that Zurich felt that taking cases of autopsy documented CTE and then retrospectively examining and trying to collect data around head impact events, sporting and non-sporting, was not a methodology that would enable us to establish there was a proven link.

SP: Some people will say that you will never prove that causal link and you need to look at exposures such as in boxing, ice hockey where punch-drunk syndrome is proven.

SK: We are monitoring the Boston Group's research really carefully. We believe that, whilst the risk... While waiting for an association or no association to become clearer, the steps we are taking in terms of managing the acute episode and the return to play in a safe and appropriate fashion are the way to mitigate no risk. OK?

SP: Do you accept that there could be a link?

SK: Do I accept there could be a link? That's a hypothetical question. Without defining 'the link' as to whether it's causal or a link by association. Do we accept there could be a link? We will have to follow the research and be guided by the research as it emerges. We will certainly be keen to engage in that research in so far as rugby can help establish any link or no link.

SP: What is your view on the credibility of the research?

SK: (*Sighs*) I think there are two questions here. The first question is that the data coming out of Boston is coming from world-acknowledged experts and is submitted for peer review. One of the approaches the RFU has always taken to scientific research is to put weight on the independent evaluation of research that's being done. In terms of the credibility of research as research the RFU acknowledges that the research is being peer reviewed. The question here is a more subtle one and it is 'to what extent can the research that has been published in this area help move forward an evaluation of a possible link between repeated head injury and CTE?' Do you see there are two questions? Again, the Zurich view as currently presented wouldn't satisfy the epidemiological criteria for establishing causality. Do you...

SP: Yes I get that. What would you say to someone who says that dementia pugilistica is accepted in medical science and boxers are more likely to develop dementia in later life? Can you explain the difference between concussions that a boxer might suffer as opposed to concussions a rugby player might suffer bearing in mind I have spoken to a number of players who believe they were concussed more than 100 times in their career?

SK: (*Sighs*) Phrase the question again.

SP: (*Silent*)

SK: The dementia pugilistica argument is something that is accepted. Mike and I are probably not sufficiently expert in this area in boxing to comment, so I am not going to comment on that.

SP: What would be a threshold for you to accept that link between multiple concussions and CTE? What evidence would you need to see? There are some experts in neurology saying they are seeing a group of players emerging in South Africa (*Kemp visibly slumps in seat and sighs again*) who are suffering serious brain illnesses, whether it be motor neurone disease, brain tumours… What would be a threshold where you would say there is a link?

SK: I can't answer that question succinctly. This is… I would need to see. I, the union, the game, would need to see the evidence emerging, evaluate it critically and then make inferences and change our position as the evidence emerged. I think it would be inappropriate to specify up front. The other real challenge here is that all the science tells you that asking players to retrospectively comment on their concussion history has huge errors involved in it. So it's like the study will need to have an element of prospectivity which means it's going to take some time to definitely answer this question.

SP: What would you say to people who say that is very convenient for rugby?

SK: I don't think it's convenient at all. It makes it difficult. Let's be very clear here. Rugby's record on risk management is mature and sophisticated and has been present for a number of years and if you look at our approach to preventing risk of catastrophic injury it is again very mature. I would argue again that our approach to mitigating risk of concussive injury is again very mature. The piece that we are missing is the awareness of the medium- and long-term consequences of concussive injury in rugby. I'm not quite sure what trick rugby is missing with respect to the CTE debate here.

SP: The fact that evidence from other sports would suggest there is a link there.

SK: Sam, can I challenge you on that?

SP: I think people struggle to understand the difference between concussion in a helmeted sport and a non-helmeted. Surely if someone is concussed they are concussed?

SK: I understand. Tell me what you understand when you use the term 'link'.

SP: That one leads into the next. As in repeated concussions lead into an increased likelihood of early onset dementia.

SK: OK. That wasn't the position the Zurich Consensus Group reached. We were both there and I have followed this debate. What evidence are you aware of which I am not aware of which makes you think that there is evidence of a link?

SP: Punch-drunk syndrome.

SK: (*Sighs*)

SP: It is widely accepted that boxers are more likely to suffer from early onset dementia. Is that not the case? Tell me if I'm wrong to believe that.

SK: Again, I don't want to talk about the boxing case. You would need to speak to someone more expert.

As I thanked the doctors for their time Kemp turned his back and declined to bid me farewell.

*

In the end the article ran to 750 words, or a page lead as we would call it, but I was left frustrated by my failure to pin Kemp down on the issue of CTE. By constantly falling back on McCrory's Concussion in Sport Group position, he had a readymade 'get out of jail free' card.

I was surprised by Kemp's apparent lack of inquisitiveness when it came to wanting to understand CTE. My concern was that a generation of players could be left unnecessarily damaged by this seeming lack of interest. I would later be introduced to an important phrase in research: 'absence of evidence is not evidence of absence', but to most sports doctors around this time, apparently it was.

*

It felt like we were now engaged with the full weight of the RFU machine. Their comms department were all over us, sending reams upon reams of information demonstrating their absolute commitment to player welfare.

I was most interested in the players' experience and had an excellent network of contacts willing to share their invaluable personal knowledge with me, often completely off the record, while Dan, who would soon be snapped up by *The Times*, was also tapping into a rich vein of information.

For his *Mail on Sunday* article published on 20 October 2013 he spoke to Professors Tony Belli and Michael Grey at Birmingham University along with former England flanker Michael Lipman.

Belli, one of the country's leading neurologists with no links at that time to sport, said:

> There is clear evidence of a link between concussion and
> dementia, but rugby is in denial about that. It was the same

argument used by the cigarette companies many years ago to deny that smoking caused cancer. We already know that people who have developed a large number of concussions over time are at risk of developing neurodegenerative conditions and that evidence is now pretty clear.

We have a large body of evidence. Most of that has come from the United States, and if you are looking for clear evidence in rugby then it might not be there, but that's only because no one has looked for it.

But the overall evidence for repeated concussion in sport [being linked to brain damage] is almost incontrovertible... Rugby is a wonderful sport with huge benefits, but at the moment there's a culture of denial.

Meanwhile, Lipman's testimony added more weight to the growing body of evidence which showed players were proactively cheating the CogSport reliant baseline test.

'I used to think those tests were a bit of a laugh,' said Lipman. 'I'd try to do as badly as I could because I knew that I was going to get concussed. That's exactly what a lot of players still do because when they get a knock, they want to be back playing. They have careers and reputations and, at the end of the day, they just want to get out there and play rugby.'

9

Even the doctors are laughing

It was becoming clearer with every passing week, every passing conversation and every incident of head injury mismanagement that professional sport had an endemic problem. And the problem, as far as I could see, was that for every publicized case where a player was either knocked unconscious or showed very visible signs of having a brain injury being returned to the field of play while under the care of doctors in a professional arena, how many more incidents were not being highlighted? And how much would the impact of seeing these incidents effectively normalized on the professional field seep into the mindset of players, coaches and parents watching games of rugby or football on a Sunday morning where almost no medical provision existed? Having started to understand the scale of the problem in the professional game, it began to trouble me deeply that there was a much broader issue around head injuries and their treatment in sport, full stop.

But the only area I could influence at that stage was the professional game. And, for the time being at least, rugby union was my world. The newspaper campaign had got off to an extremely good start and before we knew it, the Rugby Players' Association had come on board in support.

I'd learned in August that Chris Nowinski had presented his evidence to the RPA board, made up of current players, giving them a full debrief of the NFL landscape and the understanding of CTE at that time. By all accounts, you could have heard a pin drop.

Bizarrely, the RFU's head of medicine Simon Kemp sat in on the meeting while Paul Morgan, now Premiership Rugby's head of comms, and a host of RFU comms people, were also present. This felt completely wrong to me. I was not alone. Why would the players' trade union allow the most senior figures from the organizations who employed them to be present at such a sensitive and potentially critical welfare meeting?

'I very much remember Simon Kemp being there,' Nowinski would later tell me, continuing:

> One of the big breakthroughs that we had with the NFL and NFL Players' Association led to convincing the Players' Association to bring in their own independent experts.
>
> The chief medical officers of the sports organizations have conflicts, even great people have conflicts. But they're not the voice of the players, and they're not necessarily going to be as aggressive in protecting the players as the doctors who only report to the players would be.
>
> I was surprised he was there. It made me worry about the influence, or what would be said when I left the room.

For many players, this meeting was the first they'd heard about the potential for long-term problems associated with head injuries, while Nowinski also briefed on research which had shown that the cumulative effect of sub-concussive blows – where no demonstrable signs of concussion were detectable but microscopic damage still occurred – could also be a significant factor in long-term cognitive problems.

Nowinski explained the mandated and strictly policed protocols which had been introduced in the NFL including limits on contact training and independent concussion doctors at all games. To me, it seemed inevitable these very same protocols should be introduced in rugby, too.

The Bloodgate scandal had highlighted in technicolour the risk presented by a toxic conflict of interests where the best interests of a coach or director of rugby, player, medic and club, not to mention the all-important television broadcasters simply could not all be served simultaneously.

So how, in medical terms, could sport have allowed head injuries to be so routinely mismanaged and for so long? I had a long way to go before I reached any firm conclusions on this but, undoubtedly, the RFU's 'Concussion Forum' at Twickenham in November 2013 was an eye-opener.

I was among a select group of journalists invited to attend the forum, apparently convened partly in response to the *Mail on Sunday*'s campaign, on the strict understanding that reporting the bulk of the event would be off the record. I report on it now only because I fundamentally believe it to be in the public interest for me to do so.

One of the primary reasons I was able to gather so much information around such a sensitive and hitherto secretive subject was that if I said a conversation was 'off the record' then that is precisely where it stayed. Sources learned I could be trusted with sensitive information and as a result I built my knowledge base and network of contacts faster than if I'd just printed the first story that came across my lap.

So it goes against the grain reporting something which I agreed not to, but in this instance I believe it is firmly in the public interest to paint the picture of a sport-wide culture which revealed itself in that room at Twickenham that day.

If the doctors saw concussion as a source of entertainment, giggling openly as athletes were knocked unconscious, then of course the players and coaches would follow their lead. They say culture is set from the top and I have no doubt senior figures in rugby, and sport more broadly, found it amusing to see players or participants being knocked out. Fortunately, that is no longer the case. As one person involved that day would later say 'fortunately we've grown up since then'.

If people within the RFU accuse me of a breach of trust in relaying this information, in this instance, I am prepared to live with that.

Through my work I began to understand and believe brain injuries in sport are significantly underestimated public health issue and as such, they deserve to know 'why?'.

'There'll be time allocated for on the record interviews but anything on stage is under Chatham House rules,' I was told by the RFU's media manager Dave Barton in advance.

It came as no surprise that Kemp was at the heart of organizing the forum. He was everywhere. Moving chairs on stage, briefing fellow guests, checking the AV equipment.

When we arrived we were welcomed into one of the several cavernous function rooms beneath the stadium and ushered to our seats toward the back of the room. Up on stage sat Kemp alongside Professor Willie Stewart of Glasgow University and Dr Michael Turner, a name I'd noticed on a number of papers relating to sports-related concussion, including the Concussion in Sport Group.

What followed shocked me.

I had spoken to Stewart on and off the record on numerous occasions already and knew him to be a strong advocate for reform in rugby, especially when it came to the management of brain injuries. His life's work had involved studying the brains of the deceased for evidence of trauma and, at that stage, he was the only person in the UK with the expertise to diagnose CTE at autopsy.

Initially, all seemed well. Stewart spoke first, making what seemed to me a reasoned, rational but sobering presentation relating to what we knew of the long-term effects of head trauma on the brains of the unfortunate people he'd examined under a microscope over the years.

Far from sensationalizing the issue, Stewart admitted there was much we did not know when it came to brain injuries and why some suffered severe long-term consequences while others appeared to experience almost no negative long-term effects. His presentation was populated by slides showing cut-throughs of brains, coloured in certain areas to highlight the rippling effect of damage while explaining that chronic traumatic encephalopathy was essentially punch-drunk syndrome rebranded.

As the new knowledge was emerging, or should that be established knowledge refreshed, Stewart argued for a more cautious approach to head injury management, while warning CTE was 'akin to a crack in a windshield which, once done, can't be undone, unless you replace the whole windshield'. Clearly replacing an entire human brain was not an option, hence Stewart's call for greater caution in its management.

Once Stewart had finished, Kemp took the mic again and introduced Turner, making no secret of the regard in which he held him. Kemp promoted Turner as one of the most enlightened thinkers in the world of concussion management.

With Stewart back in his seat, and robbed of the microphone, Turner began his presentation.

'People have different positions when it comes to concussion in sport and Willie Stewart is the Attila the Hun of the debate.' That got the audience chuckling, not least Kemp, sitting on stage behind Turner.

'I on the other hand am Michael coming down from the mount to read his sermon.' More laughter from the crowd. More giggles on stage. Stewart, however, was unamused.

Whether or not Turner intentionally set out to belittle Professor Stewart, it seemed clear to everyone in that room that he did intend to position himself as the owner of truth, while Stewart and anyone else who challenged his narrative was, effectively, a barbarian.

My love affair with rugby began playing for Richmond minis. Here I was aged six playing for the under 7s in the Worthing Festival.

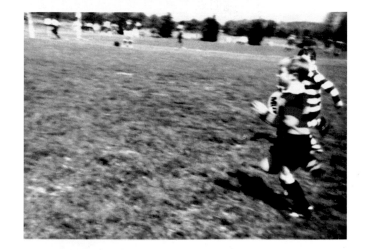

Football was also a passion. Here's me pictured front row third from right sporting a black eye I picked up playing rugby aged 16 for the 1st Seven a week earlier.

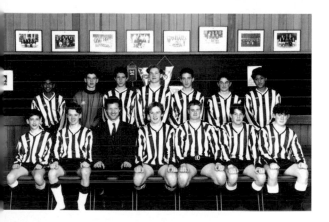

Told you I was a fan. This picture of Rob Andrew after England won the Grand Slam in 1995 was on the back page of the *Times*. I'm in the white hat cheering loudly.

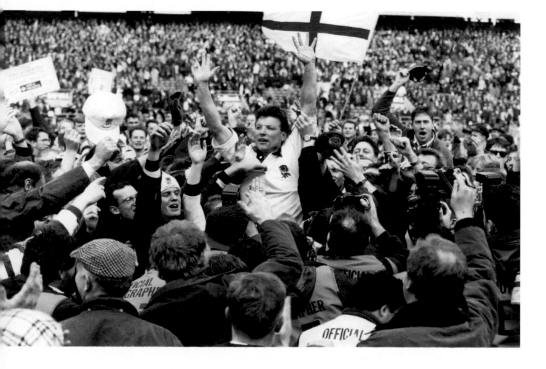

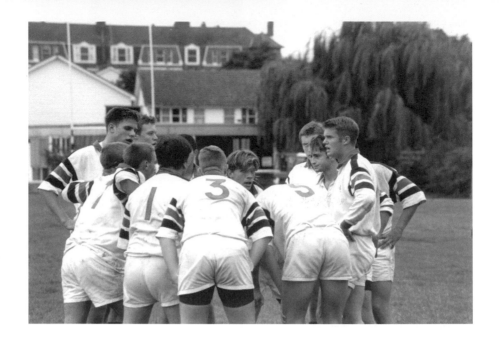

Barking orders. Captaining St Paul's School
First XV was my proudest rugby achievement.
Here's me giving a half-time team talk as we beat
London rivals Whiftgift in 1996.

With dad in 2000 in the Edinburgh University
clubhouse at Peffermill, where two years earlier
I'd dislocated my shoulder so badly it would
eventually force me to quit rugby.

Living with the Lions. After graduating in 2001,
I followed the British & Irish Lions to Australia
with my dear friend Matt Ross. He took this
snap of me with Jonny Wilkinson and Neil Back
on Manly Beach.

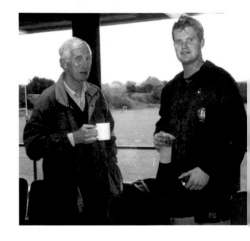

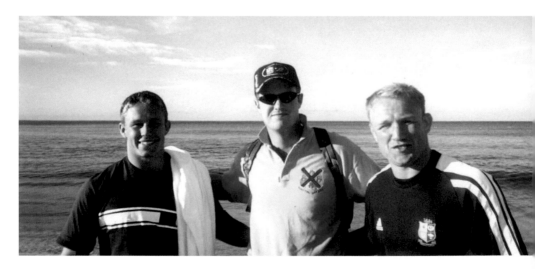

Jonah Lomu's impact on world rugby is incalculable and I had the privilege of interviewing him during the 2007 World Cup in Paris. He died eight years later, aged just 40.

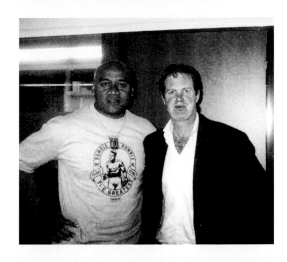

By 2007 I had serious concerns about the physical demands on professional rugby players and an increasingly lax attitude to brain injuries. England captain Lewis Moody was knocked out twice against Tonga in the World Cup but allowed to play on by Dr Simon Kemp.

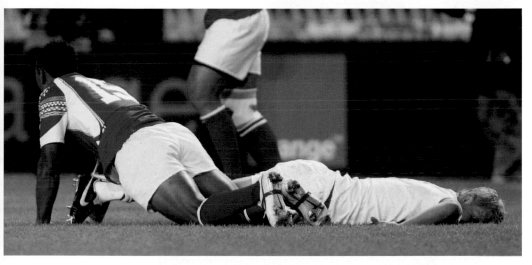

In 2009 my concerns about unscrupulous coaches' potentially toxic influence on players and doctors were realised when Harlequins director of rugby Dean Richards received a three-year ban for his role in the Bloodgate scandal. Here Leinster's backroom staff complain to referee Nigel Owens that fake blood had been used to cheat substitution laws. They were soon proved right.

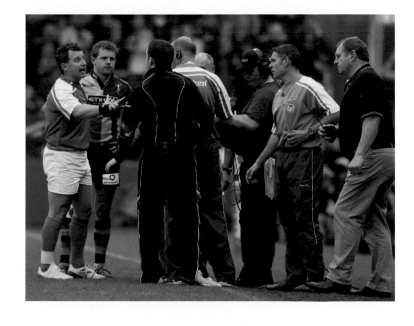

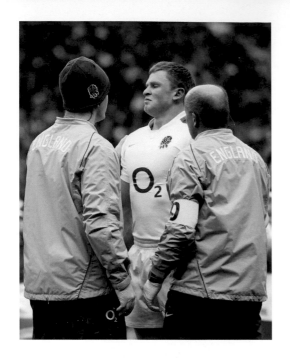

Contrary to the narrative presented by World Rugby and the RFU, it was clear by 2010 that professional rugby union was far more dangerous than the amateur version of the game, and players were routinely being allowed to play on with concussion. England winger Chris Ashton would later admit not being able to remember anything after he was knocked unconscious against South Africa.

The 2011 World Cup was desperately difficult for Martin Johnson, England World Cup-winning captain turned head coach, as scandal beset their campaign. Here I am amongst the press pack quizzing my former hero about his handling of events.

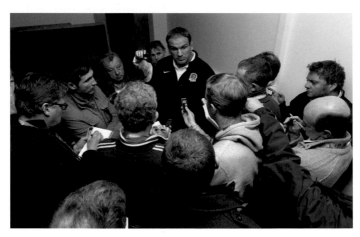

The targeting of fly halves, rugby's main playmaker, is nothing new in rugby but by 2013 I was seeing many No10s knocked out early in games. In the Premiership Final Leicester fly half Toby Flood was knocked out in a tackle but allowed to play on before enentually being substituted.

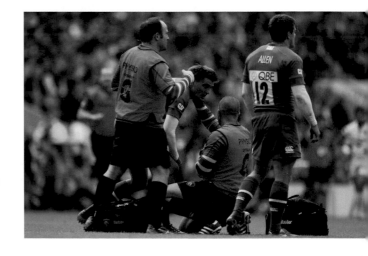

I covered the 2013 British and Irish Lions tour to Australia for the *Mail on Sunday* and witnessed first-hand the decision to allow brain-damaged Wallaby flanker George Smith to return to play after he passed a new off-field concussion test. To my shame I did not include the incident in my match report, believing concussion remained a 'nonstory'.

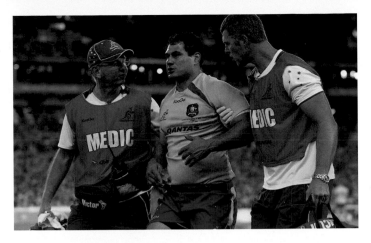

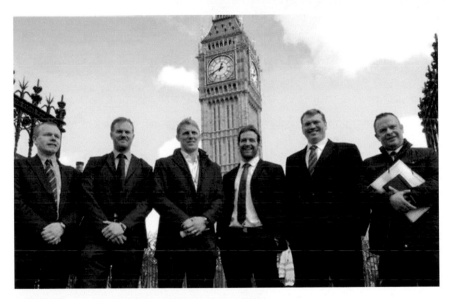

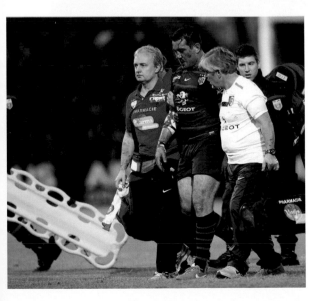

The *Mail on Sunday* concussion campaign rapidly gained the attention of politicians. Here I am pictured second from the left outside Parliament in 2013 alongside fellow campaigners (from left to right) Professor Willie Stewart, me, Lewis Moody, Rory Lamont, Chris Nowinski and Peter Robinson.

This incident involving Toulouse centre Florian Fritz, who returned to the field with a severe head injury after veteran coach Guy Noves was filmed haranguing medics and shouting at his player, was among the worst cases of concussion mismanagement ever witnessed on a sports field. The following year Noves was appointed France national team coach.

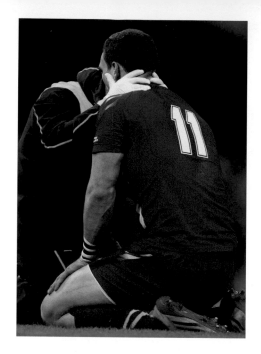

George North became an unwitting poster boy of our campaign when he was allowed to play on after being knocked unconscious twice in the same game against England in February 2015. The WRU medical team were found not guilty of any wrongdoing. I asked the WRU for permission to use images which they own the rights to of North unconscious for this book, but they refused.

Getting players to speak openly about their concussion issues wasn't always easy. With contracts at stake and fearful of being mocked, some preferred to stay silent. Over time many came to trust I would handle their story appropriately. Following a string of concussions in 2014, All Black captain Kieran Reid told me 'obviously my brain wasn't quite right. My wife is worried I guess.'

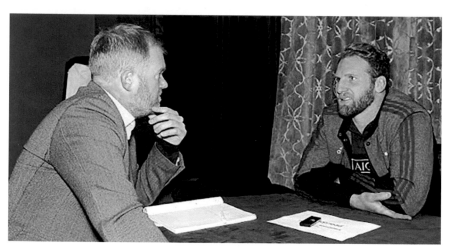

I learned of Cae Treyharn's death by suicide in the summer of 2016 and went to interview his mum Althea at her home near Pontypool a few months later. Althea was convinced head injuries Cae suffered playing rugby had caused his death and told me 'rugby killed my son'.

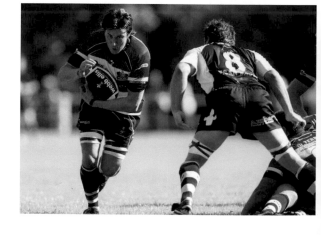

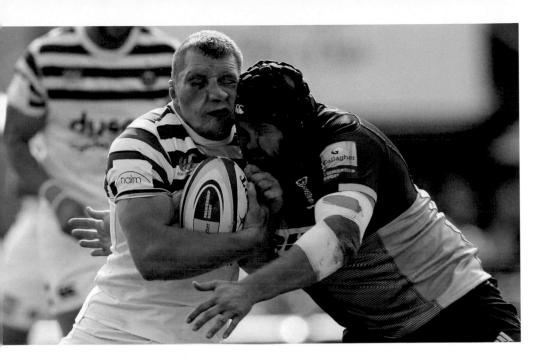

Modern day rugby players face bigger and more frequent collisions, although instances such as this – where Harlequins prop Mark Lambert accidentally clashes heads with Bath's Sam Underhill in 2018 – are now getting less frequent as overdue moves to reduce the tackle height are being properly policed by referees. For me, players like Underhill should have been afforded greater protections much sooner.

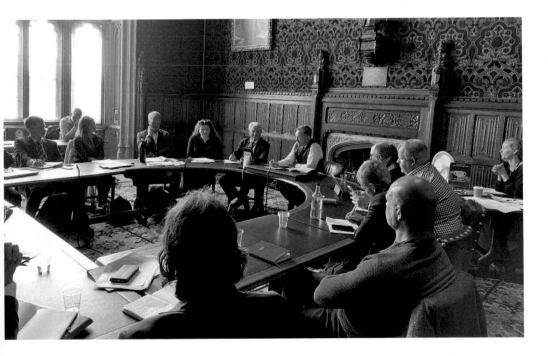

Since 2013 I have become a reasonably frequent visitor to Parliament, thanks largely to Chris Bryant's relentless pursuit of an Acquired Brain Injury Bill after I first alerted him to the concussion crisis in rugby in 2013. Here I am sitting three to Bryant's right at a meeting of campaigners and sports bodies in 2022. The RFU were notable for their absence.

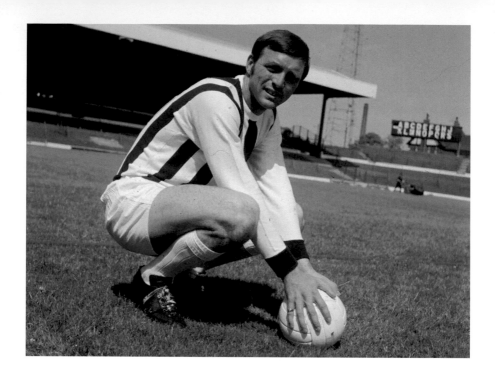

When I found out the FA had failed to carry out potentially lifesaving research after Jeff Astle was found to have died from 'industrial disease linked to heading footballs' I alerted his family, who immediately launched the 'Justice for Jeff' campaign. The following year FA chairman Greg Dyke apologised for his organisation's appalling failure and the Jeff Astle Foundation was launched.

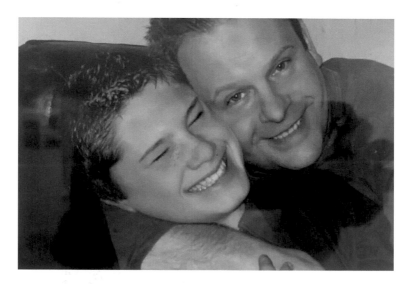

Learning about the circumstances surrounding Benjamin Robinson's death, when the coroner found he had died from second impact syndrome resulting from brain injuries playing rugby, sparked me into action. Ben's father Peter, who I first met at Parliament in 2013, has campaigned relentlessly for better concussion awareness ever since. I'm proud to call him my friend.

'No sport in the world has more concussions than mine, horse racing,' he said, 'and today, in sporting terms, this is a willy waving exercise. And my [horse racing] dick is bigger than yours [rugby].'

Much laughter in the room including from Kemp.

I turned to Andy Bull, sports writer at the *Guardian*, and asked: 'Is this guy for real?' Andy shrugged.

Andy's look of bemusement was matched by Dan's, who was sitting alongside me.

Turner, who was chief medical advisor to the British Horseracing Authority at the time, proceeded to give a video presentation in which jockey after jockey was shown falling off their horses and smashing their heads into the ground. Many in the room found it all very amusing. I didn't. I thought it was crass and inappropriate considering why we were there: to understand the extent of brain injury in sport and what we could collectively do to reduce it.

The thrust of Turner's position, as far as I could establish, was that because horse racing had more concussions than any other sport and he hadn't seen lots of 'demented jockeys', the CTE cases in America must have been to do with something other than head injuries.

He went on to compare a concussion to 'rebooting a computer', essentially suggesting the brain could be temporarily switched off and then switched back on with no lasting effects.

Years later, Turner would seek to defend his presentation style which in 2016 prompted Dawn Astle, the daughter of former England footballer Jeff Astle, who had died with dementia linked to CTE, to storm out of a room in disgust, later saying: 'You can be a jokester and an entertainer, but not when you're talking about people's lives. I just felt like he was trivializing it and he was laughing.' In his defence Turner told the *Mail on Sunday*: 'I have had a particular way of delivery over the years that gets my message over but can offend people, for which I have invariably apologized. Of course Willie is not Attila the Hun.'

With a number of media articles, including one particularly hard-hitting one by former ESPN turned ABC News reporters Mark Fainaru-Wada and Steve Fainaru, questioning the funding streams of the International Concussion and Head Injury Research Foundation which Turner co-founded with McCrory in 2016, Turner also subsequently sought to play down accusations of a conflict of interest.

> People get money from all over the place but that does not make research and researchers corrupt.
>
> The problem here is proving causation [between repetitive head injuries and CTE]. You also need to have examined 200, 300, 400 brains donated by people who never played sport and compare those to the brains of those who have. To my knowledge, there has not been a CTE study of the normal population. To produce a heading study like that is an absolute nightmare.

*

I have several other recollections from that day, not least former Newcastle, Wasps and England No.8 Dean Ryan's open hostility to the *Mail on Sunday*'s campaign, which he accused of being 'sensationalized nonsense'. When I attempted to interview him, he accused me of 'scaremongering'. I'd expected to encounter hostility that day but not from Ryan of all people. If there was one person in the room I had assumed would be an ally, it was the man whose interview in 2002 articulated his concerns about the potential long-term implications of mismanaging concussion. Here was I, attempting to shed more light on the issue, and Ryan was abusing me for doing so.

Within a couple of minutes of beginning the interview, and for the first time in my career as a journalist, I turned the tape off as the 6ft 6in, 18 stone former soldier continued his rant. I have not spoken with him since.

Another standout incident was Barry O'Driscoll having to plead with RFU director of rugby Rob Andrew to be given a platform to speak. Despite O'Driscoll's impeccable credentials and decade of experience as an advisor to the IRB's Concussion Committee, he had not been included as a speaker. Finally, after pressure from several of us who wanted to hear his position, he was given an all too brief five-minute window from the floor to flag his concerns.

At the end of a troubling day I spoke to Kemp and other doctors on and off the record. I asked Kemp why independent doctors could not be present at every professional game. His response was odd.

'It would be like turtles upon turtles, Sam.' By that I think he was asking 'where would it all end?' or implying it was some kind of never-ending race to the bottom. I'm not sure. It would take another six years before independent matchday doctors would become mandatory across the professional game in England.

I also asked a number of people about the idea of mandatory limits on training which, although limited data around concussion was available at this time, was still the source of an astonishing 335 injuries the previous season. This was well over double the number identified in 2002/03, the so-called Wild West years.

My suggestion to limit contact was dismissed out of hand.

'Who on earth is going to police that?' one delegate asked me, incredulously.

*

The campaign was by now in full swing and my feet hardly touched the ground. Player after player came forward and incident after incident occured on the field. The way I watched matches completely changed and I stopped following the ball and instead started following the injured players and observing how they were treated. The more I watched, the worse it got. I can't pretend that, journalistically, what was unfolding wasn't thrilling. I was on the inside of the story. But from a human perspective, it was increasingly difficult to comprehend how these players were basically being treated like pieces of meat.

I would later discuss this with former England hooker Steve Thompson for a BBC documentary broadcast in 2022, *Head On: Rugby, Dementia and Me*:

> ST: What you've got to remember on that is it would be 'the defence is bad so I'll tell you what we'll do, we'll just smash the hell out of you even more.'
>
> SP: Or the scrum was going backwards so you'd do 25 scrums or whatever.
>
> ST: Well, 100 live scrums.
>
> SP: You'd do 100 live scrums?
>
> ST: We did 100 live scrums.
>
> SP: I can't even begin to comprehend what that… You did 100 live scrums? Jesus.
>
> ST: We did 100 live scrums… The injuries you were seeing, but what people weren't seeing were the knockouts, the concussions. Lads would be lying on the pitch and it would just be 'oh it's all right, he's hit his head, he'll get up in a minute.' No one was there for the players. No one at all.

With access to training often strictly limited, especially with England, I sensed there was a serious issue there but couldn't prove it. Yet. I became determined to understand what neurology and neuropathology experts without ties to sport were talking about and attended lectures at the National Hospital for Neurology and Neurosurgery, St Thomas's and the Royal London hospitals among others, to find out what experts were saying. I also visited Birmingham University where I spent a day in the company of Professors Tony Belli and Michael Grey

These were not places I'd expected to find myself when I started out as a sports journalist. But there were several common themes which kept emerging when I attended these respective centres of excellence, unrelated to sport. One was that the debate over whether repetitive head injuries could cause long-term neuro-impairments had been resolved many decades earlier with the work of people such as Harrison Martland, Augustus Thorndike and the many other neurological research studies mentioned earlier, not least Boston University's. Others would emerge in the years to come. The more pertinent question was around the extent of the problem and, perhaps even more importantly, how to mitigate these risks. Reducing exposure to head injuries was universally accepted as a means by which to reduce long-term risk.

I was incredibly fortunate that Alison and Mike appreciated this was a topic I needed to immerse myself in deeply and, on occasion, they would accept me disappearing off in different directions to speak to people seemingly completely unrelated to rugby, the actual subject I had been brought onto the paper for.

The issue became the talk of the Twickenham press box, even though I was still very much a lone voice when it came to writing about CTE red flag and longer-term risks. It was clear the majority of my fellow rugby journalists, although by no means all, thought I was going over the top in the way I was reporting on concussion. Others, Dan among them, applauded my stance.

The suggestion head injuries could in some way be linked to issues like Parkinson's or motor neurone disease filled me with horror. No one involved in rugby at the time could have failed to have been moved by the memory of former London Irish full back Jarrod Cunningham's fight against and ultimate defeat by MND, but to my knowledge no one for a second suggested it could have been linked to the possibility he may have banged his head too many times.

But when former Springbok Joost van der Westhuizen was diagnosed with the disease, aged 42, in 2011, I started to ask questions. Some simple digging found other names: fellow Springbok Ruben Kruger died of brain cancer in 2010 aged 39, while in November 2014, Tinus Linee, a centre who played nine times for the Springboks without a full Test cap, died, aged 45, from MND. This may well have been a desperately sad coincidence, but some, including me, thought it entirely plausible that, with our growing understanding of the long-term risks, repetitive head injuries sustained during their playing careers could have been a factor.

*

In 2010, the Boston Group had reported evidence of a direct link between repetitive head injuries and motor neurone disease, while traumatically induced motor neurone disease had, according to medical historian Stephen Casper, been discussed as far back as the 1870s. But for some reason, sport seemed to be of the view this was all brand new science that had caught everyone on the hop. The reality was something very different. In 2017, the Boston Group presented more evidence linking head trauma in football with MND. But the powers that be steadfastly ignored them.

In an interview with Dan for the *Mail on Sunday*, Boston University School of Medicine's Professor Ann McKee said:

> I met with FIFA in Zurich at a concussion conference. I am very unpopular there. They just have a very low opinion of my work and they told me that it was very poor science.
>
> You would think they would be concerned about the players that made them wealthy. Apparently not. I really do think it's denial and deflection.
>
> They are not taking care of the players that made them such a big deal in the first place. They should be funding this research.

Naturally, those very doctors belittling McKee's work, or indeed any work revealing links with longer-term problems, were the doctors sports journalists were being briefed by and listening to. It was and is an echo-chamber of self-reinforcement. Despite this research, journalists I admired and respected overlooked it. One interview with van der Westhuizen in *The Times* in 2013 reported: 'No research has yet identified the exact causes of MND; there is no suggestion that it is related to contact sport.' This simply wasn't true.

In November 2014, I would interview van der Westhuizen myself, and I asked him whether *if* rugby had caused his disease, he would change anything.

'Not at all, not at all. I'd do it all again,' he said. 'It would not be fair to say rugby caused this but it's fair to say there could be a link.

'I broke my nose 16 times in my career which should say enough.'

Van der Westhuizen died just over two years later.

I would later learn Ryan Walker, the former Natal Sharks and Leeds Tykes player, had been diagnosed with MND in August 2013.

He died in November 2022, during the course of me writing this book, while former Scotland lock Doddie Weir passed away nine days later, aged 52, of the same cruel disease.

In the same year Gloucester lock Ed Slater retired from professional rugby union aged 33, having been diagnosed with MND, while former Leeds Rhinos scrum half Rob Burrow's battle against the disease was brilliantly and sensitively documented by former BBC reporter Ben Dirs in his book *Too Many Reasons to Live*. Today, only the most one-eyed doubt a link exists.

*

Within a few weeks of our campaign getting started, we'd made contact with Chris Bryant, the Labour MP for Rhondda, who we had noticed was supportive of some of the calls for change on social media. Bryant, a Welshman whose constituency had a high concentration of rugby clubs, understood rugby's culture well and had a personal interest in acquired brain injury. He agreed to meet me and Ben Robinson's father, Peter, at Portcullis House in late October. It was the first time I had met either man and I was impressed by them both in different ways.

Peter, a relatively short but strongly built man, had an inner steel about him. He was calm, rational and clearly a rugby lover. But he was also a father who had lost a son as the direct result of rugby's failure to get its house in order when it came to education around brain injuries. Peter passionately believed that if the message 'concussion can kill' had been writ large across every rugby clubhouse in the country, his son would still have been alive. I agreed with him and so, it appeared, did Bryant.

Peter's absolute determination to get justice for his son reminded me of a Ken Follett quote: 'When you've lost everything, you've got nothing to lose.'

We spent a good hour in Bryant's office, with Professor Willie Stewart on the end of a conference call talking us through the science, and as we left the Welshman assured us he supported our cause and he intended to pull together a cross-party group of MPs and peers to investigate the issue. There appeared to be some political traction. Having said that, it was completely uncharted territory for me, although Peter had already had success with the Scottish government for his 'If In Doubt, Sit Them Out' campaign, with apparently far more appetite in Scotland for a co-ordinated concussion message across all sports at all levels. Time would tell how it would play out in Westminster.

'Ben Robinson died playing a sport he loved because the level of awareness that concussion can cause death is far too low,' said Bryant in a *Mail on Sunday* interview.

> Coaches and players alike need to know the dangers. We
> must make sure that concussion is taken seriously at all levels

of sport, from the professional bodies all the way down to Saturday teams and schools.

I am going to do everything in my power to work with Ben's dad, Peter, and others to build a cross-party campaign to raise awareness of this important issue in Parliament.

Meanwhile, Boston University's Professor Robert Cantu, a signatory to the 2012 Zurich Concussion in Sport Group Consensus Statement, reiterated his opposition to the controversial five-minute PSCA which was still on trial in professional rugby union at this time.

'My position has never changed,' said Cantu. 'The five-minute concussion assessment period is inadequate. It's a start, but it sure better not be where they wind up.'

Our concussion campaign is proud to win support from Parliament to Hollywood... as rugby leaders agree to review 'five-minute rule'
By Alison Kervin
10 November 2013

Last week we received high-level support and a real breakthrough in the campaign.

First, the MP Chris Bryant urged Parliament to step into the concussion debate. In doing so, he cited the importance of this newspaper's campaign in the House of Commons...

Our greatest triumph, however, came on Thursday when the Rugby Football Union announced that they will consider mandatory concussion training for all players and will review the controversial Pitchside Suspected Concussion Assessment protocol.

This newspaper, in conjunction with leading doctors, believes the PSCA – rugby's 'five-minute rule' – is an ineffective way of assessing whether a player is concussed.

We are delighted that rugby's rulers now appear to agree, and believe the RFU deserve real praise for the step they have taken. But we urge them to go further. Some of the world's most influential neurosurgeons believe that there is an irrefutable link between concussion and long-term neurological problems.

Rugby, in particular, has consistently refused to acknowledge such a connection, insisting that there is no scientific evidence of a causal link between repeated concussions and the later onset of neurological problems.

We implore the rugby authorities to accept that this link may exist and to ensure, either through funding or direct action on their part, that the issue is subjected to the most stringent independent scientific research possible.

Our campaign will not stop until this important step has been taken.

Concussion is dangerous, concussion can kill. Broken bones will mend, broken brains won't. Sportsmen make themselves vulnerable every week for the entertainment of millions; we urge the governing bodies of all sports to do everything in their power to make sure they are as safe as possible while doing it.

A week later I was thrilled by the news that IRB head of medicine Martin Raftery appeared to have conceded significant ground to our demands when he went on record admitting a 'potential link' between repetitive head injuries and CTE.

I wrote in the *Mail on Sunday*:

Last night, in a huge victory for the Mail on Sunday's concussion campaign, the International Rugby Board finally accepted a link exists between repeated concussions and Chronic Traumatic Encephalopathy (CTE) – a disease associated with the early onset of dementia.

'CTE is a form of dementia, and there are studies about boxers and American football players who have suffered repetitive head injuries, so we recognize that there might be a potential link,' said the IRB's chief medical officer Martin Raftery.

The Mail on Sunday has been calling on rugby union authorities to improve their management of concussion for months after a string of high-profile incidents where concussed stars played on following perfunctory examinations.

Last night's news – albeit buried at the bottom of a statement placed on their website without notifying the media – indicates the IRB are waking up to their responsibilities.

Raftery added: 'Rugby is a physical contact sport and that is part of the fabric and attraction for those who want to play the game. However, our duty is to ensure that the sport implements the very best standards of care to protect our players.'

*

I had two more key meetings before the end of the year including an off the record briefing with RPA chairman David Barnes and chief executive Damian Hopley. As a paper, I was proud of the stance we were taking on player welfare. We'd pushed back harder than any media organization had ever previously been prepared to in calling for change, going way beyond the usual article or two by questioning policy, and driving at the heart of the issue; namely, rugby was routinely mismanaging brain injuries and the long-term risks were potentially greater than we had ever previously thought. They were not easy conversations to have, but we'd been prepared to have them.

I had been hugely supportive of the RPA as it was clear their members were the ones with most to lose and the smallest platform upon which to defend themselves. It was routinely said they 'had a place' at the table with the Professional Game Board, which manages all issues to do with playing professional rugby in England, including player welfare – but, evidently, for whatever reason, they were struggling to make their voice heard.

With Alison's blessing, and I understood editor Geordie Greig's too, I attended the meeting at the RPA's head office, by Twickenham train station. With optimism and confidence we could forge a working partnership which would, in the long term, help protect the RPA's members – the players – and protect their long-term health.

On the face of things, the meeting went well. Barnes was receptive and enthusiastic about the idea of partnering with the *Mail on Sunday*, which could essentially become the players' mouthpiece; Hopley, notably less so. I understood the RPA already had a commercial relationship with the *Sunday Times*, who sponsored their annual dinner, but this was not about a commercial relationship, it was about protecting the lives of players. In retrospect, I was spectacularly naïve. I had no hard currency to offer, just the promise, in good faith, that I would continue to be their organization's voice as I had been over the past decade. Now, with the evidence of CTE emerging, here was the opportunity for the players to seize the day. Reduce the number of games top players played; reduce the amount of contact training demanded of them; put strict rules in place to protect players from coaches and directors of rugby prone to putting undue pressure on them. Tell the truth and allow participants to make informed choices.

Just as Nowinski had a few months before, I walked them through the NFL landscape, which Barnes was already across, before explaining how I'd started to watch the game differently in the past few months, no longer following the ball, but rather watching behind it to see if players were injured and, if so, how they were being treated.

At the end of the meeting, after explaining this to Hopley, he looked me in the eye and said: 'Don't take your eye off the ball too much, Sam.'

What he meant, I understood, was that I shouldn't probe too hard.

Hopley's comment unsettled me and I probed further, quite the opposite to what he told me, and I started to understand the funding model which saw the RPA's funding come largely from the two organizations which, in my view, the players need protecting from: namely their employers – Premiership Rugby and the RFU.

To muddy the waters further, the RPA had taken on the role of negotiating the top England stars' commercial deals with the RFU when it came to appearance fees and image rights. This gave the RFU and Premiership Rugby leverage to push back hard in negotiations. Essentially, the line could be: if your members want more money, they will have to earn their pound of flesh.

I flew to Ireland to attend the IRB's medical forum in Dublin. I had the same sense of foreboding I had when I'd interviewed Kemp and England at Twickenham just a few weeks earlier and, knowing I would be coming face to face with Raftery, I was prepared for another frosty reception. I wasn't to be disappointed.

At the opening press conference, the Australian made a point of glowering at me as he addressed the assembled media. He argued that the IRB had been taking concussion seriously since 1977, and had more of a grasp of it than anyone else in the room.

But in my mind, the evidence which had played out before me over the past two decades had been that rugby union's attitude towards concussion had become less well informed and far less cautious. That was on Raftery's watch, along with the likes of Kemp, who had controlled the data collection and rugby's internal narrative in this space. I wasn't playing ball. The reason both men were so annoyed with me, I believed, was because they were losing control of their narrative. I wasn't playing ball. Public perception was shifting as a result of the campaign and rugby knew it.

I bumped into Owain Jones, who had taken over from Morgan as *Rugby World*'s editor two years previously. I'd always got on well with the affable Welshman and it was nice to see a friendly face.

'Mate, fair play on the concussion stuff,' Owain said as we sat in the foyer. 'You've gone balls out on that one, haven't you? It's like you drunk the truth serum. Telling it how it is. But I'm no medical expert, so I'll leave the news stuff to you boys.'

It was reassuring to hear some supportive words from a colleague I respected and I certainly didn't begrudge his lack of enthusiasm for writing news stories which, by their very nature, upset somebody, somewhere. All the rest, Phil Derbyshire said, is PR. For me, by that time, writing news stories had become a way of life.

That afternoon, I sat down with Brett Gosper, the highly polished, square-jawed IRB chief executive who reminded me of a character from an American drama series. When it came to concussion it quickly transpired he had a weak grasp of the facts and was effectively walked through the entire interview by the IRB's head of communications, Dominic Rumbles. Similar in age to me, I would definitely place Rumbles in the 'rugby evangelist' category. But to be fair to the former Bath press officer, he was, and is, exceptionally good at his job and he protected his boss throughout.

In particular, I quizzed Gosper about a research project I'd been told his organization was funding in New Zealand looking at the long-term neurological effects of playing rugby. The study was already several months overdue. I'd written about this a few weeks earlier and I knew Raftery in particular was twitchy.

Rugby vow: no cover up! IRB chief promises to make research results public

By Sam Peters

24 November 2013

The most powerful man in world rugby insists there will be no attempt to cover up research investigating the long-term health implications of playing the sport.

Brett Gosper, the International Rugby Board's chief executive, has restated his commitment to player welfare days after The Mail on Sunday revealed IRB-funded research into a possible association between head trauma and dementia is woefully behind schedule.

The research, and much of the current discussion around concussion, has been fuelled by the discovery of chronic traumatic encephalopathy (CTE) – formerly known as punch-drunk syndrome – in former American Footballers. That led to a $765 million (£472m) payout by the NFL after accusations they knowingly underplayed the risk of concussion for years.

The IRB are funding research into rugby, which is being undertaken at Auckland University of Technology by the governing body's chief medical officer, Dr Martin Raftery.

They were initially meant to publish their findings last September but are still 'several months' away from completion because of a failure to attract enough former players.

Gosper says that when the research is finally completed there will be no attempt to hide anything – regardless of what is found.

'Will it be published? Of course,' said Gosper in an interview with The Mail on Sunday. 'We're not a cigarette company. We will make transparent whatever research comes out of it. You've got to be absolutely transparent on what we know and we will share that with the rugby community.

The Mail on Sunday concussion campaign has led to rugby's administrators agreeing to introduce mandatory concussion awareness training for players, coaches and referees.

Last week, it was reported the Rugby Football Union intend to form a working group, led by operations director Rob Andrew alongside head of medicine Simon Kemp and development director Steve Grainger, to investigate the possible link between concussion and CTE.

It is understood that the group will include a legal representative but it is not yet clear if independent mental health experts will be invited to participate.

'This group is being set up primarily to assess the legal threat posed to the union by concussion,' said one well-placed source.

An RFU Council member described the formation of the group as a 'good business decision' and, last week, the IRB admitted for the first time that there could be a link between concussion and CTE. However, Gosper is adamant rugby has taken enough steps to prevent similar litigation.

'The NFL settled because they felt they were in a vulnerable position,' he said. 'We don't feel in a vulnerable position. We feel we are taking every action possible, given the current knowledge, to ensure there are safeguards in this area. Rugby has done that historically and things are evolving as knowledge evolves.'

Gosper has called for mandatory concussion education to be introduced by all unions around the world and he wants players, coaches and match officials to 'recognize and remove' players they suspect are concussed.

*

By the end of 2013, like most of the players, I needed a rest. But not before two more English professional players – Geoff Parling and Dave Jackson – experienced their own concussion nightmares.

I interviewed Championship star Jackson, Nottingham's top try scorer of all time, who had experienced almost identical problems to Berry, Moody, Hazell and others with concussions becoming ever more frequent through the latter stages of his career. In the end a consultant warned him: 'One more hit to the head could kill you.' Like all those who'd gone before, Jackson held no resentment towards the sport he'd played since he was a young man, although, on Championship wages, he was in a trickier financial position than some. It's important to remember professional rugby players are not especially well paid. The top Premiership stars around this time could expect to earn around £250,000 a year from their clubs, with bonuses for international appearances and endorsements. But some professionals in the Championship earned a fraction of this, some barely £20,000 a year, but the risks they were taking with their bodies were extreme. One injury could see their ability to do their job ended in an instant.

But while many players were now coming forward willingly to share their stories, others were frustrated by the heightened focus on head injuries.

England and Leicester lock Parling, who suffered a succession of concussions between 2013 and 2016, was among a group of players who resented the relative health of their brain being speculated over. After suffering a concussion in training and being ruled out of England's opening November Test against Australia, Parling wrote in his *Metro* column in 2013:

> So, last Tuesday I decided to tackle Billy Twelvetrees' knee with my head. A bad thing to do. Although I wasn't unconscious, I was what is classed as concussed. Blurred vision, a headache and a bit of dizziness, but still I did my best to try and convince the doc I was fine.
>
> I was desperate to play a part in the game against Australia and convinced myself I would be OK to do so by the time last Saturday came around.
>
> Thankfully, I had a doc who recognized some of the symptoms immediately and took the decision to pull me out of the game.

I did my best to convince him otherwise. I'd just found out I would have to watch the game from the stands and had lost a chance to represent my country. The doctor took that chance away from me. But he was right.

While this was eminently sensible, Parling's next offering troubled me, as he not only questioned the six-day return, claiming it reduced players' willingness to declare concussions, while also showing a worrying lack of grasp of what a concussion actually was.

> Player welfare should be paramount. I don't understand why parents and coaches would take a risk with kids. Yes, we seem to wrap kids in cotton wool nowadays, accidents happen, it's part of growing up. But if a kid takes a knock to the head, why take the risk?
>
> I do worry, however, about the flip side – the 'mandatory rest period'. Sometimes we get a knock on the head and we are fine to carry on playing. Will mandatory rest periods (a minimum of six days) force players to hide these knocks as they worry about being pulled from games when they don't need to be?
>
> What we need is common sense from all parties. A good doctor will know the difference between being dazed and concussion. At professional level we don't need to get to the point where players miss games or leave the field after picking up a bit of a bang, as they will then hide injuries and stay away from the doctor's office.

To me, this was symptomatic of the RFU's seeming inability to bring clarity to their messaging. On the one hand, Parling supported the increased focus on the issue because it was so serious, but on the other he didn't want to miss games. On the one hand, kids should be protected. On the other, professionals should be allowed to carry on. Parling's position was confused and confusing. Much like the RFU's.

10

Head games

If I'd have known how deep the concussion problem ran and the lengths the sport's governing bodies would go to to suppress the story, would I have immersed myself to the extent I did? Would I have been prepared to sacrifice a successful career involving subsidized global travel, prime seats at the biggest games, free food and booze and access to some of the highest-profile sports stars on earth?

I'll answer that when this book is published and I'm sitting by a river or lake somewhere without internet connection or a rugby field within a 100-mile radius.

For this uncomfortable truth to be revealed, someone had to reveal it. And, for whatever reason, that person was me.

I'd never had the remotest interest in working in PR. Spoon-feeding company lines to complicit journalists in search of an easy life. To my mind, a journalist's role is not just to follow the news, but to lead it. To challenge, probe, disagree and confront difficult subjects. Set the agenda. Shine a light. Always ask one more question. If anyone taught me that, it was Peter Jackson.

But there's no point leading the pack if no one follows and it was heartening in 2016 when the *Telegraph* launched their Dementia in Football campaign, in direct response to the *Mail on Sunday*'s campaign. Mike was furious about what he saw as them ripping us off, whereas I took their campaign to be a case of 'imitation being the highest form of flattery'. And at least it lasted longer than the *Sun*'s Concussion Campaign, which 'launched' in September 2016, furiously calling for football to introduce new rules 'right now'. After one story, the campaign was never heard of again.

Without question, the media has been complicit in burying the truth about concussion. Think how it works. Sport is played. Fans pay to watch and for analysis. Sponsors pay media and sport organizers for exposure and access to eyeballs. Players get paid. Media gets paid. Sport gets paid. Everyone is happy. Well, happyish.

While the relationships can be uneasy, no one wins if one or the other comes crashing down. And that was the argument people used for suppressing the concussion story: it will kill the sport. It is a lazy consensus based on the assumption everyone needs to keep the commercial ship sailing no matter what the cost. Growth, growth, growth. I've heard that somewhere before.

Concussion, performance-enhancing drugs and illegal gambling are among sport's most challenging subjects. Partly because they involve calling out cheats or liars and questioning people's ethics, while potentially putting an entire sport in the dock. Legal action had been threatened in rugby for several years, with Cillian Willis bringing something of a test case, heard in court in 2019, when he alleged clinical negligence against Sale's medical team for allowing him to play on following a series of concussions in an LV Cup game against Saracens in 2013.

Willis claimed he sustained two head injuries in one match and, in breach of IRB and Premiership guidelines, was allowed to play on both occasions, despite showing clear evidence of concussion. He was eventually withdrawn early in the second half but the damage had been done. He never played rugby again.

Sale settled without admitting liability and this paved the way for a much bigger case four years later. My reporting of it also set me on a collision course with Sale's director of rugby, more of which later.

But while the Willis story was clearly an important one, I seemed to be the only reporter in England tracking or writing about it. Why?

Journalists naturally feel loyalty to 'their' chosen sport. Many of the older reporters I looked up to had covered the transition from amateur to professional rugby and knew only too well how dire rugby's financial position was and its need to stay relevant to drive investment. Many had close ties with clubs and schools where rugby was played. No doubt many agreed with others who argued, largely behind my back, that my seemingly relentless concussion and injury focus risked turning the game soft. Others could see the commercial threat it posed

I could understand this position but, unlike me, they weren't looking at the data or speaking to the individuals and their families behind it. It was easy to take a hard-line position if you never bothered to speak to those who were actually living with the effects of brain injury. Or worse, those living with the effects of a death in their family caused by brain injury.

Time after time I concluded, in the face of criticism, that if the game was damaging players' brains and bodies, it was my duty to report it. And the more rugby's authorities said 'look the other way', the more determined I became to do precisely the opposite.

I found myself repeatedly butting up against the people I believed were enabling a culture which downplayed the risks and allowed brain-damaged players to carry on. Many 'old school' coaches, who'd played most of their rugby during the amateur era, either didn't understand what they were asking of their players, or didn't care. Medics were either too weak, too compromised, or both, to put their feet down.

By suggesting rugby was no less dangerous today than before it turned professional, an idea so absurd it insulted everyone who had even the remotest understanding of the game, it legitimized putting more and more physical demands on the players through longer seasons and more intense training, while encouraging the endless pursuit of power and brawn, to the detriment of skill, spatial awareness and creativity. That presentation of the narrative was, in my view, causing untold damage to the current and future generations of players.

*

In February 2014, with the publication of the latest injury audit, the RFU and Premiership Rugby were at it again. And the media complied. Despite concussion now being the most common injury in professional rugby, the line pushed out was that there really wasn't a problem.

The 2012/13 audit figure of 6.7 concussions per 1,000 playing hours was more than double the figure reported in 2003/04 but still way short of what I believed the true figure to be. Kemp told reporters:

> My sense is that with players' increased awareness and better
> diagnosis, we are likely to see in all sports including rugby a
> rise in reported rates. Eight to 10 years ago a player may not
> have realized the significance of feeling sick or a headache after
> a clash of heads. Within professional rugby there has been a
> well-regulated programme seeing a re-setting of the bar as to
> what the lowest threshold is that constitutes a concussion.

Kemp, meanwhile, hailed as good news the results that while injuries in matches overall had remained stable during the last decade, the number of recurrent injuries had dropped significantly.

He added: 'That is testimony to the increasingly effective rehabilitation. If you have an injury now this is not a question of people patching you up but getting you back to pre-injury levels or even stronger. It's a really positive story.'

Again, the suggestion was that players were being given more time to recover from injuries, which went against all previous statements and the knowledge that players were constantly under pressure from themselves and coaches to return faster than ever. Kemp himself had told the *Financial Times* this just a few years earlier.

Meanwhile, I was alerted to a spike in injury-enforced early retirements in the English Premiership which suggested my concerns were founded in fact, rather than wishful thinking. By speaking to players directly, frequently off the record, I also learned of a growing issue around insurance payouts. Despite the RPA acting as the exclusive commercial representative of the England team since 2004, the average professional player's contract was desperately flimsy and lacking protections from the ever present threat of a career-ending injury. Scandalously, clubs had the right to terminate players' contracts if they were sidelined by an injury for more than six months. This clause was intended to mean six months of continuous injury but some clubs in England and Wales chose to abuse it.

One such club was Llanelli Scarlets who sacked Wales and British Lions winger Dafydd James when he suffered a serious neck injury in September 2008. He waited 10 weeks to undergo surgery only to be told in March the following year, when he was declared fit to return, his contract was no longer valid because he had been sidelined for 26 weeks.

It was an appalling state of affairs adding to players' mental burden while leaving many not only physically damaged but also financially desperate overnight. It also placed far too much power in the hands of directors of rugby, who controlled playing budgets. The RPA managed to negotiate an extension of the clause to nine months of continuous injury around 2016, but with insurance still desperately hard to come by, despite the presence of some of the world's biggest insurers such as Gallagher as sponsors, players remain horribly exposed.

*

With help from RPA insiders, fearful of speaking out publicly over threats to their funding, I learned that the number of players retiring prematurely during the 2013/14 season was about to treble in the space of four years: from 13 in 2010/11 to close to 30 in 2013/14.

I contacted Hopley, who agreed to be interviewed at Twickenham in early March. Outside the stadium I bumped into Kemp. By now, there was an uneasy impasse between us. I think he'd realized I wasn't going away.

I told him about the story I was working on highlighting the spike in early retirements, assuming, as a doctor, he would be as concerned as I was.

'You can't print that,' he said. 'There is no data to support that. You mustn't print it.'

I thanked him for his unwanted editorial advice before telling him I was going to print it and extracting myself from another excruciatingly awkward encounter to go and meet Hopley.

We did run the story that weekend with the headline 'Rugby's obsession with size and power is forcing the game to the brink of crisis', with comment from a broad cross-section of the rugby world, which supported my premise that radically bigger collisions on the field were now manifesting in shorter careers, more concussions and worse injuries than during the amateur years.

I highlighted the combined weight of the two centres, Jamie Roberts and Luther Burrell, in England's opening Six Nations game against Wales, of more than 34 stone, which would see them collide at a force equivalent to a 60mph car crash.

The article also directly challenged the RFU's injury figures suggesting only five players with 'unresolved injuries' in 2012/13 had retired, with information I had gathered suggesting the figure was actually more than four times that number at 22. That figure was set to rise again to almost 30 in 2013/14.

While acknowledging that medical provision at the top level was

'light years' ahead of where it had been during the Wild West early
professional days, Damian Hopley said:

> 'There is a cumulative effect of playing rugby for 10 years at
> the top level and it's getting harder and harder for players to
> cope with playing year in, year out for a long period of time.
> It's a very worrying statistic for any professional sport.
>
> 'I've no doubt there will be more retirements this season.
> We talk now about two players per club per season retiring
> early through injury. Five years ago it used to be one player per
> club per season. That shows the severity of the problem.
>
> 'The game has caught up with a lot of players and it's now nigh
> on impossible to perform at the top level for as long they used to.'

Premiership Rugby director Phil Winstanley disputed our
retirement figure, but said: 'Basic physics dictates that larger
forces travelling at higher speeds are going to inflict more
damage in the short and long term.'

Our investigation found that the average weight of
the England team in 1994 – a year before the advent of
professionalism – was 14st 5lb (91.2kg). The England team
that took on Ireland in 2014 averaged 16st 6lb (104.3kg) while
the Wales team that played France the same year weighed on
average 16st 7lb (104.8kg) a player…

With concussion rates also showing a clear year-on-year
rise from 3.1 per 1,000 playing hours in 2005-06 to 6.7 per
1,000 hours in 2012-13, it is clear that, as Hopley describes it,
the 'beautifully brutal' nature of modern rugby, which attracts
huge television audiences and packed stadiums every week
during the Six Nations, will inevitably have long-term health
implications for its participants.

Hopley said: 'I was at the Scotland game and I met up with
two former players who, between them had four new knees and

two new hips. With all due respect to rugby in the Seventies, it wasn't the same intensity that the players face now.

'My concern is longer term and one of the things we are talking to the RFU and the clubs about is 'What are we doing for these guys five, 10, 15 years after they've retired?' This is about the game looking after people who have given so much to it. It's a duty of care we must have for all of our players.'

With eight England players, including Dan Cole, sidelined ahead of the Six Nations, a relatively small number compared to other post-World Cup campaigns, once again injuries were dominating the narrative. England head coach Stuart Lancaster diplomatically told us that the relationship between clubs and country medical teams was working: 'We need to keep reassessing the volume of rugby the top players play. Clubs are very good in managing the rotation of players but eight injured players is more than I've ever known.'

For the same article I interviewed former Scotland captain Rory Lawson about the ongoing issues facing 300 professionals being denied payouts from Manchester-based insurance fund Shepherds Friendly, writing:

> The dispute centres on the insurers' insistence that players making claims had pre-existing degenerative conditions when they took out the policy. One source has predicted a 'tsunami' of court cases as more and more injured players retire only to be denied payouts to cover lost earnings.
>
> Lawson said: 'When I got injured I went to see a specialist and he told me I needed to think seriously about not playing. He was talking about a wrist replacement or wrist reconstruction. So I stopped playing.
>
> 'I spoke to Dean Richards at Newcastle and it was a very straightforward case of 'How much is it going to cost the club? Right, here's your severance. Goodbye'. I did all

the paperwork and sent it back to Shepherds but got an email to say my claim had been declined. They said I was injured at the time I took the policy out and that this was a degeneration of that injury.'

Shepherds said in a statement: 'In assessing a claim it is imperative that full and accurate disclosure is made to us of all information in these areas so that fair decisions can be made.'

The RPA, RFU and Premiership Rugby currently contribute to a joint fund, which has no connection with the Shepherds scheme, to help cover players. But out of English professional rugby union's estimated turnover of £280 million only £800,000 is set aside for player insurance. An estimated £2m is paid to fund dinners and other social events for the anachronistic RFU Council.

Premiership Rugby director Phil Winstanley said: 'The Joint Professional Players' Insurance, which is the personal accident policy offered by Premiership Rugby, the RFU and RPA, is paying out more money than it ever has previously.'

But he added: 'There is no evidence that exists that injuries increase in line with body weight.'

Hopley, mindful of the need to preserve the physical nature of rugby, said: 'You don't want to take anything away from rugby's sheer gladiatorial nature. But you often watch a game and think, 'How on earth do these guys get up after that hit?'

'It's important to stress just how much good is going on in English rugby. It's not all doom and gloom. But we need to give the players more security in a sport that is, by its very nature, beautifully brutal.'

The RPA's Restart charity, which offers practical careers advice as well as confidential counselling and insurance advice to current and retired players, has seen a steady rise in those requiring long-term medical support.

The same weekend, the *Mail on Sunday*'s campaign became the first sports campaign in history to be nominated for the Hugh Cudlipp Award at the UK Press Awards – named after the legendary *Daily Mirror* editor. The prize, organized by the *British Journalism Review*, recognizes 'excellence in popular journalism and can include popular campaigns and investigations in any national newspaper' and our nomination commended us for 'seizing upon a sports story the potential of which escaped its rivals', adding 'the paper's vigorous campaign influenced rugby's governing bodies to make safer the way life-threatening head injuries were dealt with.' It was, unashamedly, a proud moment.

A week later, I found myself sitting alongside Kemp and other senior representatives from a variety of sports in Parliament, along with Lewis Moody, Peter Robinson, Chris Nowinski, Rory Lamont, Willie Stewart, cross-party MPs and peers and others concerned by sport's relationship with brain injuries.

It was telling that Bryant chose to highlight the Hugo Lloris case when talking to the media. He knew football got headlines. The Tottenham goalkeeper had been knocked unconscious in a collision with Everton's Romelu Lukaku in November the previous year. After several minutes of treatment and dialogue with the Spurs medical team the France international had returned to the field.

'The truth is that concussion can kill and too few coaches, players and parents know enough to protect players, especially in collision sports,' Bryant said.

> Following the head injury Tottenham goalkeeper Hugo
> Lloris sustained at Goodison Park in November, I promised
> to establish a cross-party campaign in Parliament to raise
> awareness of this important issue.
>
>   In my constituency every young lad plays rugby. For many
> of them it's the only way out of very deprived backgrounds,

becoming a star. In those kinds of communities it's so
important to get education down to that level.

We're going to get a cross-party group to produce a report.
But I'd much prefer to see a formal inquiry by Parliament
done along the lines of the congressional hearing in the States
because that's when you get all the evidence rolled out.

That evening, a number of those present at Parliament,
myself included, attended the London premiere of *Head Games*,
featuring insights from Nowinski, Stewart and other neurological
experts and which the Six Nations committee had tried to block
the BBC from releasing footage from, claiming it was being
'sensationalized'.

'We approached governing bodies from most of the major sports
bodies around the world and it was only when it came to rugby that
we encountered any resistance,' *Head Games* producer Steve Devick
told me. 'The Six Nations said we were sensationalizing the subject
and they wouldn't be releasing it. Eventually, they saw sense and
the BBC were really co-operative. But it had looked as if we weren't
going to be able to use footage which had been broadcast. It made
it look like they had something to hide.'

A Six Nations spokesperson denied the claims: 'We weren't being
obstructive but wanted to be clear about the context the footage was
being used in.'

The film told the story of the NFL's concerted attempts to
play down concussion risks by controlling the narrative around
data collection about injuries. It identified men such as former
rheumatologist turned NFL doctor Elliott Pellman who had no
previous experience or training in brain injuries or neurology and
who spent many years actively playing down the risks associated
with repetitive head injuries, while leading the NFL's Neck, Spine
and Brain Committee. Pellman eventually resigned in 2016, the same

year the NFL acknowledged a link between head injuries and CTE. To me, rugby was behaving in an almost identical fashion.

While the film focused on the NFL, it made a compelling case that all contact sports, especially rugby union, were lagging badly behind the curve. It also covered the case of rugby league player Barry Taylor, the first rugby player found to have CTE post-mortem.

All the experts argued against the narrative being peddled by some that the sport was somehow safer than ever before.

Several of those who appeared in the film led a panel discussion afterwards and invited questions and contributions from the audience. At one point, two burly figures in black tie walked down to the front of the stage and took the microphone. At first I thought they were security staff before realizing, to my astonishment, one of them was current England and British Lions prop Alex Corbisiero. He took the mic.

'As a player, you feel like you have very little say or control over how you can actually change the game. In rugby, we play 30-plus games a year. We do contact all through the week in training and then take minimal time off in the summer before we are back into contact training and the season,' he said, visibly emotional.

'Our concussion protocols can be laughable at times. CogSport is the last hurdle people need to go through, but you can pass that concussed or not concussed. I don't think it's an acceptable guideline. I don't think there is a single rugby player who hasn't had concussion or a sub-concussive blow.'

At 25, Corbisiero had suffered more than his fair share of injuries. He had just been ruled out of the Six Nations with a serious knee injury, while his fellow black tie-wearing speaker Jon Fisher was a journeyman professional whose contract with London Irish had also been prematurely terminated following a string of concussions.

*

The week after Corbisiero's public outcry, which we published, the RFU announced a 'new concussion management standards and education initiative'. As with so many of their press releases, it said everything and nothing, although the apparently arbitrary extension of the routine minimum stand-down following a confirmed concussion to 19 days for adults in the amateur game and 23 days for Under 19s once again gave the impression a professional's brain had miraculous powers of recovery or was less valued than an amateur's.

*

In June 2014, I met Peter Robinson and his wife Carole along with Dawn Astle, her mother, Laraine, and sister Claire across the road from Parliament on the steps of Portcullis House to hear the findings of the cross-party report titled 'Concussion Can Kill'. The lack of representation at the hearing from the RFU, apart from someone in their legal department, did not bode well and it was bitterly frustrating when the chair of the group, hereditary peer Lord Addington, began by effectively apologizing for the title.

'Concussion can kill? That's a bit strong, isn't it? I think the important thing to remember here is that we have an obesity crisis and we do not want to put people off playing and participating in sport.'

The report was not entirely toothless, however, labelling the PSCA 'insubstantial' while Bryant accused rugby's authorities of 'turning a blind eye' to concussion and adding: 'We are convinced that the divergence between the protocols in different sports and therefore the different messages that are sent out is quite dramatic.

'I'm conscious in Wales that the WRU [Welsh Rugby Union] seems utterly complacent about concussion in Welsh rugby. There is nothing on the WRU website which refers to concussion at all.'

But Lord Addington's opening remarks had set the tone for a lacklustre presentation which, although no doubt largely well intended, lacked bite. Immediately, any hope of a Parliamentary inquiry, which I believed was required to get this all out in the open, was lost.

The following year, as listed in the Register of Lords' Interests, Lord Addington, captain of the Parliamentary rugby team, accepted a series of gifts from the RFU in the form of tickets to the World Cup pool game against Australia and a ticket to the semi-finals. He also attended the Challenge Cup final as a guest of the Rugby Football League the same month and was a guest of the Football Association (FA) at the 2019 FA Cup final between Manchester City and Watford.

*

Sure enough, within days, there was yet another brain injury scandal.

Florian Fritz, a tough-tackling centre, capped 34 times by France, was a linchpin for French giants Toulouse. They were playing high-rolling Racing Metro in a Top 14 quarter final in front of a full house. Midway through the first half, with the home side 6–3 down, Fritz carried the ball up to the defensive line. As he was falling to the ground, having been tackled legally around his legs, his forehead smashed into the knee of the covering François van der Merwe.

Initially, television commentators Alastair Eykyn and Peter Richards were not overly concerned. But upon viewing a replay, Eykyn's tone changed.

'This is worrying times. Florian Fritz, scythed down in the tackle. He doesn't look too sharp right now. Looks like he collided absolutely with the knee from van der Merwe. Ouch.'

Richards, only recently retired, immediately thought of the tactical implications for Toulouse, whose coach Guy Noves had selected only two three-quarters on his substitutes bench out of eight.

'This could be interesting. Toulouse opting this evening for a six, two split on the bench. Only two backs on the bench.'

As Fritz staggers to his feet medics attempt to stem the blood streaming from a deep gash on his forehead. He is disoriented, pushing doctors away and apparently in a state of semi-consciousness as he's led off.

Blood fills his eyes, one of which is completely closed, the other barely open. Initially at least, he is unable to speak. He has, without question, suffered brain trauma.

PR: He's not in great shape at all. He's all over the place. He needs to come off. Absolutely he wants to stay on. He is a warrior. But the physio is having to physically drag him off. I'd be surprised if we saw him again this evening.

The bandage Fritz has on his forearm is by now soaked in blood continuing to gush from his head. He nears the touchline. Dazed, confused and angry, he lashes out again at the Toulouse medical team, as they attempt to usher him towards what should have been the safety of the touchline. These are all classic signs of a brain injury.

AE: For his own health and safety he needs to be removed and kept on the touchline. No matter how much he wants to continue.

Fritz collapses on the ground.

AE: Florian Fritz is in a world of bother.

A stretcher is brought out.

AE: He's collapsing on the touchline. Remember not so long ago he had a nasty motorbike accident, hurting his shoulder, his finger. It was a very near thing.

At this point, Toulouse head coach Noves, a former France international and one of the most decorated coaches in the history of rugby, appears on camera for the first time. He is agitated. Gaël Fickou, one of only two Toulon three-quarters, readies himself to replace his stricken team-mate.

AE: If you're going to have a replacement, this guy is not half useful. Gaël Fickou can come on in his place.

Back to replays of the incident.

AE: That is a sickening blow. Connecting flush with the knee of François van der Merwe.

More slow-motion replays.

PR: It's not too pleasant to see. The French director loving the replay on that. That isn't something you want to see too many times. As I mentioned, what a tough guy. He'll want to walk himself off the pitch.

Fritz appears to have regained a semblance of composure and is able to walk gingerly from the field with the assistance of two medics. But his match is over, without question.

PR: This guy is Toulouse through and through and he would want to play his part in a Toulouse victory tonight so it's sad to see him go.

As Richards is speaking, Noves can be seen approaching Fritz. Ignoring the medics, he goes straight into his player's field of vision, pressing his face close to the stricken star's while barking instructions. He proceeds to follow his bloodstained charge down the tunnel.

Minutes later, a close-up of Fritz being tended in the medical room. Noves is standing by the door. His already agitated state is heightened and he is addressing both the medics and Fritz directly.

AE: Nice to see Guy Noves, the Toulouse coach, taking a keen interest in his welfare.

Eykyn is reasonably assuming Noves is showing normal human compassion. But this is not normal.

Suddenly, the experienced broadcaster realizes to his disbelief what is playing out in front of him and the live television audience.

AE: He can't possibly be asking him to go back on the pitch, surely?

But that is precisely what he is doing. Noves gestures the brain-damaged player out towards the playing field.

PR: It's a time limit thing. He's only got 10 minutes. He's going to give it a go. I don't know if that's courageous or stupidity.

AE: It's bonkers. Surely that can't be right for the player. An extraordinary decision. Pete, I've got to ask you about this. This just does not seem right to me.

PR (initially lost for words): Well, it's difficult to say, Alastair, what state of mind Florian Fritz was in but when we saw him no more than 10 minutes ago, collapsing on the pitch.

AE: He was staggering around like a drunk after a night out.

PR (at one point laughing awkwardly): Yep. Well, time will tell. Other than the obvious health and safety aspect of the player's welfare.

AE: Well, there are many people who will applaud his bravery, and of course we will do that, but we've got to think about the long-term implications. Are there concussion protocols in France similar to those employed in the Aviva Premiership?

PR: Yes, absolutely. But what I'm thinking more with a big open wound on his head is how keen is he going to be to put his head over the ball and into tackles.

Moments later, a close-up of Fritz's forehead, glistening with the Vaseline applied by the doctors to help stem the bleeding and protect 20 or so stitches from ripping in the contacts he's been sent back out to take.

Almost a year since the George Smith case, and four years after Bloodgate, it was astonishing to witness Noves harangue the Toulouse medical team knowing he was being filmed. Noves's response to the incident was typical of rugby's 'old school' culture around this time, as he declared: 'I have been knocked out, played on and was fine; as you can see, I am still standing here'. This perfectly encapsulated the culture around this time and was precisely what I believed needed to be driven out of rugby. But old habits die hard and, as the saying goes, culture eats protocol for breakfast.

I felt sick. Naïvely, I genuinely believed that by then our work had helped change rugby's culture and had been encouraged by what I was seeing in the English Premiership, where conversations around adding a video concussion spotter to a team's matchday medical team felt like a move in the right direction.

But the Fritz case, which once again saw no one held to account, felt like a quantum leap backwards.

'Seeing that incident feels like a massive slap in the face for our family,' Peter Robinson said in the *Mail on Sunday*. 'We have worked tirelessly to try to raise awareness of the dangers of concussion and feel like we have made progress. But seeing the Fritz incident makes you feel like rugby is still in the Dark Ages.'

Noves escaped without even a token punishment. Two years earlier Fritz had received a three-week ban and was fined 15,000 euros for an illegal tip tackle on Tom Varndell. I found it perverse that a player could be punished for that, but a coach and his medical team receive no punishment for an act I believed to be more extreme than anything Richards had done during Bloodgate.

The following year, Noves was appointed coach of the France national team. When it came to concussion, it appeared only players were accountable.

Just days after the Fritz incident, former England player Shontayne Hape, who I'd got to know well when he was involved in Martin Johnson's squad around 2010/11, spoke to Steve Deane of the *New Zealand Herald*.

He told him: 'Growing up playing league in New Zealand, everyone got knocked out at some point. Everyone got concussed. I can't think of a single guy I played with who didn't. You just got up and played on. We were told to be Warriors. It's the nature of the sport. Harden up. That was the mentality. I was brought up with that.'

Nothing too new in that, but when Hape contrasted his experience in league to union, my ears pricked up.

I reckon I'd have been concussed 20 times by the time my professional league career ended with a switch to English rugby. That was nothing compared to what was to come.

After playing for England at the rugby union World Cup in 2011 I joined London Irish for the 2011/12 season.

Halfway into the season against Gloucester I copped a knee to the head and was knocked out. I told the club's medical staff I'd copped a head knock, but didn't admit the full extent of it, that I'd blacked out. The next week against Harlequins I copped another knock. It was a pure accident. Our lock Nick Kennedy kneed me in the temple and it put me straight to sleep. Concussion on concussion. That was the big one for me, the worst I've ever felt.

The following day I was to undertake some head questionnaire tests relating to how I was feeling and my symptoms, and the results were shocking – some of the worst they'd ever seen. They stood me down for eight weeks, which was the protocol.

I've always loved music. DJ-ing is my hobby and I have my own turntables and gear at home. But the effects of the concussion meant I couldn't bear to listen to music. The sound was too much. Sunlight was a problem too. I had to stay in a blacked-out room for days. I'd bike to training and by the time I'd get there my head would be throbbing and I'd have to go

home to rest. My tolerance for my three young kids was zero.
I was always angry around them, couldn't even last a minute
without getting cross and losing my cool.

My relationship with my wife Liana suffered. She was left
to manage the three children and household on her own, while
I tried to get my head right.

Hape also turned the focus on the CogSport tests, relied upon to
provide a baseline marker for players.

In England it is a standard procedure for all players to perform
a computerized pre-season head test. There are a few different
versions of the test used around the world, but they are all
basically the same thing... The problem with the test is that
players can manipulate it by under-performing so that later if
you have a head knock and you have to beat it you normally
can. In my league days the boys all beat the test and everyone
kept on playing...

When I got knocked out the first time at Montpellier I just
said 'oh nah I'm fine'... That first French concussion came in
my fifth game, against Toulon. I clashed heads with someone in
a ruck. I felt terrible, but decided to bite the bullet. I was on the
biggest contract of my career, so there was a load of pressure
to deliver. You don't want to let anybody down. You have to be
out there playing.

I played the next week and got knocked out again... It was
just a slight tap but it got me in the wrong place. This time
I was really worried. They rested me for a week. That's the
French rest. Normally you'd have two–four weeks of doing
nothing. In France it was 'OK, we'll rest you for a week and
you'll be fine'...

I was back to having constant migraines. I was pretty much
in a daze. Things got so bad I couldn't even remember my PIN

number. My card got swallowed up twice. My memory was
shot.

Dosing up on smelling salts, Panadol, high caffeine sports
drinks and any medical drugs like that to try and stop the
dizziness, fatigue and migraines was the only way I could get
through trainings and matches.

I went through the next four or five months like that. Pretty
much a zombie.

Hape admitted he hid symptoms but explained why he felt the
need to do so.

There was constant pressure from the coaches. Most coaches
don't care about what happens later in your life. It is about the
here and now. Everyone wants success. They just think 'if we
pay you this you are going to do this'.

Players are just pieces of meat. When the meat gets too old and
past its use-by date, the club just buys some more. You get meat
that's bruised or damaged, the club goes and buys some more.

I wasn't thinking straight... Somehow I got through 11
games but by then I was falling apart. I would try not to get
involved in rucks because I was terrified of getting knocked
out again. My performances were terrible and eventually I was
dropped... I was just happy I was going to give my head a rest.

I had three weeks of no games but heading into my
comeback match I was knocked out at training. It wasn't even
a head clash. One of the boys just ran a decoy line and bumped
into me and I was knocked out. When you are getting knocked
out and no one is even touching your head you realize things
have got pretty bad.

But I still didn't tell anyone. I played the match and got
knocked out in the first tackle. I tackled a guy and I was out.
Asleep...

After the game I knew I had to do something. I phoned my mum and my agent. They said I had to put my health first. At a team meeting our coach Fabien Galthié, a former French halfback, grilled me for lying in the ruck and giving a penalty away. I didn't want to admit that I was there because I had been knocked out. It was humiliating. Galthié was blowing me up in front of my team-mates and I just held my tongue.

Afterwards he came to me to talk about my performance. I was like 'I'm over it, I have to come clean'. I told him the reason I had given away the penalty and my performances had been below par was because I was knocked out and suffering from concussions. He couldn't believe it.

The club sent me for scans... I was told to count in my head while doctors monitored my brain function... The specialist showed me on a chart the average score for someone with a normal brain. My score was just above someone with learning difficulties. The specialist explained that my brain was so traumatized, had swollen so big that even just getting a tap to the body would knock me out.

He referred me to another top specialist in Paris but he was very clear – I had to retire immediately.

Shockingly, this still wasn't enough to convince Galthié and Montpellier.

Back at the club I broke down in tears telling Galthié.

I had been told I couldn't do what I'd been doing all my life. I was gutted. The club was shocked.

But even then they tried to overrule the medical advice. They said they'd rest me for a couple of months and see if I could recover...

I'm not telling my story because I want sympathy. I'm telling it because this is an issue people, particularly young

players, need to know about. More people need to speak out
about it, tell the truth if they are suffering. Most players won't,
though, for fear of being thought of as soft or because of the
financial pressures.

Rugby and league have come a long way in dealing with
concussion but there is still a lot further to go.

Recently I watched a quarterfinal between Toulouse and
Racing Métro. Florian Fritz got knocked out, blood pissing out
everywhere. He was totally in Lala Land. He came off and a
medic came out of the tunnel and told him to get back on. He
did but he was in no [fit] state. I see stuff like that all the time.
It's what I used to do.

The combination of the Fritz incident and the Hape article
jolted me back into action and reminded me how far there still
was to go.

I wrote another article implicating the CISG in a sport-wide effort
to deny the long-term risks of concussion and listing their failings.

The article highlighted delays in the IRB's AUT study, which was
now eight months overdue.

Around this time I also learned that the *British Journal of Sports
Medicine* – now edited by Karim Khan – had declined to publish Doug
King's groundbreaking research into concussion in rugby league.

Everyone I spoke to about the study believed it to be robust,
ethical and worthy of publication. Everyone except the *BJSM*, that
was. A pattern was emerging.

My latest article for the *Mail on Sunday* was the first I'd
written specifically questioning McCrory and the CISG's conflicted
relationship with sport.

The former Australian rules medic [McCrory] – who refuses
to speak to the media – has carved out a position as the most
influential doctor in sport, and is salaried by, amongst others,

the Australian Rules Football League and National Rugby League.

But, despite routinely denying any significant long-term risks associated with concussion and dismissing sports links to CTE, The Mail on Sunday can find no record of McCrory publishing original research into CTE in the past decade.

'Let me say to you the incidence of this condition (CTE) is vanishingly rare,' McCrory said at a FIFA conference last year. 'Something like 0.0001 per cent of people who play American Football develop CTE. It is almost zero.

'It's fair to say there is increasing scepticism around the world as to whether this condition actually exists or not and that might seem very strange and provocative to say because if you listen to the media you get a very different story.'

McCrory's claims are at odds with research in the US – which was buried by the NFL – which found a 19 times increase in dementia in former American Footballers while a 2005 study in Turin – involving more than 6,000 participants – found former soccer players are up to seven times more likely to develop motor neurone disease than the wider population.

McCrory has so far failed to disclose any evidence to support his claim that just 0.0001 per cent of players develop dementia. He has also refused repeated requests from this newspaper for an interview.

I quoted Chris Nowinski's reaction after learning McCrory had once again looked to undermine the Boston findings, which he labelled 'questionable': 'The only people in the world who reject our findings are medics employed by sports bodies.'

In the face of plenty of hostility myself I took comfort when contacted, as I often was, by highly regarded doctors from inside and outside sport.

One, a senior maxillofacial surgeon in Ireland with a keen interest in rugby, wrote:

> Sam, I have followed your campaign with serious medical
> interest. Your approach has been relentless and correct. Player
> welfare in all sports is the overriding concern.
>
> I hope you continue your campaign despite the sordid
> protectionism of the sporting bodies and indeed some of
> my 'colleagues' who quite frankly continue to defend the
> indefensible.
>
> Keep up the good work. You are winning. Right will out.

A few weeks later, Germany defender Christoph Kramer was knocked out in the World Cup final and played on for another 15 minutes. After the game, which I watched in a bar in Nottingham with some journalist friends midway through the Trent Bridge Test between England and India, Kramer revealed he had almost no recollection of the match.

We joked that at least by covering cricket I'd get a break from writing about concussion. Less than a fortnight later Stuart Broad, whose column I was ghosting, suffered a badly broken nose when a bouncer from India fast bowler Varun Aaron smashed through his grille.

Two months later, Australia opening batsman Phillip Hughes, aged 25, died two days after he was hit on the back of the neck by a delivery which caused a cerebral haemorrhage in a Sheffield Shield game between New South Wales and South Australia. The coroner found 'no failure to enforce the laws of the game contributed to his death' and that 'neither the bowler nor anyone else was to blame for this tragic outcome' but the incident shook cricket to its foundations.

The following year, Broad invited me to ghost-write a book which recounted his glorious contribution to a winning Ashes summer.

Like everyone in cricket, Broad was deeply moved by Hughes's death and spoke with rare insight about head injuries in cricket.

He told me of the frequency at which batters were hit on the head in the nets as they practised against 90mph short-pitched bowling intended to intimidate.

It was telling, when it came to the book's final edit, that almost all the mentions of concussion were redacted by the England and Wales Cricket Board's communications department, who had final editorial control over their centrally contracted player.

The ECB's secrecy was representative of a sport-wide anxiety around concussion. Two years later, concussion substitutions were introduced in cricket, while the sport is now far more proactive than previously about players being removed from the field following a head injury.

*

That summer, my friend and colleague Ian Stafford left the *Mail on Sunday*. I was sad to see him leave and would miss his mischievous sense of humour on the road. The paper had lost a brilliant journalist with a sense of perspective on life I respected. But when Alison asked if I would replace Stafford as rugby correspondent, I of course accepted.

After 12 years in journalism, I'd landed my dream job. Aged 36, I was ready for the correspondent's job.

With a home World Cup approaching, I was also keen to rebuild some of the bridges if not completely burnt by my pursuit of the concussion story by this stage, then mildly toasted.

As correspondent, I naturally felt more pressure to promote the sport. I was aware of the commercial challenges facing rugby and that people's jobs could be jeopardized if I continued reporting on concussion in this way. I was also conscious of turning readers off with the relentless nature of my reporting.

For my own mental health, I also craved less conflict.

Inevitably, from time to time I questioned if I was doing the right thing. Many people accused me of attacking rugby, with even some of my closest friends asking 'Are you going to kill rugby?'

But in the end, I chose to keep going. For me, it was literally a matter of life or death. Of commerce over people. Even some of the players thought I was going too far.

'Mate, I get it. The concussion stuff is really important. But do you really have to write about it every single week?' former England wing Ugo Monye asked me.

Players were hardwired to get up and go again and it was drilled into them in military terms that if they were not part of the defensive line, they were as good as dead.

Even England head coach Stuart Lancaster was guilty of militarizing the language. His regular references to war heroes and tales of valour on the battlefield jarred with me a little.

In a bid to imbue a sense of patriotism – or pride in the shirt – which he felt had been absent under Martin Johnson, Lancaster instituted, among other things, a series of defensive awards named after Arthur Harrison, a Royal Naval officer and the only England player to be awarded the Victoria Cross. The players loved it and I've no doubt Lancaster was well intentioned. But dying for your country on the battlefield was one thing, dying on the rugby field, quite another.

In October 2014, Dr Phil Batty, who had joined the RFU from Manchester City FC in 2012, left his position as England team doctor to become consultant sports physician at the Isokinetic Clinic, which, outside English football's training base at St George's Park, is the only FIFA-approved sports medical centre in the country.

In an interview with the *Independent* two months later, Batty contradicted his former employer's position when it came to injury risk in professional rugby.

'Rugby is a collision sport and you cannot deny there has been an increase in injuries,' Batty said.

'It used to be that the forwards wouldn't be quick enough to catch the backs but now, with greater emphasis on fitness training, they are and then you can get serious collisions. That, in very simple terms, is what has happened to club rugby.'

It was common sense. But it was revealing that, whether he meant to or not, Batty's position directly contradicted Kemp's.

As rugby correspondent, I was in conciliatory mood when I filed an interview with Lewis Moody that September, one year since the campaign launched, hailing rugby's changed culture around concussion. Despite the Fritz incident a few months before, it was undeniable that rugby, in England at least, had finally started to move on concussion. I honestly believed then that another case like Smith's or Fritz's would never again be seen in England.

The tangible sense of progress continued in October when the RFU along with Premiership Rugby and the RPA announced that all players, coaches and referees in England would have to undergo online concussion training.

At the press launch at Harlequins' Twickenham Stoop ground, where Bloodgate had played out six years before, it was announced that the Pitchside Suspected Concussion Assessment was being rebranded as the Head Injury Assessment (HIA) and doctors would now be given 10 minutes, as opposed to five, to assess players.

With the introduction of an 'independent' concussion review panel and medics being given more access to television footage, this felt like progress. Kemp had also noticeably softened his position on the potential link between head injuries and long-term neurodegenerative problems.

'What we say in the module, which is consistent with the IRB's position, is that with concussion, you may be at increased risk of developing neurodegenerative problems,' Kemp said at the launch, where the RFU, Premiership Rugby and RPA all showed a united front.

Kemp did, however, remain reticent about comparing rugby's experience to the NFL.

'I don't think this has all been informed by what's happening in the NFL,' he added. 'We have been working with Premiership Rugby on a concussion management programme since 2004. We brought in baseline testing across the board in 2004. We have been at this for a long time.'

I pressed Kemp on the looming threat of legal action following the NFL case and mounting evidence rugby had been slow to respond.

'That's not a question I can answer,' he told me.

> What we are trying to do is to put in a system of provision that protects player welfare and minimizes reputational, legal and participation risks to the game. We are approaching this in a very structured way, disclosing and working with players, coaches and referees and just trying to do the right thing about an important issue.
>
> What we are doing is principally being driven by player welfare. Player welfare is the No.1 priority of the IRB and RFU. Yes, we have had one eye on what's happening in North America and I was over there with [IRB head of medicine] Martin Raftery to have a meeting with the NFL and other sports in August.
>
> Yes, we have sought legal opinion on our module, yes we have sought independent medical opinion on our module, but this is not a defensive response. This is about trying to manage an injury well. You need a lawyer to answer that question which is why I don't think we can.

But despite Kemp's words, some players remained seriously concerned about long-term consequences. A source at the RPA who told me: 'A group of recently retired players are seriously concerned. If they develop long-term problems and can show they were misled about the risks then they will pursue legal action. No doubt about that.'

Those words proved prophetic but, despite those concerns, I was, for the first time in years, optimistic rugby was finally travelling in the right direction.

Then George North happened.

11

A tale of two valleys

The next two years would be bookended with stories about brain injuries affecting two brilliant young rugby players from south Wales. The first, a household name, lived to tell the tale. The second, a hero in his hometown of Pontypool, did not.

By the time we'd reached the start of the Six Nations in 2015, the *Mail on Sunday*'s concussion campaign had been running for almost 18 months. The nonsensical notion that concussion was a 'non-story', as many contended had been emphatically debunked. The campaign had led the sports news agenda, been shortlisted for a long list of industry awards, including the highly respected Hugh Cudlipp Award, and catapulted concussion in sport onto the front pages as well as the back.

Concussion was not just a story. It was *the* story.

Whereas before I'd been almost a lone voice, now everyone was covering the story, grudgingly in some cases. The RFU and World Rugby (as the IRB became in 2014) had instituted a raft of policy changes and player welfare-driven safety measures, while the sport's two most influential doctors, Raftery and Kemp, now admitted there 'could' be a link between repetitive head injuries and long-term neurodegenerative issues. It was a subtle but significant shift.

There would be more changes to come over the next few years, some of them radical. After decades of denial, a genuine attempt to understand and ultimately reduce concussion appeared to be under way. One thing which still had not happened, however, was for a coach or medical team to be held accountable when breaches of protocols occurred.

Sadly, hopes that heightened scrutiny would end malpractice disappeared in the first game of the 2015 Six Nations when Wales hosted England in Cardiff on a Friday night.

This time the incident, or incidents, involved Wales and British Lions winger George North. Twice he was knocked out in the game. Twice he was allowed to play on. In the first incident, late in the first half, North dived for a ball on the ground, only for his head to meet the foot of England lock Dave Attwood as he attempted to hack the ball forward. The 18 stone lock's size 13 boot smashed into the side of North's face and left him prone on the floor.

The player, concussed against New Zealand the previous November, was attended by Welsh medical staff but played on.

Twenty minutes into the second half, Richard Hibbard – the same player who accidentally collided with Smith in Sydney 18 months earlier – attempted to tackle England full back Mike Brown but in doing so clashed heads with North, who again collapsed on the ground.

'That looks to me as though he is definitely concussed,' commentator Brian Moore said at the time.

Not to the Welsh medical team, though, who would later insist they had not been able to view video footage of either incident so hadn't realized North had lost consciousness on both occasions.

Moments before the final whistle, I received a text from a supportive friend in the television commentary box urging me to look at video footage of both incidents. When I did, I was speechless.

And while the Wales medics may have missed the incidents, unfortunately for the Welsh Rugby Union (WRU), more than 7 million BBC viewers witnessed them both, live on HD.

It was exasperating to see. Despite all the new policies, rhetoric and press releases about player welfare, here was another example of a brain-damaged player allowed to play on not once, but twice.

I got down into the mixed zone beneath the stadium, where the media interviews the players, and asked around to see who else had seen the North incidents. Amazingly, some reporters still couldn't see the news when it was staring them in the face. One agency reporter, who I won't name to spare his blushes, told me: 'North is not the story.' I told him he was wrong.

My article pulled no punches and gave both barrels to the Welsh medical team for what I believed was a clear failure in their duty of care to the player.

World Rugby launch probe into WRU's handling of George North's head injury after winger appeared to be knocked out during Six Nations loss to England
By Sam Peters
7 February 2015

Wales were on Saturday night coming under mounting pressure to explain why medics allowed George North to carry on playing against England after the winger appeared to be knocked unconscious twice during Friday night's RBS Six Nations opener.

World Rugby, the sport's governing body, issued a statement requesting a 'full report' from the WRU to explain the circumstances surrounding the decision to allow the 22-year-old to remain on the field despite television pictures clearly showing him slump motionless to the ground after suffering a 61st-minute head injury.

North had earlier passed a Head Injury Assessment (HIA) after being accidentally kicked in the face by England lock

Dave Attwood in the first half, when he also appeared to be out cold temporarily.

World Rugby guidelines state any player who is even suspected of losing consciousness should immediately be removed from play to avoid the risk of the potentially fatal 'Second Impact Syndrome'.

North, who missed last autumn's win over South Africa with concussion, was left dazed following the initial incident and, while Wales coach Warren Gatland defended his medical team, the decision to let him play on has drawn stinging criticism.

The WRU insisted on Saturday night correct procedures were followed, although they admitted the second incident had not been picked up by medical staff at ground level, despite TV footage being available to them.

A WRU statement read: 'While George is currently symptom free, retrospective video review of the second incident identified the mechanism of injury which was previously unsighted on the field of play. This review has warranted the medical team to manage the player as concussed although the player currently has no signs and symptoms. He will now undertake a graduated return-to-play protocol with multiple follow-up cognitive and physical tests.'

Gatland said immediately after the match that he had not seen the second incident, although his attempt to trivialize the concussion suffered by prop Samson Lee in the same game by saying: 'He should be OK, he's got a pretty thick head,' suggested a worryingly cavalier attitude to the issue.

'The medical team definitely wouldn't have allowed George to go back unless they were 100 per cent confident that he was OK,' Gatland said. 'He seems fine at the moment.'...

World Rugby intend to employ independent matchday

doctors at this year's World Cup whose job will be to alert team medics to suspected concussions in a bid to avoid a repeat of the North incident.

'In an ideal world we'd have independent doctors at every single professional rugby match but it always comes back to cost,' said one well-placed source.

The point about cost rankled. Kemp had raised it with me at Twickenham in 2013. But if player welfare really was rugby's 'number one priority', cost should not have come into it. The unions could find tens of thousands of pounds each season to waste on unwanted and polluting pre-match fireworks alone. Why not spend that on employing and empowering more doctors?

Not only were players more prone to picking up secondary injuries once they'd been concussed, due to problems with their balance, they were also more likely to make an error in the heat of battle. This was evident with North, who missed a glaring second half tackle on Jonathan Joseph which led to an England try.

In an increasingly fast-moving and complex game, where attacking plays could often be planned multiple phases down the line, while defensive organization and tactical awareness had never been more important, I struggled to understand why coaches didn't see the value in players being mentally sharp at all times. It was obvious players should come off, simply from a performance point of view. But it still wasn't happening.

On 3 February 2015, three days prior to the North incident, the *Oxford Handbook of Sports-related Concussion* published a paper by Paul McCrory, Michael Turner and others titled 'Does "Second Impact Syndrome" exist?' in which they wrote:

Second impact syndrome is a condition believed by some people to be a consequence of recurrent sports concussion. The only evidence to support its existence is anecdotal and, if it does exist, it is rare. The fear of this condition has driven the promulgation of concussion management guidelines and, more worryingly, the recent trend towards government regulation of the clinical management of concussion in the United States. Diffuse brain swelling following a single head injury, a well-recognized condition, is more common in children than in adults and usually has a poor outcome. It is posited that the so-called second impact syndrome simply represents diffuse brain swelling mistakenly attributed to repeated concussion.

The North incident was unrelated to this paper but it was telling that the description of the 'trend towards government regulation' as 'worrying' inferred sport was capable of getting its own house in order. Sadly, when it came to brain injuries, the evidence to support this was vanishingly small. Meanwhile, by appearing to cast doubt on the existence of second impact syndrome, this undermined the case for extending return to play times.

Contrary to the agency reporter's assertion that North 'wasn't the story', the story ran and ran. It was messy and difficult and reporting on it upset a lot of people. But that, to my mind, was no reason. Countless people told me to back off. Not for the first time, I did the opposite.

The North incident will be remembered in history as one of rugby's worst examples of concussion mismanagement and was yet another spur in the campaign when things had been dying down. But it only drew attention because it was on live terrestrial television.

Contrary to my hope these incidents were a thing of the past, they continued. In January 2015, Leicester's Argentinian prop Marcus Ayerza was concussed but allowed to play on, having passed the newly branded HIA, prompting Barry O'Driscoll to email Brett Gosper and Martin Raftery, copying in a number of interested parties, including myself, James Robson, Chris Nowinski, Tony Belli, Michael Grey and Willie Stewart. He wrote:

In the recent Leicester/Bath Premiership rugby match on 4th January, Marcus Ayerza received a head injury and there was patent suspicion of concussion.

He was taken off the field for 5.5 mins. His return was greeted with expressions of surprise by the commentators who declared their suspicion of concussion and explained their reasons for this to the millions watching.

The new 10 min Head Injury Assessment (Ayerza was off for 5.5 mins) replacing the failed 5 min 'bin', was to be strictly applied to potential concussion only; i.e. when there are no signs, no symptoms and no suspicion... just the potential for concussion. All collisions where there is any sign, symptom or suspicion of concussion were to be removed.

In my original letter to the CEO of World Rugby, followed by my resignation over 2 years ago, I expressed my concern that performing clinical trials on rugby players' brains in such a cavalier fashion is to be abhorred.

Predictably, the incidences of failure of this baseless experiment continue apace in elite rugby, providing worrying examples to our young talent, their parents and to the world.

There will be a price to pay by rugby but more significantly and tragically, by so many young men who we in rugby are potentially abusing.

Two weeks after the North fiasco, in England's Six Nations game at Twickenham, Mike Brown was knocked unconscious in an accidental head-on-head collision with Italy's Andrea Masi. Brown required almost 10 minutes of treatment and was administered oxygen before being taken from the field on a stretcher.

After the game Stuart Lancaster was quick to reassure us about Brown's health, telling us: 'He is talking fine now and seems OK. It helps that it is two weeks and a day [until the Ireland game] but we will take him through the return to play protocol.'

Spotting an opportunity to demonstrate they were 'leading the way' on concussion, and no doubt relishing the WRU's discomfort over North, the RFU invited the media on a tour of the stadium's medical facilities before an interview with Brown, who was picked to play against Ireland a fortnight later, was circulated among rugby's written media on condition we carried an RFU promotional message stating how seriously they took concussion. It was an unusual move but we grudgingly agreed.

As it turned out, Brown was not fine and he pulled out on the morning of the Ireland game, still experiencing post-concussive symptoms. He wouldn't play again that season.

Just days before Brown had been knocked out, the RFU's latest injury audit showed concussion rates for the 2014/15 season were continuing to trend upwards – now at 10.5 per 1,000 playing hours, more than three times where it stood at its lowest recorded point in 2005/06 (3.1 per 1,000 playing hours) – and it remained the most frequent injury reported by professional players.

It was growing increasingly difficult to maintain the pretence that the professional game was no more dangerous than before. Kemp, certainly, appeared less confident in his assertions, although he insisted the dramatic rises we were seeing in concussion rates were purely down to better reporting of it, thanks to the RFU, of course. 'We think reported concussion will continue to rise with greater awareness and focus,' he said.

> To give the figures some context, 87 per cent of players didn't report a concussion last season.
>
> Our figures are reported figures when historically there has been an underreporting of concussion across all sports. Concussion is one of the most difficult injuries to diagnose. You can scan other injuries, but at the moment there is no gold standard diagnosis for concussion. It relies on checking symptoms and cognition, so it's a challenge.

Everyone believes it is underreported and where the graph point finishes, nobody will be able to predict.

The severity of injury in training, measured by the number of days players were sidelined, also continued to rise from a low of 33 days absent per 1,000 playing hours in 2003/04 to 73 days absent per 1,000 hours by 2013/14. The frequency of training injuries also continued to trend upwards with the overall figure of 414 injuries now eclipsing the 2002/03 figure of 159.

The audit report also saw matchday injury severity increase from 73 days absent per 1,000 playing hours in 2012/13 to 91 per 1,000 hours. While statistically this in itself was not overly significant, the anecdotal stories of more and more severe injuries were supported by the fact that the number of injuries which required more than 84 days' absence – which could also be described as 'career-threatening' – had also doubled from three in 2002/03 to six in 2013/14. Over the next five years that figure would double again.

Kemp, as usual, sought to play things down. 'That [2012/13] increase could either be because the injuries are more severe or because the medical staff are managing players more comprehensively and are taking longer to return them to play,' he said. 'We have good evidence that injury care is becoming more comprehensive and conservative based on the fall in injury recurrence.'

Once again, I could barely believe my ears. To suggest rugby doctors were suddenly taking a more conservative approach to injury stretched credulity. All the evidence I had seen or heard first hand or anecdotally was that medical departments were constantly looking for new treatments, medicines and methods to speed up players getting back on the field. Kemp had said so himself in his *Financial Times* interview in 2009.

Willie Stewart, by now one of World Rugby's advisors on concussion, cut to the chase when I interviewed him for the *Mail on Sunday*:

'The underlying trend over 10 years in professional rugby has seen a year-on-year increase in concussions.

'I do not believe this has anything to do with greater awareness of concussion. Instead, it reflects a steady rise in concussion rates over 10 years as on-field collisions have got bigger. People are more aware because the problem is much greater than it ever used to be.'

If the trend continued, concussion rates in professional rugby union would soon eclipse those seen in professional boxing (17.5 per 1,000 playing hours), while the issue of sub-concussive blows, the symptomless repeated rattling of the brain which Chris Nowinski first raised to the RPA board in 2013, was not going away. Just a few years earlier, I would have considered any comparison between rugby and boxing, in terms of risk, absurd. Now, having studied the data and witnessed the action, I concluded it was entirely reasonable.

Unfortunately for rugby, the medical care afforded players was nowhere near that afforded professional boxers. In light of the Michael Watson v Chris Eubank fight in 1991, boxing's authorities had been forced by law to make radical improvements to safety procedures and medical provision after Watson was left severely brain damaged due to an absence of appropriate medical provision ringside.

'If George North had been a boxer he would have been removed from the arena after his first concussion and taken for neurological assessment,' said Stewart.

'A brain-injured boxer would have stood down for a minimum 28 days. I would say the level of brain injury in professional rugby has now become unacceptable.' I agreed.

And headgear wasn't and isn't the answer.

Over the past century American football had invested hundreds of millions of dollars in new helmet technologies but with no evidence whatsoever they reduce the effects of whiplash or the rotational impacts on the brain. Meanwhile, World Rugby research into protective headgear in rugby has routinely shown that, while lacerations and abrasions are lessened by wearing some products, concussions definitely are not. Some studies have shown concussion incidence actually increased with headgear as players acted more recklessly.

It was becoming increasingly obvious to me that the only way to be sure of reducing concussion exposure was to play and train less frequently. This, of course, did not sit well commercially or with those indoctrinated into believing you needed to 'toughen up' during the week.

North, like Brown, faced an extended spell on the side lines.

The Welsh winger returned to club colours, only to be knocked out again in late March following a collision with Wasps No.8 Nathan Hughes, who was subsequently shown a red card by referee Craig Maxwell-Keys for what he deemed to be reckless action in goal.

The incident raised difficult questions over 'intent' and provided more ammunition to the uneducated 'game's gone soft' brigade.

Wasps captain James Haskell tweeted, 'astounded would be an understatement', while former Leicester Tigers fly half Andy Goode said it was 'shocking', and Harlequins and England prop Joe Marler called it 'an absolute joke'.

At the conclusion of what had been another bruising Six Nations campaign, not just for the players but also for rugby's medics, Kemp defended the HIA protocol, telling Reuters:

> When I started as a team doctor you were making assessments in a break in play on the pitch with a player who wasn't concentrating on the assessment because he wanted to get back to playing.
>
> You don't usually feel any pain with a concussion so it has to be taken out of the player's hands
>
> It's much easier to persuade a player not to return in that cool 10 minutes in a medical room than on the pitch halfway through a game and it is the medical professional involved, not the coach.

And what we've seen is fewer concussed players remaining on the field. The message is very simple – 'recognize and remove'. If you have any suspicion you remove the player.

It's the same message for the professional game as the community game.

Same message. Same brains. But still gross errors were being made and evidently brain-damaged professionals allowed to play on. This set the culture for the rest of rugby to follow.

These were traumatic times for North. Never before had a rugby player's brain health come in for anything remotely close to this level of scrutiny. Not only did he have to cope with the very real effects of the head injuries, he also had to deal with a public debate over what had happened.

By now, it was obvious social media was playing a vital tool for those of us with concerns about concussion to share stories, identify issues which had previously been overlooked or swept under the carpet and piece together a bigger global picture which had previously gone unseen.

With access to old research papers and the ability to scrutinize previously buried studies, a light was being shone on a hitherto murky and inaccessible world.

While I had enormous sympathy for players who found it invasive having their injury records and concussion histories publicly opined upon, this was the new world we were living in. For me, greater transparency and scrutiny could only be a good thing.

With the UK media historically unwilling to touch concussion, I simply don't believe the vital research and stories of mental decay in the NFL would have ever seen the light of day here, had it not been for social media. Whereas in the past campaigners could be swatted away after one article in the paper, with social media, this was no longer possible.

Barry O'Driscoll called for North to be stood down until the end of the season, while even Wales coach Warren Gatland, so flippant about Samson Lee's 'thick head', admitted concerns over the 23-year-old's longer-term future. He told the *Sunday Times*:

> I had a meeting with George's agent and said if I was being purely selfish I would say: 'George, don't play in the last few (Premiership) games, get yourself right for the World Cup.'
>
> Because if he gets another knock he's going to have to be out for six months or a year. If he picks up two or three more of those in the next year that's going to finish his career, isn't it?
>
> That is a concern, but I can understand Northampton being desperate to get him back playing.

*

In May, three months after Lancaster described him as 'fine', Mike Brown gave his first interview to my colleague Nik Simon at the *Mail on Sunday* when he admitted considering retiring.

'I try not to think about how my body will be in 20 years' time,' he said.

> Concussion symptoms are much worse than having a dodgy knee when you retire. It's your brain, and you don't want to be facing depression and constant headaches.
>
> It's something you've got to look after. You don't want headaches all the time. You reach the stage where just a tap on the head can knock you out. When you're a sportsman it's sometimes hard to remember all of those risks.

This was dangerous territory for World Rugby, whose showpiece World Cup was to be held in England later that year. The last thing the sport's governing body needed was a high-profile concussion incident at their main event.

I had some sympathy with both World Rugby and the RFU who, unlike other sporting bodies, had proactively attempted to track injuries in their sport and, albeit belatedly, implement changes to reduce them.

But the reality, we all knew, was that concussion would always be part of rugby. It always had been. But no one at the top had been honest enough to admit that or warn the players about the potential long-term implications. Or indeed admit the problem was worse than at any point in the sport's history.

Whereas in the past on-field medical calls were rarely questioned, especially in the amateur days when medics and physios were almost always volunteers, the spotlight was now falling on the very people who once carried the 'magic sponge' onto the field. Professional rugby couldn't have it both ways. If it was going to claim 'player welfare is our number one priority', I was determined to hold them to account.

And if the marketing people wanted to cash in on the big hits and gladiatorial nature of modern rugby, what were they doing about the inevitable consequences?

With huge sums found for marketing, lavish lunches and dinners for the RFU Council, and stadium improvements – including close to £70 million spent on developing Twickenham's east stand ahead of the 2015 World Cup – the relative pittance spent on player welfare and medical budgets was shocking. Immoral even.

'To go for a scan was an expensive thing to do,' Thompson's World Cup-winning team-mate Ben Cohen told the BBC's *Head On* documentary in 2022.

'Are they willing to spend that money? How many times were we in that position when it was like "OK, I don't think it's that, it's going to cost a fortune to send you for a scan for that." I remember that three or four times myself.

'It [concussion] wasn't managed properly.'

It concerned me how heavily World Rugby still leant on the CISG, but through their head of communications Dominic Rumbles they had an impressive and unflappable figure at the heart of their operation.

From early in the campaign, Rumbles sought to keep me close. He always responded to messages and was polite and informed. All good qualities for someone charged with communicating their organization's position. While the calibre of some Premiership clubs' media departments was shockingly amateur, Rumbles never hid when a difficult story broke. He was proactive and I admired the fact he always fronted up, even though I often disagreed with his position and his evangelistic promotion of rugby occasionally jarred.

Meanwhile, rugby continued to tinker with its laws in a bid to draw in ever greater crowds. Most of the time, they were just more confusing. With television revenues eclipsing all other revenue lines, rugby needed to compete in the entertainment space which, despite what some diehards believed, was not a 9–9 draw involving 200 rolling mauls and 40 reset scrums. A good game was a fast game which unfortunately, from a player perspective, came at a cost.

In May 2015, with the World Cup looming, World Rugby's Law Representation Group, led by former Scotland flanker John Jeffrey, met in London with a 'view to ensuring the enhancement of player welfare, the maximization of enjoyment for players and fans, while making sure the sport can continue to develop at all levels around the world'.

Having successfully tweaked the scrum engagement laws the previous season to reduce neck injuries, there was a belief among some that introducing law changes around the tackle, where most concussions occurred, could reduce spiralling concussion rates. Kemp had first said to me back at Twickenham in 2013 that he believed the tackle height should be lowered.

Once again, tensions arose between 'maintaining the fabric of the sport' and the Law Representation Group saying it would 'further consider proposals regarding the tackle, ruck and maul with a view to maintaining a fair contest for possession while also enhancing player welfare'. Yet again rugby wanted to have its cake and eat it.

*

In the background, I'd been monitoring the desperately slow progress of World Rugby's head injury and player health study at AUT, and on 18 July 2015 the findings were finally published. But by deciding to publish before the research had been peer reviewed, the sport's governing body broke all normal research protocols. According to one researcher I spoke to, this was a 'very dangerous gamble', adding that the report was 'no longer worth the paper it's written on'.

As soon as I read the headline of an extraordinary 1,600-word press release – 'World Rugby welcomes long-term health study outcomes' – I was concerned about a whitewash.

The press release reported that the study did 'not provide definitive links between rugby and long-term cognitive health issues', while burying far down the text that 'ex-sportsmen who reported four or more concussions during their sporting career performed worse on some, but not all, measures in the neuropsychological test used in this research, reported more injuries during sport, had more hospitalizations for injury and rated their current health lower'.

In other words, players who suffered four or more concussions were more likely to experience poor long-term mental and physical health outcomes. This, by anyone's definition, was cause for concern.

The primary finding of interest, and the reason the study was apparently commissioned in 2012, was to determine if retired rugby players experienced worse neurological outcomes than those in the wider population. The answer, from the research, was emphatically yes. But you would not have known it from the press release, it was an exercise in burying bad news.

The research added to a growing body of evidence supporting

the work of Thorndike and many others as far back as the 1950s which showed between three and four diagnosed concussions were enough to cause significant concern and require a lengthy, potentially permanent removal from contact sport.

But, rather than report this, World Rugby attempted to divert attention by listing a number of points.

- Player welfare and concussion research continues to be a major priority for World Rugby and member unions.

- Further research recommended into potential links between rugby and long-term cognitive health.

- Sports should identify and highlight not only the injury risk associated with sport but also the potential benefits to general and neuropsychological health that are associated with sports participation.

Brett Gosper, Martin Raftery, NZRU senior scientist and research associate at ATU Ken Quarrie and International Rugby Players' Association CEO Rob Nichol were all quoted, welcoming the report's findings.

Remember Gosper who, two years earlier, had told me: 'We're not a cigarette company. We will make transparent whatever research comes out of it.'

But instead, World Rugby did precisely the opposite, stating: 'World Rugby's number-one priority is player welfare and our strategies regarding concussion education, management, prevention and research are at the very top of our agenda. We welcome the findings of this study, and while the study does not provide any definitive conclusions, we are alive to all potential risks and will continue to prioritize research in this very important area.'

Thankfully, on this occasion, some media outlets, at least in New Zealand, spotted the real story and ran with it. Apart from me, the

UK media hardly touched it let alone challenged their presentation of the findings.

It was also telling that while the great and the good of World Rugby were quoted, there was one key voice missing: lead researcher Patria Hume.

It would later emerge in an article titled 'Rugby Research Caught in the Breakdown', published in the *New Zealand Herald* in June 2016, Hume almost refused to attend the press conference held shortly after the release went public. Thankfully, she chose to put her misgivings about how her data had been misrepresented by World Rugby and NZRU to one side and spoke to the media in Auckland.

'We've got to go through that scientific process, but what I'm saying is that, as a scientist, it's irresponsible for people to say there are no long-term brain health issues,' she said.

'Because all indications so far from the analysis we have done indicates that there possibly are for the rugby players and for people who have been concussed more than four times.

'You also need to consider that potentially there may be some long-term health effects. Ninety-four per cent of elite level rugby players experienced one or more concussions, that's a lot.'

Twelve months later Hume would tell the *New Zealand Herald*'s Dylan Cleaver: 'World Rugby and NZ Rugby did not give approval for the full report and all the results to be released.' It also emerged that a statement she had intended to read out had been vetoed by the two organizations.

Here is what she would have said: 'Proportionately more rugby players had worse brain health scores. To better address the implications for player neurocognitive health we believe players should be aware of the potential increased long-term risk of cognitive impairment from concussion so they can make informed choices about engagement in sport and return to play following injury.'

Massive alarm bells should have been ringing around the sport.

They certainly were for Peter Robinson who, without prior knowledge of World Rugby's report, told the *Belfast Telegraph* that year:

> There are far too many people who have an interest in telling sport what it wants to hear.
>
> It's like the tobacco industry in years gone by. It's time to start listening to the brain injury experts, not the sports experts.
>
> Coaches who put children who've suffered brain injuries back on the field should be booted out of the sport. If they are willing to risk children's lives for the sake of winning, they are in the sport for the wrong reasons.
>
> People talk about hard decisions and taking a kid off during a game is supposedly a hard decision. But for me a hard decision is whether to switch a life support machine off or donate your kids' organs after they've died. They're the real hard decisions.

Peter had been commenting on a study, authored by Kemp, Patricios and Raftery, which called into question the effectiveness of the six-day Graduated Return to Play by reporting that players who suffered a concussion had a 60 per cent higher chance of sustaining another injury that season.

*

Back in England, Premiership teams continued to mismanage concussion, with England star Anthony Watson the latest high-profile player to play on after being hit high in a tackle by Owen Farrell.

The previous week Newport Gwent Dragons centre Ashley Smith, 28, had retired following a 'series of concussions', prompting my friend and colleague Steve James to write: 'For this, undoubtedly, was the season in which it became clearer than ever that concussion is now rugby union's greatest problem.'

From a personal point of view, it was also gratifying to read Steve's praise for the *Mail on Sunday*'s campaign in our rival the *Sunday Telegraph* when he added:

> The statistics show that the number of concussions increased significantly this season – up 59 per cent in the Aviva Premiership. Although there is debate about whether this is because more are now reported or simply because the game, with the breakdown now a frenzy of hostility and collision, has changed so much (I think it is a combination of the two), the fact remains that high-profile games rarely seem to go by without a nasty concussion.
>
> The incidents involving England's Mike Brown and Wales's George North during the Six Nations merely highlighted that. The Premiership final last Saturday continued the trend with Bath's Anthony Watson sustaining a blow to the head from Owen Farrell that eventually ended his afternoon.
>
> However, that Watson did not leave the field immediately for a head injury assessment also shows there is still some considerable distance to be travelled before this issue is dealt with satisfactorily.
>
> Crucially, though, matters are improving. Steps are being taken, and knowledge and understanding are progressing. For that we have to give a good deal of credit to a rival rag, The Mail on Sunday, and to their rugby union correspondent, Sam Peters, who has relentlessly probed and questioned in his ongoing concussion campaign.

Much more importantly, World Rugby knew I was back on their case. I'd wanted to give them the benefit of the doubt but their actions around the AUT research had reminded me how duplicitous some within the sport were prepared to be to protect the game's reputation at all costs.

And in a bid to show how much they cared about players and concussion they started leaking me stories including details of their plans for the World Cup where, according to insiders at the governing body, there would be:

- Sanctioning and possible suspension of team doctors found to have breached concussion protocols through an 'untoward incident review panel'

- Independent pitchside doctors and neurologists with no affiliation to either team's union with the right to overrule team doctors

- Baseline cognitive testing for every participating player and compulsory medical screening

- Identification of high-risk players with a history of concussions

- Assembly of a sport-wide group looking at law changes to reduce concussion rates

- Real-time television replays available for all pitchside medics to assess head injuries

The long overdue introduction of independent doctors for World Cup matches, although not across the professional game, undoubtedly had a positive impact. I lapped up the stories. What self-respecting journalist would do otherwise? But I was also conscious of the risk of getting too close, too cosy to World Rugby. I knew they were deploying the 'keep your friends close and your enemies closer' principle. By accepting the stories they were feeding me at face value, I was running the risk of doing their bidding for them. I had no intention of doing that.

But despite some progress around awareness, I feared there would inevitably be another medical howler when the spotlight

fell on the home World Cup. As it turned out, the biggest shocker
came when England became the first host nation in history to exit
in the pool stages. Lancaster and his entire coaching team were
sacked as a result.

Amazingly, the tournament passed off well on the concussion
front and finished in a manner which truly left me believing progress
had been made when Australia's star player Matt Giteau was
concussed in the final and removed from the field. No fuss. No
shenanigans. Off he went. It simply would not have happened four
years before and set the best possible example to young players
watching.

In February 2016, another study, commissioned in part by the
RFU and Premiership Rugby and written by Kemp, Raftery and Jon
Patricios, the leading South African sports medic who had, in 2013,
confirmed to me his belief that CogSport tests were routinely cheated,
found that players who returned to play after a concussion were 60
per cent more likely to sustain a subsequent injury in the same season
than those who had not. The conclusion was that Graduated Return
to Play protocols, which permitted a six-day return to play following
a confirmed concussion, were inadequate.

But while he was prepared to take the lead in defending rugby,
when it came to presenting injury data Kemp was less prepared to
take the lead in advising players about what it actually meant. Asked
if players should be worried, he told *The Times*: 'I think the players
really need to answer that. We have shared the study with the RPA
board.' Kemp could say this with the knowledge that the RPA would
not push back too hard. They never did.

Hopley, though, was more prepared to make an assessment:
'Clearly this data is of considerable concern. We have to be broad
in our thinking. This may well have an impact on the way we play
the game. It may be that in the longer term there is an impact on the
Laws of the game.'

With the report finding that concussions were rising, while more than 50 per cent occurred in the tackle, it was becoming inevitable that further law changes would be required.

12

'Not a rugby man'

I'd covered the career of Courtney Lawes from the time he broke into Northampton's first team aged 18. The epitome of the modern-day forward, a dynamic carrier, brilliant lineout operator and far better footballer than widely credited, his USP is his ability to hit. And hit hard.

At 6ft 7in and 18 stone, Lawes is not a monster by modern professional standards. But he is and always has been a monster hitter. Toby Flood, on the receiving end in the Premiership final against Northampton in 2013, was just one among his victims. Lawes's work-rate, appetite for making destructive tackles across the field and willingness for self-sacrifice have made him one of English professional rugby's greatest servants.

Born in Hackney, Lawes moved to Northampton with his family aged four and attended Northampton School for Boys, where Steve Thompson had also been a pupil. Lawes took up rugby aged 13 and was quickly scouted by Saints, remaining at the club ever since. His loyalty is beyond question.

But to me that loyalty and willingness to put his body on the line left Lawes vulnerable to being chewed up by professional rugby's machine.

By 2016, six years after his international debut, it was clear his body was creaking under the strain of what was being demanded of him. Part of the problem, I believed, was that he was working under coaching regimes with regressive attitudes towards player welfare. Northampton's forwards coach Dorian West had watched Chris Ashton be knocked out for England in 2010 and had simply said, 'Rugby is rugby.'

But while I had West's card marked, I knew little about Eddie Jones other than the 30-minute chat I'd had with him to ghost his column for the *Daily Mail* the morning after Japan beat South Africa in the World Cup the previous September, and the rumours coming out of Japan about his relentless appetite for work and the extreme demands he placed on players.

I'd also covered Saracens when Jones had a brief spell as their technical director in 2006 and, following his appointment as England coach in late 2015, one contact at Saracens told me.

'He's the best I've ever known at managing up and worst I've known when managing down.' I took that to mean that Jones was expert at impressing those up the chain but, if you played under him, he could make your life a living nightmare.

By now, the notion that professional rugby's training methods were somehow less demanding or reckless than in the early Wild West days could be filed away under a growing list titled 'wishful thinking'. In fact, according to the data, the opposite was true.

By 2013/14, the number of training ground injuries had risen again to a record 414 while also getting more severe (average days absent per 1,000 hours in 2003/04 were just 33, while in 2013/14 this was up to 73). It seemed utterly ludicrous, madness even, to be beating up players so severely during the week. But despite my protests, nothing was done. And Jones was about to make things much worse.

It didn't take long for rumours to start about the demands the Australian made of his staff. One member of the backroom team told me they would routinely receive emails at 4 or 5 in the morning and if a response hadn't been sent within a couple of hours, Jones would be standing outside their hotel door demanding to know why.

Nicknames were made up which undermined staff, and players would tell me of some of the most physically demanding sessions they had ever experienced. Training ground injuries, and bad ones at that, happened with alarming frequency.

'I went through a phase of dreading going away [to an England training camp], and I know other England players felt similarly,' Dylan Hartley would later write in his book *The Hurt*.

> It wasn't something that was discussed openly, because it is such an individual issue and no one wanted to be seen to be speaking out of turn, but we were honest in privately sharing the strain. Two words recurred when we talked among ourselves: 'I'm fucked'.
>
> We probably didn't feel that different to some of the coaches, who were told one day they didn't have a good enough relationship with us, only to be told the following day they were too close to us. We were bonded by the ripples in Eddie's character and constrained by the ludicrous convention that athletes, like Victorian children, should be seen and not heard.

I didn't like what I was hearing, but with a long-term contract supported by a hugely impressive unbeaten start on the field, no one wanted to read about the dark side to Jones's methods. Besides, for a correspondent, the risk associated with running such stories at the start of a coach's tenure had a chilling effect on the truth. The constant threat of being denied access to player interviews or press conferences mean sports journalists tend to play ball. Think 'I scratch your back, you scratch mine'.

England's players tolerated Jones because they had to. But it was obvious Lawes was struggling. By the age of 28, he'd already contended with, in no particular order, a chronic groin condition, grade three medial ligament damage to his right knee (twice), multiple concussions, grade two ligament damage to his left knee, a stress fracture to his shin, double shoulder reconstruction, ankle surgery and a dislocated shoulder.

The Sunday newspaper reporters interviewed him on the record before England's Six Nations game against Italy in February 2016.

He said: 'It is tough but it is what you get paid to do. You have got to be professional and do everything you can to stay on that field for the season.'

With an unpoliced limit of 32 matches per season, I asked Lawes how much more effective he would be if he only played 25.

'If you play less games,' he replied, 'you are not going to be anywhere near as battered and you have a lot more time to rest and work on things you want to work on. You would be a considerably better player but part of the challenge is how well you manage yourself through the season.'

Like Wilkinson, and countless others, Lawes also routinely experienced 'stingers' – a severe burning pain or shock which shoots down the arm as the result of nerves being stretched and compressed in the neck and shoulder. He was also choosing to delay surgery to 'get through' the season. This was fairly routine and again illustrative of the rugby's culture of short-termism.

After the interview, held in the controlled confines of Pennyhill Park, with an RFU comms person perched on his shoulder, I collared Courtney alone in the corridor as he headed for his room.

'Mate, I'm really struggling,' he told me. 'The fixture schedule is complete madness. Everybody knows that. Coaches, players, staff. But no one can do a damn thing about it.'

He also made his lack of faith in the RPA clear, while admitting he feared for his career if things didn't change soon. I felt for him. On the surface he had it all but the toll it was taking on him as a human being was evident. And Lawes was far from alone. Almost all the players I spoke to around this time felt completely powerless to effect any reduction in their workload.

'I was a commodity, and I understood that,' former All Black, Newcastle Falcons and Toulon tighthead prop Carl Hayman told Michael Aylwin in the *Guardian* a few years later, having been diagnosed with early onset dementia and probable CTE.

'It's like that scene in *Saving Private Ryan*, when the guy tells the bloke with shell shock: "When you accept you're dead, you can function as a soldier."'

By 2015/16, as the games piled up and rugby's season stretched deeper into each summer, while the rush to get players back on the field quickened and hard taskmasters like Jones and Noves were appointed to top national coaching positions, I would argue player welfare standards had never been lower in the history of professional rugby union.

A few weeks later, the RFU announced concussion rates had risen for the fifth year running in 2014/15 and stood at the highest ever recorded rate of 13.4 per 1,000 playing hours. With an increased spotlight on the issues, the figures were beginning to reflect reality.

But while the true extent of rugby's concussion crisis was becoming clear, it was also clear how little was being done to limit game exposure or training. Every time a commercial challenge or shortfall emerged the answer was always: play more games. The notion 'less could be more' was sneered at along with any suggestion that by delivering better spectacles and a better fan experience, rugby could become a 'better product'. Professional rugby was locked into a terminally short-term attitude I was convinced could lead only to long-term decline, and serious damage to players' health.

It was obvious to me by now the RPA were powerless. There was no sense players could influence change. The lack of awareness of their power, if they had chosen to pull together, was desperately frustrating for those of us who could see how badly they were being taken advantage of. The RFU and Premiership Rugby had the players' union precisely where they needed them.

Aged 27, a 'mentally drained' Alex Corbisiero, that heroic voice in a tuxedo at the *Head Games* premiere back in 2013, announced he was taking a year out of rugby to rest his battered mind and body. He would never play again.

*

Back with England, Wasps uncapped 24-year-old flanker Sam Jones arrived at their Brighton training camp late on Sunday evening, 2 October. He had played 80 minutes of Wasps' seven-try demolition of Harlequins before driving almost 160 miles from Coventry to Brighton.

The next morning, having missed the safety brief the night before, the uncapped youngster was thrown into a one-on-one judo session with Maro Itoje, a player whose physical prowess meant his more experienced colleagues avoided him at all costs in contact training. Young Jones, desperate to impress, didn't hesitate. Within seconds his career was over, thrown onto the mat by a blameless Itoje, suffering a complete ankle dislocation, spiral fracture of his fibula, ruptured medial knee ligaments and 'significant' damage to his ankle cartilage.

Witnesses have since told me Eddie Jones initially believed his young charge was 'faking it' and vocalized his doubts.

He needn't have worried. Sam Jones never played rugby again, let alone for England.

So perhaps it should have come as no surprise when I clashed with Eddie Jones in the press conference ahead of England's Six Nations game against Ireland in February after he'd made a series of comments relating to the Irish fly half Johnny Sexton, who'd been concussed against France the previous game.

'I'd just be worried about his welfare if he's had whiplash injuries,' said Jones. 'I'm sure his mother and father would be worried about that. If you're saying a guy has got whiplash then he's had a severe trauma.

'Maybe they used the wrong term but if you've had severe trauma then you've got to worry about the welfare of the player. Hopefully, the lad's all right on Saturday to play.'

In the pre-match press conference at Pennyhill Park, the *Telegraph*'s Julian Bennetts and I found ourselves on the wrong end of a tongue lashing from Jones, irritated by us asking questions about England's plan to target Ireland's playmaker.

'We target players all the time, that's part of rugby, is it not?' he snapped, adding:

> Are we supposed to not run at one player? Is there some sort of special law? Hang on, hang on, he's got a red dot on his head.
>
> I'm not saying Sexton is a weak defender but we're going to be targeting players in the Ireland side. We want to win and you win a game of rugby by attacking their weak points. To say that's unfair is just ridiculous. It's been happening since Adam and Eve were around. You think they're not going to send [Robbie] Henshaw at George Ford at the weekend? Give me a break.

That Six Nations proved uncomfortable viewing as Sexton became the unwitting focal point of concern around concussion in rugby in Ireland. Just as North had in Wales.

While I sympathized with players not wanting their medical records being part of public discourse, I also figured that historic silence and lack of transparency was part of the problem. The alternative, I reasoned, was for concussion to be buried again. At least now the media spotlight demanded more honesty from medical teams, coaches, players and administrators.

I'd highlighted so many examples by now and called out so much poor practice, many of my journalist colleagues who'd been sceptical at the beginning were now onside, although there were times it still felt like a fairly solitary journey.

On countless occasions I asked myself why I was doing this. And the answer always came back to Ben Robinson and the deep-held belief a generation of players, including the likes of Lawes, Thompson, Hartley and Lipman, were being damaged irreparably before our eyes. Had I become a pariah by this stage? Possibly. But I'd come too far to turn back now.

I certainly wasn't alone in thinking the extreme changes rugby had undergone were to the detriment of the spectacle and the players.

'Rugby today is nothing like the game I played,' wrote former amateur British and Irish Lions captain Willie John McBride in a foreword for the book *Saving Rugby Union: The Price of Professionalism*, published in 2020.

> There is an injuries crisis in rugby. You look at every
> international game that is played. How many do you see that
> are injury-free? I believe every player should be playing for 80
> minutes unless he has to leave the field injured. I played for 14
> years and never left the field in my life…

*

On 2 March 2016, 70 doctors and health experts wrote an open letter that was widely published in the media calling for a ban on contact in school rugby, highlighting government obligations under the UN Convention on the Rights of the Child to inform children about injury risks.

One of the signatories, Allyson Pollock, a professor of public health research and policy at Queen Mary University of London, said: 'Parents expect the state to look after their children when they are at school. Rugby is a high-impact collision sport and given that children are more susceptible to injuries such as concussion, the absence of injury surveillance systems and primary prevention strategies is worrying.'

Eric Anderson, a professor of sport, masculinities and sexualities at the University of Winchester, said: 'School children should not be forced to collide with other children as part of the national curriculum for physical education. A more sensible approach is to play tag rugby.'

There was a predictable backlash from the rugby community who again felt under attack. World Rugby's lead research scientist Ross Tucker took to Twitter, where he was prolific, to pour scorn on the researchers, who, while he may not have agreed with them, had presented a credible and reasoned position.

Tucker ranted: 'I don't know who these doctors & academics are, but I'd like to thank them for reminding me I generally dislike them.'

In further tweets he sarcastically described the research as 'genius academic thinking' which was, according to Tucker, who it is reasonable to assume had not read the report which had only been released a few hours previously, strategically 'irrelevant' and 'impotent'.

I had some sympathy with the demands for reform of school rugby but felt the call for an outright ban to be a mistake. It polarized opinion and prevented people engaging in sensible debate even if, in light of what we were learning from America and here on our own doorstep about the cumulative risk of multiple exposures to head injuries, there was obvious merit in radically reducing children's exposure to them. Meanwhile, while physical activity is obviously a good way to reduce obesity, the overall cost to the NHS of cumulative fractures, concussions and other sports-related injuries, has never been published, to my knowledge. Sports governing bodies, no doubt, would prefer it to stay that way.

I had long believed that if English youngsters spent more time working on skills, spatial awareness and speed, it would be to the benefit of the game as a whole. In New Zealand, touch rugby is part of the culture. In 2011, I'd walked across the playing fields of Otago University from my hotel on the way to the ground in Dunedin ahead of a World Cup game and was amazed at the number of touch rugby games going on. It's a brilliant, fun sport which teaches kids, and adults, the skills required to manipulate opponents and create space on the field. Something which has been lost in the power-obsessed 'gym monkey' environment of the modern professional game where collisions are prized and space denied.

I certainly don't believe rugby should be compulsory in schools, while a delay in introducing contact training until children's bodies and brains are better developed is patently common sense. Ultimately, just like professional players, amateur youngsters should be allowed to make an informed choice about the risk they're being exposed to and, below the age of 16, it's hard to see how this is possible.

I write this in the full knowledge I lived for contact from the age of six and would have screamed blue murder at that age, had anyone tried to stop me playing. But that's the point, I suppose: I was six.

Allyson Pollock's group reasonably highlighted the complete absence of injury data in school rugby. On the one hand rugby's authorities doggedly stuck to their line of only making 'evidence-based decisions' while insisting the sport was overwhelmingly 'good' for kids with no actual evidence or data to prove or disprove this. The idea rugby is 'character building' is impossible to prove either way. And what defines character, anyway? Subservience? Willingness to play through pain? Acceptance of suffering? Tolerance of malpractice for 'the greater good'?

While the 2016 Six Nations became something of a circus around Johnny Sexton, there was also a flurry of media coverage when Turner and McCrory launched the International Concussion and Head Injury Research Foundation. Reportedly backed to the tune of hundreds of thousands of dollars by two of the world's most powerful sports organizations, the NFL and Godolphin, the global thoroughbred breeding operation and horse racing team founded by Dubai's ruler Sheikh Mohammed bin Rashid Al Maktoum. It would, we were told, deliver the 'biggest research project ever undertaken into the long-term effects of head injuries'.

Around this time, Turner played down concussion risks when interviewed for Sky Originals documentary *Concussion: The Impact on Sport*.

> I come from the camp that concussion is a non-problem,' he
> said. 'It is a transient difficulty for your brain from which you
> make a 100 per cent recovery. I never believed it inevitably led
> to CTE and it was a huge surprise to me when I first heard
> Bennet Omalu speak about it in the States.
>
> The fact he had five cases and there are tens of thousands
> of retired NFL players, it should be evident that five cases is
> not enough. Ann McKee with her 180 cases published, these
> are clearly tiny numbers overall. What they did show was that
> quite clearly some people don't do well long term after being
> involved in those sports.

I was stunned to hear one of global sport's most influential doctors describe concussion as a 'non-problem'.

It begged the question: if it's a 'non-problem', why do anything at all? Why have any protocols in place and why remove players under any circumstance?

In a different interview, Turner repeated the line that concussion and our scientific knowledge of it was all new and evolving fast:

> It becomes more of an issue as we learn a bit more. The problem
> at the moment is we don't have a clear idea of what the risk is,
> which is why there's so much unknown about the condition.
>
> Before we accepted that concussion, or we thought at least,
> concussion was a self-limiting problem like rebooting your
> computer, you just have a concussion, your lights go out for
> a short time and once you're rebooted again you're back to

normal and there's been no damage. That can happen again and again and again. There's now evidence that concussions can lead to long-term problems and concussion is a common injury in a lot of sports…

Once we've done a bit more research and had 10/20 years of managing concussion, we'll be in a much better position to advise people what they should be doing if they sustain concussion…

To educate people you have to explain to them what the risks are and if you don't know what the risks are you tend to fall into two camps. You're either a scaremonger by saying this is an incredibly dangerous sport or you're a flat earth person by saying actually there is nothing wrong with the sport, we've been doing it for hundreds of years and there's no evidence that you've got any trouble.

It's very difficult for governing bodies at this stage to advise people. All you can say is there appears to be a risk that you may suffer long-term damage to your brain if you suffer concussion and the research we're doing and other people are doing that's as far as you can go at the moment.

This was of course precisely what sport needed to hear. We don't know the risk so let's wait and see. Another 20 years bashing brains together wouldn't do anyone any harm, would it?

When asked about Turner's involvement with research looking into CTE, campaigner Dawn Astle said: 'I wouldn't let him anywhere near that. No way, never in a million years. That's probably why [the NFL] has chosen him, to discredit everybody and say, "Oh, it [CTE] doesn't exist."' And all the while, players continued to pay the price.

At the previous Six Nations I'd bumped into Kemp at Pennyhill Park, England's team hotel, where he'd shown me two graphs. One represented the peaks in performance expected by England's strength and conditioning coaches, the other the peaks expected by the clubs. A third represented a Lions tour year. The graph resembled a mountain range with a series of peaks at different times of the year.

Kemp explained that the respective strength and conditioning teams had completely different expectations of the players on their watch, with different peaks demanded at different times of the season. The players were caught in the middle. Kemp was showing me, as if it needed explaining, why so many of England's top stars were injured before every single Six Nations and autumn campaign. This was, of course, a problem of rugby's own making.

In late September 2016, I flew, along with the *Mail*'s chief sports photographer Andy Hooper, to Geneva before heading 55 miles west to Oyonnax in France, where we would be interviewing 19 stone former Canadian lock Jamie Cudmore who was in the preliminary stages of legal proceedings against his former club Clermont Auvergne.

As we drove high into the hills I told Hooper what I knew of Cudmore's story. I knew he had been allowed to play on following a series of concussions in the build-up to and during the Champions Cup final the previous season, including the semi-final win over Saracens which I had covered, and recounted a massive clash of heads between him and opposition No.8 Billy Vunipola.

I could tell Hooper, one of the most experienced sports photographers on the circuit, was deeply sceptical about the job we'd been sent on but he nodded agreeably nevertheless.

We were welcomed into Cudmore's home in the sleepy French town by Jamie and his wife, Jen, eager to talk about the Rugby Safety Network she was helping to establish with her husband. Like so many players' spouses and partners I met through this period, Jen was seriously concerned about her husband's health and was at times demonstrably anxious about what the couple had experienced together. In many ways, she reminded me of the spouses of war veterans I'd interviewed and got to know in the past whose partners would later be diagnosed with post-traumatic stress disorder.

The Cudmores' story was another cautionary tale, as Jamie would reveal over coffee in their newly appointed kitchen.

> There was a huge head contact with Billy and myself going head to head at a ruck. It's an accident of rugby, two guys arriving at the same time at the same height. We were both on our hands and knees and I remember saying, 'Jeez, that was a good one'.
>
> Billy said, 'We'll be good, bro', and sort of staggered off. I remember being on all fours and figured I might as well wait for the docs to come on and maybe go off for a bit of blood. At the same time I was just trying to recover because I knew I'd taken a really big knock.

According to Cudmore, despite failing an HIA after the incident, team doctors allowed him to play on.

> When I got back to the changing room they started to stitch me up and then after that they put me through the HIA. The usual questions, remembering five or six words and answering them back to the doc.
>
> I had no chance. I probably remembered one of the words and I remember clear as day, I can see his face now, saying, 'No, you're done... c'est fini.'
>
> I was distraught. It was a semi-final and I wanted to be on the field. You work all year to be in those games. I was upset. The doc could see I was upset and told me to relax, take my boots off and get in the shower.
>
> So I walked back into the changing room and I hadn't even got my boot off when I heard the door open and the doc come back in and say, 'Jamie, Jamie, how are you? Sebby [second row

partner Sebastien Vahaamahina] is not good. Can you come back on? You gotta come back on.' I was like, 'Yeah, sweet', and tied my lace and went straight back out.

Incredibly, despite demonstrating an array of symptoms in the ensuing weeks which should have immediately ruled him out of the final, a willing Cudmore played at Twickenham against Toulon in the final, when a familiar pattern played out.

Two or three minutes into the game I hit Chris Masoe and their other prop behind him at the same time and was just sparked straight out. It was a normal tackle leading with the shoulder. There was no contact with my head. But the force of the impact sparked me straight out. My body just went limp.

I went off, did the HIA and a new doc we had figured everything was all right and I went back on. Towards the end of the game I had a clash of heads with Juan Smith and cut myself. I went off and started vomiting in the changing room. I didn't know about second impact syndrome. I didn't know I could have died.

[Clermont wing] Benson Stanley was in there as well. I remember talking to him after and he asked me how I kept on playing. I said I didn't know but I just kept going. He also asked me, 'How could the doc let you back on?'

I definitely worry about the future. I don't want to be one of those guys who is 65 but can't remember anything.

Jen gave her side of the story next.

I was in the stands with Jamie's dad, Richard. We'd had a week of hell after the Saracens game with Jamie not able to sleep and constantly telling me he had this cloudy, cotton sound in his head. I knew it was not normal, but had to rely on the doctors.

For the game in London we had to rely on the doctors

to take care of him. We saw Jamie go down in the final and instantly wondered if he would go off. He did, which was good. But then he came back on and that's when I just lost it. I'd had enough. I was freaking out, standing up and everyone else was telling me to sit down. They were watching the game and I was freaking out because my husband was not well.

Before we knew it he was down on his hands and knees again. I was shouting, 'Richard, I need to go', and he was saying I needed to have faith in the medical staff. But it had been going on for two weeks and it was starting to look to me as if they were trying to kill my husband for a trophy.

Clermont would later brand Cudmore a 'traitor' who was 'trying to create a buzz' from going public with his concerns.

On the drive back to the airport the next morning, Andy's position had changed. 'I've got to admit I wasn't convinced about this whole concussion story before, but I totally get it now,' he told me. Personally, it was good to hear. Gradually the penny was dropping.

*

By October 2016, Eddie Jones's training methods were getting completely out of hand, with no one prepared to intervene on the players' behalf. While they were winning, it seemed, anything went, even though players continued to drop like flies. After England had been tactically outmanoeuvred by Conor O'Shea's Italy at Twickenham in February 2017, in what would later be described as 'Ruckgate', I was also genuinely concerned by the physical appearance of some of England's backroom team, including defence coach Paul Gustard and forwards coach Steve Borthwick, when we interviewed them at Pennyhill Park days after the game. It was clear they, as well as the players, were experiencing the brutal reality of life inside Jones's England. If things went wrong, there was always a price to pay.

Even an outcry from club owners and directors of rugby, increasingly concerned about Jones's methods, got short shrift.

With Lawes among 11 players already injured ahead of a warm weather training camp in Portugal, three of them, Sam Jones (broken leg), Anthony Watson (broken jaw) and Jack Nowell (calf) injured at the Brighton camp, Jones was defiant.

As I reported in the *Mail on Sunday* on 29 October, he said:

We won't be sipping beers in Portugal. There is nothing to change. Injuries are part of rugby.

I had a good meeting with the directors of rugby. We had two unfortunate injuries at the camp – that is part of rugby – and out of that [meeting] came a couple of things that need to happen.

We need to communicate better with the clubs and a better and more rigorous medical in and out of the clubs and in and out of the international side. I think that will help player welfare.

One morning in October I received a call from Saracens' excellent head of comms Matt Hennessey telling me club captain and former Springbok lock Alistair Hargreaves was retiring with immediate effect, due to ongoing problems with concussion. I was not surprised. I'd witnessed Hargreaves knocked out in an innocuous-looking training incident a few weeks earlier and knew he was struggling following five concussions in two seasons.

I had also been impressed by how Saracens had looked after him. Saracens were not everyone's cup of tea and I was as aware as anyone of the unsubstantiated allegations that they were breaching the salary cap, but I couldn't help but be impressed by the open-minded, family-friendly environment I encountered on the many visits I made to their St Albans training ground.

Hargreaves lived just down the road from me in north-west London and we met at a favourite pub in Queen's Park, where he recounted a now all too familiar tale. He was smart, eloquent and hugely impressive.

'Retiring was a really emotional decision but not a hard one,' he told me.

> The medical advice was that they couldn't guarantee I'd be safe in the long term. I'm 30 years old and have had a great career, loved every minute of it, but I've also got a lot to look forward to in life after rugby.
>
> My wife and I had discussions after the last incident 11 months ago [when he was knocked out against Worcester]. We made the decision that if it happened again then the writing was on the wall as it would be moving into dangerous territory.
>
> I took a knock in training and ended up feeling really bad for about four days. Typical concussion symptoms. Headaches, feeling dizzy. It was terrible. I left training knowing I'd been in my last team huddle.
>
> If I carried on playing, the risk, without being overly dramatic, was there to my long-term mental health and not being there for my family. The risk was outweighing the reward.

Like most players, Hargreaves did not have a bad word to say about the sport he played and loved. But his was another cautionary tale about the risk endemic in playing professional rugby, even at a club as progressive as Saracens was.

While growing weary of the road and increasingly sceptical about sport's desire for change, there was still great joy to be found in the company of my colleagues and trips to some of the world's great rugby destinations. One of the many oddities about being a sports journalist is that your rivals are also your friends. Time spent on the road, away from families, creates a common bond through shared experiences few members of the public can dream of. On one such trip, a group including me, Adam Hathaway, Jonny Fordham from the *Sun* and Stephen Jones from the *Sunday Times* took the Eurostar from King's Cross on a Friday morning in October to Paris. We jumped in a taxi across town to Gare du Lyon to make one of the most glorious train journeys on the planet down to Toulon on the south coast, arriving in the early evening.

The weekend was one of the most memorable of my career as we enjoyed great company, incredible food and drink in the under-rated French harbour town which had become home to a large number of English exiles, notably Jonny Wilkinson, while also covering one of the best Champions Cup games I can recall: Saracens beating the three time champions 23–31 at the Stade Mayol.

We drank late into both nights before returning on the TGF, worse for wear but happy with our lot, on Sunday morning. It was one of many occasions I felt honoured and privileged to be doing a job I loved, in the company of colleagues I considered friends.

But the problem was, every time I began to feel optimistic and believe there could be a positive future for the game, another incident would occur which made me question why I was promoting a game which at the professional level I had long since believed had sold its soul.

*

I first read about Cae Trayhern in the summer of 2016 when it was reported that the former captain of Pontypool had died aged just 37. Having learned about the tragic cases among NFL players such as Webster, Seau and Duerson, I was on alert for rugby suicides. Back then, there was a strong narrative, arguing mental health issues such as depression and suicidal tendencies in former athletes could be put down simply to the loss of status, camaraderie and structure which goes hand in hand with retirement. Having been placed on a pedestal all their lives, afforded a small army of support staff and been told when to be where and why, it was only natural the loss of that would hit them hard. Or so the argument went. And it was the usual suspects who peddled this line.

But, with evidence of increased incidence of suicide in former blast victims in the military, domestic abuse survivors and within the prison population, where a history of head injuries is also common – figures according to the Disabilities Trust finding in 2019 that 64 per cent of female prisoners at HMP Drake Hall reported a history indicative of brain injury, while a 2020 study by Exeter University found 60 per cent of male prisoners in the UK reported having had a head injury – it made sense former sports stars, exposed to massive amounts of brain injury, would also be at heightened risk.

Trayhern was a hugely talented No.8 who narrowly failed to make a career as a full-time professional but achieved hero status in the small, rugby-obsessed town of Pontypool with a population of less than 30,000, just down the road from where he was born.

Cae's mental health deteriorated rapidly after he retired in his early thirties and in 2016 he was admitted to hospital in Ystrad Mynach believed to be suffering a nervous breakdown.

Just a few months later, on 10 June, Cae, the previously happy, outgoing young man with everything to live for, killed himself. By the time he died, he was virtually a recluse.

Gwent coroner David Bowen said Cae's death was 'the result of his own unassisted act intended to end his own life. There have been suggestions the concussions he suffered in his rugby career may have played a part in the deterioration of his mental health. I make no comment on that other than it is a concern of the family. Whether it was an effect in this case I cannot say.'

After the inquest, Cae's devastated family released a statement describing their 'wonderful' son, brother and uncle as an 'honest' and 'magnificent' man who was 'loving and kind'.

Cae loved animals, his dogs especially were very dear to his heart.

We will miss him for the rest of our lives and cherish our own special memories of the wonderful times spent with the great boy that we have lost.

God bless you my darling, you are safe now.

*

The following week, I convinced Cae's mum, Althea, to allow me to visit her at home. This is the article I wrote.

Why I believe Rugby killed my son
By Sam Peters
3 December 2016

Cae Trayhern was famous in the rugby-obsessed south Wales colliery village where he grew up. Handsome, outgoing and a gifted rugby player renowned for his bravery on the field, Cae fulfilled his childhood dream when he moved down the valley in 1997 to pull on Pontypool's red, white and black hooped shirt for the first time.

He was just 19. Fourteen years, 178 games – 54 as captain – and 'at least' 11 concussions later, Trayhern hung up his boots for the last time, a legend at a club that 30 years earlier produced the famous Wales and Lions front-row trio of Faulkner, Price and Windsor. Cae Trayhern was Ponty through and through.

On June 10 this year, on a warm summer's afternoon, Trayhern took his own life. His distraught mum Althea and her husband Paul found him, alone, in his house in Blackwood. He was just 37.

A young man with seemingly everything to live for, Trayhern's life spiralled helplessly out of control in just four years after retiring from rugby. He had become devoutly religious, was unable to sleep, suffered severe memory loss and saw visions of Jesus. The once bubbly leader of men was beginning to isolate himself.

'Cae's personality changed completely after he stopped playing,' his mother Althea tells The Mail on Sunday. 'He began to lose control, his workload got on top of him and things started unravelling. He was losing control and afraid.

'Cae had always done OK at school without excelling. Then, all of a sudden, he started reading the Bible and was able to quote from every part of it. I was shocked. It was as if one part of his brain was compensating for what was going or gone. It was really strange.

'He knew something was going on in his head. He said to me, 'Mum, there's something going on'. He'd come to my house crying and saying, 'I can't cope'.

'He became more and more isolated. Cae was changing and I knew he'd had all those concussions. If we weren't watching and he got a concussion, he wouldn't tell us. It was just part of the game for him.'

A fitness fanatic who did not smoke, take drugs or drink to excess, Trayhern was an organized, diligent and compassionate young man who bought his first house at the age of 21 and worked as a gas fitter before suffering a radical personality change in what turned out to be the final years of his life.

Althea has no doubt his brain was irreparably damaged by the head injuries sustained during a career where he put his body on the line every week as an openside flanker who played once for elite Welsh franchise Newport-Gwent Dragons.

'We used to go to watch him play whenever we could,'

says Althea. 'When he was concussed, even at the time, I would think, 'Oh my God, how can he come out all right after this? Is that natural for people to be unconscious one day and then all right the next day?'

'It always bothered me. It was terrible watching sometimes. One time when he was playing for Birmingham he needed to be airlifted to hospital after being knocked clean out. I wanted to get on the field but my husband held me back. To see them with the ambulance around him... oh my God, it was terrible.

'People ask me, 'How much of a role do you think concussion played in Cae's death?' And I have to say I think it played the most significant role. I'm not saying it was 100 per cent the cause but it was definitely a contributing factor. There's no doubt the concussions he suffered when he was playing were the biggest factor in his death. I will bang on about that until the day I die.

'That answers everything for me: why he was the way he was, how he was getting worse, how he realized there was a problem, everything.'

Today, Trayhern's family are convinced he suffered from the degenerative disease Chronic Traumatic Encephalopathy (CTE) found in the brains of dozens of deceased American football players and former soccer players, including former England international Jeff Astle.

But, unlike in the United States, where advances in medical science have seen more than 100 former NFL stars – including Mike Webster, Frank Gifford and Ken Stabler – posthumously diagnosed with CTE, there remains very little understanding in the UK of a disease once referred to as punch-drunk syndrome.

'I'm not looking for blame, I'm looking for a reason for what happened to my son,' says Althea. 'CTE explains it. I understand mental illness can be sparked by any number of things, but it wasn't like that with Cae. There didn't seem to be any reason for his decline.

'Two weeks before Cae died he was assessed by a team of mental health experts. I raised my concerns with one of the ward nurses at the unit that Cae had had all these concussions when he was younger. I raised them with the coroner later on. But no one listened. Anyhow, how could they find something [CTE] when they don't even know what they're looking for?'

With only two neuropathologists in the United Kingdom trained to identify CTE, and no test currently available for people while alive, they found themselves unable to prove their suspicions as the coroner last week found the cause of death to be 'asphyxia'.

No autopsy was carried out to examine Cae's brain for signs of damage. His mother adds: 'It's a shocking state of affairs when you have people suffering in this way and yet no one is taking it seriously enough to even formulate a test that can be done to check for CTE in players playing today.

'There are scans for every part of your body, but when it comes to the most important part of your body – your brain – there is nothing at all. It's scandalous really. I firmly believe Cae could just be the tip of the iceberg.'

Althea has no intention of following in the footsteps of other affected families such as the Astles, who set up the Jeff Astle Foundation in memory of their late dad.

Having lost her first son Shane aged 26 in a car accident 20 years ago, Althea has now lost her youngest, Cae.

But she does have a clear message for sport's core of highly paid doctors who continue to deny a link between head injuries and CTE.

'The only reason I'm talking now is because I am so convinced there is a link there and a link between Cae's concussions and his suicide,' she says.

'I don't think concussion is like rebooting your computer. I think it's like killing part of the information you've got in that computer. I've lost my best friend as well as my son.'

Listening to Althea provided me with yet another timely reminder of why I was doing this. Whenever I began to consider if it was time to ease back on the campaign, another hidden story presented itself which demanded telling. Cae Trayhern's was among the saddest I encountered. He was six months younger than me. I couldn't imagine the suffering his friends and family were enduring. Althea believed rugby had killed him. For me, that uncomfortable truth needed telling.

Althea was describing a textbook case of CTE. What happened to Cae was utterly heartbreaking and I'm not ashamed to say I cried on the train back from Newport to Paddington. Just as I had the first time I read about Ben Robinson.

I filed the story on Friday evening for Sunday's paper before heading to Twickenham on Saturday to cover England v Australia in the final game of the autumn series. England won, to complete an impressive autumn on the field under Jones, but as night fell and the Sunday Jacks in the media centre pumped copy across to their respective desks, I was told I needed to see something.

I looked over at a colleague's laptop and saw a video clip of George North lying face down, apparently unconscious, in the Franklin's Gardens mud.

'He played on,' someone said.

'You are fucking kidding me?' I replied.

He wasn't. Apparently, North had passed an HIA, which he obviously never should have undergone, before being allowed to play on.

BT Sport pundit Ugo Monye was incredulous: 'George North should not be on the pitch, it's as simple as that. If there is any suspicion that someone has lost consciousness you should be taken off the pitch. You should not take any further part in the game.'

It was utterly exasperating. How many more times were we going to have to call this out? I took another deep breath and went again, writing a news piece stating Northampton's medics had 'no excuse' for leaving North on, especially with the access to video footage.

Northampton issued a statement that night:

> George was attended to by the Northampton Saints medical team rapidly after landing on his side following a challenge in the air by Adam Thompstone.
>
> George was communicating immediately with attending medics and complaining of neck pain. Significant neck injury was excluded on the field but on review of video footage pitch side, the team followed World Rugby protocols and used a Head Injury Assessment given the potential mechanism for head injury.
>
> George was fully assessed by the doctor and passed fit to return to play. Northampton Saints places the highest importance on player care and their safety is the club's primary concern.

North also put out a statement on social media saying: 'I am OK. I landed on my neck and was worried about it. Thanks to the medics for checking me out properly.'

But the whole affair looked awful.

It was an unhappy coincidence for Northampton we'd already chosen to run the devastating interview with Cae Trayhern's mum, Althea, in Sunday's paper. To see images of the stricken North, face down in the mud, alongside a story headlined 'Rugby killed my son' made for brutal reading.

It made it look even worse for Northampton, who later claimed their medics had not had access to the same footage as the BT Sport commentators. The next day I called a friend at BT Sport who insisted this was untrue.

*

The following week, with Saints under investigation, I was forwarded the recording of an exchange between their long-serving director of rugby, Jim Mallinder, and a group of journalists before a press conference in which he questioned whether I was a 'rugby person' and described the *Mail on Sunday*'s campaign as 'scaremongering'. I'd heard it all before. To some extent I sympathized with Mallinder's frustration at the lack of coverage of some of the positive things rugby was doing to try to address the concussion problem, and there were times I truly believed the sport was making a serious effort to address it. And it would obviously be completely wrong to suggest all medics were corrupt, all coaches were bullies and all players trying to cheat the system. I also did not believe any of the Northampton medical team had wilfully ignored North's symptoms. But even with me constantly beating the drum, progress was agonizingly slow and egregious mistakes were still being made in plain sight. I was all for the carrot approach but, when it came to medical protocols designed to protect players, rugby's authorities seemed completely unwilling to use the stick. A player could be hit with a hefty ban for a high tackle or swearing at the referee but no one seemed accountable for allowing a clearly brain-damaged player to play on. Why not? It was unfettered free-market rugby and its greatest assets – the players – were tanking.

And while flagrant breaches of protocols were taking place, I would keep calling them out. Besides, despite what others thought, it was not my job to act as an extension of professional rugby's PR department.

I wasn't at all surprised by Mallinder's hostility but it was disappointing to be talked about behind my back without any right to reply. I could only imagine how many conversations of this type were going on around the game. But 'not a rugby man' was a low blow and I can't pretend it didn't sting. Those who knew me knew how nonsensical it was.

It had become glaringly obvious that the only way to effect any kind of change was to relentlessly pressure the game's authorities. If that dissuaded parents from letting their children play, I was genuinely sorry, but to me, the problem was brain-damaged players being allowed to play on, not me reporting it. As long as that kept on happening, I believed I owed it to families like the Robinsons and the Trayherns, not to mention future generations, to keep going. If that meant I was 'not a rugby man', so be it.

Before the North findings were made public in December 2016, I asked Kemp if he still had faith in the HIA.

> I can't remember where it was constructed but it's been adopted by World Rugby and therefore it's World Rugby rules and regs,' he told me. 'I certainly think it's demonstrable that it's seen an improvement in levels of awareness, understanding and analysis. I'm talking about the system as a whole.
>
> What we're looking at in this other case [North] is whether it was applied in the ways one would have wanted it to be applied. The system as a whole has been pretty successful in terms of awareness, preventative situation about removing people, carrying out analysis.

It surprised me to hear Kemp try to distance himself from the construction of the HIA. My understanding had always been that he was heavily involved in formulating the protocol. Fortunately, RFU chief executive Ian Ritchie clarified this position a few weeks later when he told me: 'Anybody who has been involved in the creation of the HIA, and Simon has been pivotal, absolutely wants to see it work.'

When the verdict from the Concussion Management Review

Group (CMRG) finally arrived, more than three weeks after the incident, any hope of a watershed moment vanished.

'The CMRG's view is that there was sufficient evidence to conclude he should not have returned to the field,' the review read in yet another statement of the blindingly obvious.

> Northampton Saints medical team has accepted North may have lost consciousness and therefore should not have returned to play.
>
> In addition and although not a determining factor, the CMRG is aware that the player appears to have had no residual effects in the short term. For these reasons the CMRG will not be imposing any sanction against the club or any of its individuals as a result of this incident.

Instead, the CMRG published a nine-point plan supposedly to ensure it would never happen again.

Apparently, clubs would only be punished if the player showed 'residual effects'. How long after the brain injury? Five minutes? Five days? Five years?

Northampton's defence of not having complete access to the camera shots was accepted in full, while the panel concluded that 'the welfare of North was always at the centre of Northampton's actions and does not consider that the medical team (or the club) failed to complete the HIA protocol nor intentionally ignored the player's best interests'.

Alistair Hargreaves took to Twitter, labelling the findings a 'disgrace' and a 'depressing day for rugby'.

'It's a step backwards. There needs to be accountability,' he added. 'In the review there wasn't any hint of condemnation of the fact North was allowed to go back on to the field. There needed to be a statement showing how seriously matters like this will be taken if the protocols aren't followed. We've missed that chance.'

Predictably the RPA stopped short of criticizing the report. 'That George was permitted to return to the field was a significant failing,' they said in a statement.

'While we feel sanctions would have sent a clear message about the gravity of concussion mismanagement, we welcome the recommendations outlined in the report. These must be adopted and all concussion processes kept under constant review to ensure this does not happen again.'

But of course, it would happen again. Three weeks later, Sale Sharks, already facing a legal challenge from former scrum half Cillian Willis and whose director of rugby Steve Diamond had said a few weeks previously: 'All you need now is a slap on the head and they'll have you off for 13 minutes', allowed a clearly concussed TJ Ioane to play on.

This time the 'independent panel', containing lawyer and doctor Julian Morris, RFU director of professional rugby Nigel Melville and Premiership Rugby's rugby director Phil Winstanley, who incidentally played 55 times for Sale between 1997 and 2000, concluded: 'While a case could have been made for the player's removal for an HIA following the incident, the group felt the decision for the player to play on and be monitored was consistent with the range of current practice and current interpretation of the criteria for requesting an HIA. The decision to instigate the HIA then becomes a clinical judgment call of the doctor at the time. No further action will be taken.'

Within days, World Rugby moved again. This time issuing a 'zero tolerance approach to reckless head contact'. Once again, responsibility and accountability for rubgy's concussion crisis landed on the players' shoulders.

While there was a predictable backlash from the 'game's gone soft' brigade, World Rugby, reasonably in my view, were working on the basis that if referees were empowered to uphold the laws protecting a player's head in contact, coaches and players would soon adapt their behaviour accordingly. This had certainly been the case with tip tackles, which had largely been eradicated by now.

The governing body increased sanctions for reckless high tackles and instituted a new framework to measure what was adjudged to be a high tackle. The aim was to 'effectively lower the acceptable height of the tackle'.

Michael Aylwin wrote in the *Guardian*:

> World Rugby's new directives for punishing high tackles come into effect this weekend, but in truth they have left it up to coaches and players to figure out for themselves how to adapt.
>
> To call it a law change is the first disingenuous step from World Rugby. This is actually a ramping up of punishment for an existing offence. The threshold for a high tackle remains the line of the shoulders. World Rugby has instituted two new categories for a high tackle – 'reckless' and 'accidental' – together with rhetoric that tries to define each. But a high tackle remains a high tackle, and both the reckless and accidental manifestations have long been penalized.

Seven years earlier, attendees at a World Rugby medical conference had unanimously agreed with a study published in 2008 entitled 'Injury Risks Associated with Tackling in Rugby Union' co-authored by, among others, Colin Fuller of Nottingham University, Tony Ashton from the Boarding Schools' Association and Simon Kemp. It found 'stricter implementation of the Laws of Rugby relating to collisions and tackles above the line of the shoulder may reduce the number of head/neck injuries.'

A memo to referees following the conference also stated:

> The participants at the Medical Conference generally recognized that tackles above the line of the shoulders have the potential to cause serious injury and noted that a trend had

emerged whereby players responsible for such tackles were not being suitably sanctioned.

The purpose of this Memorandum is to emphasize that as with tip tackles, they must be dealt with severely by Referees and all those involved in the off-field disciplinary process.

It is recognized, as with other types of illegal and/or foul play, depending on the circumstances of the high tackle, the range of sanctions extends from a penalty kick to the player receiving a red card. An illegal high tackle involving a stiff arm or swinging arm to the head of the opponent, with no regard to the player's safety, bears all the hallmarks of an action which should result in a red card or a yellow card being seriously considered.

Referees and Citing Commissioners should not make their decisions based on what they consider was the intention of the offending player. Their decision should be based on an objective assessment (as per Law 10.4(e)) of the overall circumstances of the tackle.

In truth, the 2017 directive was just about empowering referees. But now, with cameras everywhere and an eye on any hit to the head, people were beginning to wake up to just how many head contacts there were in every game of professional rugby. But again, I feared that without addressing the elephant in the room – CTE – World Rugby would never convince the large number of sceptics in the 'rugby family' why these changes were needed.

Despite World Rugby's promise of 'zero tolerance' on high tackles, progress remained desperately slow. I found myself once again running out of steam, weary from almost four years of campaigning. With our first baby on the way and after 15 years on the road reporting sport around the world, I felt my race was almost run. I'd had some amazing experiences, met some incredible people and built lifelong friendships. But the past three years had been hard. Really hard. I felt as if I was butting up against people all the time as my frustration at the slow pace of change continued. At the start of 2017, more than ever, I was beginning to wonder how much longer I could keep doing this for.

In March, yet more evidence emerged that professional rugby was, in effect, holed below the waterline. Initially, World Rugby's announcement promising an 'optimized global calendar' providing 'certainty and sustainability' over the decade beyond the 2019 World Cup promised to finally provide a playing framework which did not involve beasting the top stars to within an inch of their lives for most of the year.

Unfortunately, far from reducing the players' season, England's top stars were now being told they could expect to play for 11 months a year. A hard-earned guarantee of what was still a woefully inadequate five-week break between seasons, up from four, which the RPA had claimed as a triumph the previous year, went out of the window.

The RPA, Hopley especially, had been completely outmanoeuvred.

Gloucester winger and RPA board member Charlie Sharples said the move had 'no benefits for players', while another, Christian Day, told me: 'A 10-month domestic season is frightening enough but with the prospect of an international season then becoming 11 months with a summer tour it begins to stretch the boundaries of what's possible. If you add in the five-week rest period, which the RPA fought really hard for as a mental and physical recharge for the players, it basically means there is no off-season. It is an incredible ask of our elite players.'

Talk of strike action was back on the table for players in England, but mercifully, Premiership Rugby were forced to climbdown for their plan to extend their season deep into the summer, but they had revealed their true colours.

The constant treadmill had caught up with me. Much as I enjoyed the company of my fellow journalists on the road, the thought of leaving Debs for several weeks to cover a Lions tour in New Zealand just a few weeks after our daughter was born in April 2017 was not an option.

After six years at the *Mail on Sunday*, three of them as rugby union correspondent, I resigned, aged 39.

13

Justice for Jeff

Soon after the *Mail on Sunday*'s concussion in rugby campaign got under way in 2013, my friend Jim Holden, chief sports correspondent at the *Sunday Express*, approached me in the press box at Lord's following a press conference. Jim congratulated me on the work I'd done so far reporting on concussion in rugby and told me I'd still be writing about it in another 10 years. He was only half joking.

Jim asked if I was aware of the case of former England and West Bromwich Albion footballer Jeff Astle.

'Wasn't he the guy who died from heading the ball?' I replied.

'He's the one,' said Jim. 'I wrote about it a lot at the time. Nothing's happened since. You should take a look.'

Like many sports fans of my generation, my first recollection of Jeff Astle had been from watching his regular appearances on the 1990s cult BBC comedy series *Fantasy Football League*, hosted by Frank Skinner and David Baddiel.

I knew Astle had been a professional footballer for West Brom but, such was the relentless lampooning he received for missing a sitter against Brazil which saw England knocked out of the 1970 World Cup, viewers could be forgiven for not realizing he was actually one of the greatest English centre forwards of all time.

Following Astle's death, aged 59, in January 2002, I'd been shocked to read reports suggesting his premature death from dementia was linked to heading footballs during his career. According to Dr Keith Robson, who examined his brain, repeated head injuries sustained during his playing career had seen Astle die from an 'industrial disease'. In essence, Astle's job caused his death.

As a diehard sports fan, this obviously wasn't something I wanted to hear. But I also remember being reassured when various footballing representatives explained confidently that this was a historic problem caused by heading heavy leather balls, which in Astle's day were often soaked in water to make them even tougher to head in training. Meanwhile, the FA's promise to 'leave no stone unturned' in a bid to understand the extent of the problem was also comforting.

Jim's suggestion I'd still be writing about the issue in 10 years irked slightly. The implication was that I'd also find myself butting up against a relentless series of obstacles which would prevent change occurring. I'd had conversations with respected friends in rugby who believed the same thing.

'It's all very worthy, mate, but where are you going with it?' my friend and travelling companion Adam Hathaway asked me when I sought his opinion around the same time.

Undeterred, I carried on.

Inevitably, as a rugby correspondent, my focus was on the sport I covered and which, to my mind, had changed beyond recognition in the past two decades, turning what had previously been described as a contact sport played predominantly by physically big men, into a collision sport played by giant athletes. But, having played and watched most sports growing up, I was fully aware rugby union was not the only sport involving a concussion risk.

A few weeks after I'd started writing about concussion in rugby, Tottenham Hotspur goalkeeper Hugo Lloris was knocked unconscious in a collision with Everton's Romelu Lukaku at Goodison Park. After several minutes of treatment and dialogue with the Spurs medical team the France international returned to the field.

Spurs later said Lloris was cleared to resume by the medical team but the game manager André Villas-Boas insisted he had made the call.

'It was a big knock, but he looked composed and ready to continue,' said Villas-Boas. 'Hugo seemed assertive and determined to continue and showed great character and personality. We decided to keep him on based on that. The call always belongs to me.'

Clearly, rugby wasn't the only sport where doctors could be influenced by coaches.

Previously, the incident would have gone unreported by a UK football media who had shown even less appetite to tackle the head injuries story than rugby's, despite the Jeff Astle case.

But our spotlight on the issue in rugby had had an effect. The Lloris incident made back page news across almost every newspaper.

Previously low-profile brain injury charities were also being afforded an overdue platform.

'When a player – or any individual – suffers a blow to the head that is severe enough for them to lose consciousness, it is vital they urgently seek appropriate medical attention,' said Luke Griggs, spokesman for brain injury charity Headway.

'A physio or doctor treating a player on the pitch simply cannot accurately gauge the severity of the damage caused to the player's brain in such a setting as there may be delayed presentation of symptoms.

'By continuing to play, the player may have caused greater damage to his brain. He should have been removed from the game immediately and taken to hospital for thorough tests and observation.'

Football was obviously not immune to incidents of concussion mismanagement, although judging by the Lloris incident, coaches felt brazen enough to meddle in what should have been a purely medical decision.

The incident actually provided me with a welcome reason to move the focus away from rugby, where I knew many of my friends and contacts were uncomfortable with the relentless spotlight I was shining on the issue. I had some sympathy with those at the RFU who pointed to the injury data collection as a genuine attempt to understand the scale of injuries in their sport. Other professional sports, notably football, had far less transparency, partly, no doubt, because clubs saw it as too commercially sensitive to share injury data with the sport's authorities.

I'd been aware of former Rangers defender Fernando Ricksen's diagnosis with motor neurone disease in October 2013 and was directed to a study carried out at Turin University and published in 2005 which examined more than 7,000 former professional footballers and found a 6.25 times higher incidence of MND in former professional footballers than would have been expected in the wider population.

One football club which at that time was leading the way was Barnet FC. The club's chairman, Tony Kleanthous, invited me to their impressive training facility in north London to discuss the recent £2 million deal he'd done with Toshiba to bring a range of high-tech scanners and imaging equipment to the club, as a part commercial, part community driven venture he insisted would make the club the most medically progressive in the world.

I also sat down with player-manager Edgar Davids, the former Netherlands and Barcelona midfielder who had been signed the previous summer. For an hour we discussed his concerns over football's approach to concussion. I wrote in the *Mail on Sunday*:

> The furore surrounding Tottenham manager André Villas-Boas's decision to allow goalkeeper Hugo Lloris to return to the field after being knocked out a fortnight ago further focused public attention on football's mismanagement of head trauma.
>
> The issue highlighted the pressures that can be exerted on medical staff by coaches keen to keep their best players on the field.

Dutch football legend Edgar Davids said: 'Sometimes pressure is applied and that's why it's so important to have good doctors around you. Footballers may play professional sport but first and foremost they are human beings.

'The threat of legal action is always there. The decision always has to be in the hands of the medical department.'

Davids is manager at forward-thinking Barnet, where a £2m sponsorship deal will transform part of the club's Hive Stadium into a hi-tech medical centre with cutting-edge CT and MRI scanners, ultrasound and X-ray facilities, staffed by top London neurologists.

Their director of football, Paul Fairclough, who as manager of the England C team is also concerned with the grassroots game, said: 'We pay scant regard [to concussion] in football. It's a case of the physio coming on and saying 'Follow my finger', then 'Oh, you're all right, son, get back on'. It's criminal. There will be fatalities if we carry on the way we are.

'It's going on all over the country, managers bullying physios to keep players on the pitch. I see things going on at lower-level football that frighten the living daylights out of me. We've got to take it more seriously.

'We're in that culture of where there is blame there is a claim and it will happen eventually [litigation] and it would devastate a club.'

The Lloris case took our campaign to another level, bringing football squarely into focus and reminding any sport where head injuries occurred they were no longer immune from media scrutiny.

The conversation I'd had with Jim Holden at Lord's about Jeff Astle stuck in my mind. Following the incident with Lloris, I decided to investigate further.

I dug out several articles from around the time of his death as well as from November 2002, when the South Staffordshire coroner Andrew Haigh gave his verdict. Dr Keith Robson, the neuropathologist who examined Astle's brain, said:

> I found that most damage to the brain was at the front of the head. I found there was considerable evidence of trauma to the brain similar to that of a boxer. It is quite probable that it was heading a heavy football that caused it. I remember as a small child how heavy it was to head a leather football. The chronic nature of the trauma could occur naturally but without further investigation it is not possible to say. From the evidence, the persistent heading of the ball could be a factor in the loss of Mr Astle's faculties and his behaviour.

Commenting on signs of the early stages of Alzheimer's disease, Dr Robson added: 'It is unlikely that he would have developed the condition so young if he had not headed a football repeatedly. He may not have even developed the condition.'

One *Times* article had the unequivocal headline 'Heading footballs killed Jeff Astle, coroner says'.

> His prowess at heading a football made the England centre-forward Jeff Astle one of the most celebrated players of his generation, but his gift ultimately killed him.
>
> A coroner ruled yesterday that Astle, who played for West Bromwich Albion, died of an industrial disease after 20 years of heading a heavy leather ball. The inquest was told that he suffered from degenerative brain damage, mostly to the front of the head.
>
> The Professional Footballers' Association believes that this is the first time that a coroner has said that heading a ball can kill.
>
> Astle's wife, Lorraine [sic], hailed yesterday's verdict as 'justice', while football clubs braced themselves for the

possibility of a welter of compensation claims from retired players.

Those claims, it would transpire, never came. Not because of a lack of evidence that thousands of former professional footballers were suffering early onset dementia, with a far higher incidence than in the wider population, but more because of the heavy-handed legal tactic deployed by the FA against families, most of whom were not wealthy enough to pay their own legal fees.

In early 2003, the FA's lawyers Addleshaw Goddard sent a letter to Astle's widow Laraine, warning against pursuing legal action against the FA. The letter stated:

> Mr Astle participated in many forms of football from childhood until his retirement from the game in 1977. During that time, it is reasonable to assume he played with many types of balls, in every conceivable condition and also experienced the exigencies of life, both on and off the field. He would have had, for example, many occasions when his head would have been hit other than when heading the ball, in matches to which the Laws applied, such as clashing heads with other players, hitting the ground, being kicked... We also note that Mrs Astle was only aware of 'changes' some 20 years after Mr Astle stopped playing.
>
> Furthermore, even on Dr Robson's evidence, there was neurological disorder, changes consistent with Alzheimer's Disease and a genetic predisposition to disease.
>
> We consider any suggestion by you of a claim to be flawed, misconceived and without foundation.

Another element of the *Times* article caught my attention. It read:

> There have been recent conflicting psychological and physiological studies on whether heading the ball, even the

modern type, can damage the brain. In the Netherlands one study found that Dutch football players scored significantly lower on tests that measured visual and verbal memory compared with swimmers or track athletes.

Consequently the Football Association last season set up a study, costing £116,000, to examine the structure and functioning of the brains of 30 youngsters in professional academies. Under the direction of Dr Myles Gibson, a leading neurologist, the players will be subjected to regular scans and neurological tests. Most players head the ball 800 times during a professional season, with the total increasing to 1,500 for defenders.

Alan Hodson, the FA's head of sports medicine, said: 'This is a prospective study which will monitor the careers of youngsters over a long period.'

With the FA's legal warning accompanied by the promise of this study, the grieving Astles understandably decided against pursuing a prohibitively expensive claim for compensation.

The *Guardian* reported that Brendan Batson, the managing director of West Bromwich Albion, said that the FA and the Professional Footballers' Association (PFA) had begun a joint 10-year project to learn more about how heading a football affected young players' brains. He was quoted as saying: 'We cannot do anything about what has gone on in the past, but maybe we can do something in the future.'

According to the *British Medical Journal* (BMJ) in 2002: 'The English Football Association and the Professional Footballers' Association are conducting a 10 year study into how heading a ball can affect the brain. The study... began last year, with 30 players aged 18–19 who are likely to go on to have long careers in professional football and will include players from defence, midfield, and striker positions.'

Laraine, along with her daughters Dorice, Dawn and Claire, had no reason to believe the FA and PFA would not deliver the potentially life-saving research. They didn't know at that time Dr Gibson had promised studies into the issue in the past including a prospective study in 1997/98 which had not materialized after Dr John Rowlands, GP and family friend of legendary England international Joe Mercer, who died of dementia in 1990, voiced serious concerns at a meeting with PFA chief executive Gordon Taylor in 1996.

'I believe this was the first time he had heard of such a problem,' Dr Rowlands told the *Daily Mail* in December 2020, the year it was revealed that seven of England's 1966 team, including my relative Martin, had either died from or been diagnosed with early onset dementia, and the year after Professor Willie Stewart's FIELD (Football's InfluencE on Lifelong health and Dementia risk) study found former professional footballers are at a 3.5 times higher risk of dying with dementia than the wider population. The study looked at over 7,600 former Scottish professional footballers and compared them to 23,000 people in the general population.

'He was extremely helpful and offered to help us get it off the ground but told me that we needed funding from elsewhere, from the likes of the FA,' said Rowlands.

Encouraged by the promise of funding, Rowlands pressed on.

'I contacted Myles Gibson, a lead neurosurgeon and adviser to the FA who wrote that a retrospective study wouldn't be helpful, but said they'd be carrying out a prospective study in the 1997/98 season.'

The Astles did not know they were far from the only football family affected. Nor did they know that in 1999 Exeter City club doctor David Kernick had called for heading to be banned outside the box in a paper published in the *BMJ*.

'There can be few global health proposals that cost nothing, are easy to implement and have the potential to confer benefit on such a large number of people,' Kernick said.

According to newspaper reports at the time, 'the Football Association's medical committee is poised to launch a monitoring programme.'

'What happens now depends on how seriously the football authorities take my paper,' Kernick said.

With all these historic promises of research and monitoring programmes, I felt sure I would find some interesting information, if anything to put families' minds at rest, when I came to look at the results. There was just one problem. There weren't any results. The more I looked, the less I found. Following weeks of digging, I began to seriously doubt if the FA's research had ever been carried out.

On 28 March 2014, I contacted Dr Gibson himself, who was now 87. I asked him about the FA study he was tasked with leading after the Astle case and he told me: 'It was totally separate from the Jeff Astle case. This was on its own. It wasn't involved in it [Astle case] in any way.' Dr Gibson also insisted the study was ongoing and would be published 'fairly soon'.

I couldn't believe my ears. I knew the research hadn't been carried out. I knew Dr Gibson had been the FA's most senior advisor on neurological matters for many years. I knew he had been tasked with leading the study soon after the coroner's findings on Jeff Astle. We both knew the research hadn't been carried out but, here we were, playing out a charade.

I spoke to Roger Lacey on the *Mail on Sunday*'s sports desk. We agreed the Astle family deserved to know the study had not been completed, as did the countless other families who had pinned their hopes on the FA and PFA seeing it through.

I managed to track down Laraine Astle's phone number. I took a deep breath and rang her. I explained I'd spent almost a year researching head injuries in rugby. I explained my work had led me into looking at incidences of dementia in ex-professional footballers and I had some information about the research promised following her husband's death. I asked if she would agree to meet.

The next morning, I drove 110 miles from London to the small former colliery town of Netherseal, near Burton-on-Trent in the East Midlands, just a few miles down the road from where my brother Tom and I had spent many happy summers playing cricket in Nanny's front garden. I parked outside a smart but unassuming detached house in a reasonably new development with tidy front gardens and neatly trimmed hedges. There was a sense of English order about the place.

I was 20 minutes early and sat in my car nervously playing out how the conversation could go.

At 10.30am on the dot I knocked on the door. A kind, gentle face greeted me. It was Laraine. She asked me in and offered me tea. We walked in through the hallway, pictures of Jeff adorning the walls and corridors.

'By the time he died, Jeff couldn't even remember who I was,' Laraine said.

Soon after I'd arrived, the doorbell went and one of Laraine's daughters, Dawn, was at the door. She immediately struck me as tough, determined.

I explained the work I'd been doing, the discovery of CTE in ex-American footballers and my battle with rugby's authorities. I explained I was gravely concerned that other sports, including football, were systematically downplaying the findings of studies into the long-term effects of head injuries. I told them about the Concussion in Sport Group and I explained I believed football, which helped fund the CISG, had spent decades ignoring the risks. I told them I did not believe the research they thought had been carried out following Jeff's death had ever been completed.

'I'm really sorry but unless I've missed something really obvious, I can only conclude it's been kicked into the long grass,' I said.

I'll never forget the look on their faces. They've subsequently told me they were expecting me to tell them the results of the research and were utterly shocked when I told them it simply didn't exist. It transpired later that the 'groundbreaking' study had been quietly shelved less than five years in due to problems tracking all the participants. No one had seen fit to tell the Astles, or anyone else.

**England star Astle died from the 'industrial disease'
of heading footballs... 12 years on his widow is still
waiting for the FA to deliver on their promises**
By Sam Peters
15 March 2014

Laraine Astle sits beneath a framed black and white picture of her husband Jeff scoring the winning goal in the 1968 FA Cup final at Wembley for West Bromwich Albion against Everton.

As she talks, a mounted wooden clock on the living room wall ticks relentlessly.

Most of the time the 69-year-old is composed but occasionally, inevitably, her voice cracks and she wipes away a tear at the burning injustice she still feels 12 years after a coroner found Jeff died, aged 59, from 'industrial disease' caused by heading footballs.

'Jeff was known as the best header in the game,' Laraine says from the modest house in the sleepy former pit village of Netherseal in South Derbyshire she shared with Jeff in the years before he died from dementia in 2002.

'Players have said to me that in every practice session the ball was sent into the middle for Jeff. Free kicks, corners... they all went to Jeff's head. On average he scored a goal every other game and he must be the only player to have scored more goals with his head than his feet. I don't think there's another player alive who has done that.'

By the time Jeff died, a broken shell of a man, he did not even know he'd been a professional footballer, let alone one of the finest of his generation. By the time Jeff died he couldn't remember his grandchildren's names, a single one of the 174 league goals he'd scored or the five England caps he'd won. He never forgot his wife's face though.

'Jeff had a fantastic memory,' says Laraine. 'We'd go somewhere once in the car and from then on he'd always remember the way. He used to joke with me that I'd get lost down a one-way street but he was so observant and remembered everything.

'When he was about 55 I started to notice he was forgetting more and more simple things and made him go to the doctors for a check-up. It was clear straight away he had a problem. I asked the doctor if there was anything that could be done but she said, 'Almost certainly not'.

'From that split second I knew our lives would never be the same.

'Towards the end I'd show him a photograph of him scoring a goal in the FA Cup Final and say, 'Do you remember that photograph, Jeff?' and he'd say, 'No'. I'd say, 'That's you there, you scored the winning goal in the Cup Final'. He'd say, 'Did I?' I'd say, 'Yes, it was 1–0 and you went in the record books as the first player to score in every round on the way to the final' and he'd say, 'Was I?'

'I'd ask, 'Do you know who you played for?' and he'd say, 'Did I play for Fulham?' I'd say, 'No, darling, you played for West Brom'.

'Everything he'd won in football, in the end football took away from him.'

Following his death, and aware who Astle was, a quick-thinking doctor at Burton District Hospital referred his body to Queen's Medical Centre in Nottingham where one of the world's pre-eminent neuro-pathologists, Dr Keith Robson, carried out a post mortem.

When he inspected Astle's brain, Robson discovered levels
of catastrophic damage more usually associated with boxers
and at the resulting inquest the Coroner, Andrew Haigh,
deemed it beyond reasonable doubt Astle's death had been
caused by his excellence in the air.

At the time, the Football Association promised a 10-year
joint study with the Professional Footballers' Association to
investigate any possible association between heading footballs
and an increased prevalence of neuro-degenerative illnesses
among retired professional players.

To date, not one single piece of FA research has been
published, and The Mail on Sunday can find no evidence of the
study ever being carried out. Similar promises were made in
2003 following the publication of research involving more than
7,000 retired Italian professionals at Turin University in Italy
which found significantly higher incidences of motor neurone
disease – also known as Lou Gehrig's disease – among the
study group.

'I'll never forget when Dr Robson stood up to give his
findings in court,' said Laraine. 'He said, 'Every slice of Jeff's
brain had trauma in it. It resembled the brain of a boxer's as a
direct result of heading footballs'.

'After the inquest the FA promised research but what
they've actually done is swept this under a carpet for 12 long
years. Where are the answers they promised? I've never seen
any results. Where is the research they said they'd carry out?

'Not many people would ask that question 12 years later
but that's what we're asking because it's affected our lives
because it killed my husband. We know damn well they didn't
do it [the research].

'The FA said to me on the phone soon after the hearing, 'If
we do anything for you it will open the floodgates to others'.

What a thing. Could they say that to Yorkshire miners that if they paid them out because of the dust in the mines they'd have to pay the Nottingham ones, the Durham ones? You don't do that. If their job has killed them or made them poorly then you do what you can to help them.

'I know of seven players from the Port Vale team of the 1950s have gone on to develop dementia. Is that coincidence? And it's not just Jeff's generation they're failing, it's future generations too. There are six and seven year olds running around heading footballs on a Sunday morning. What is that doing to them?'

To compound matters for Laraine, 69, and her three daughters Dorice, 49, Dawn, 46, and Claire, 35, the FA, who initially promised to support them in the wake of the coroner's findings, appear to have washed their hands of any responsibility.

The only correspondence the family received, apart from the offer of two tickets to an England friendly, was a menacing letter from the FA's solicitors Addleshaw Goddard a year after the inquest – which The Mail on Sunday is in possession of – warning against any legal action.

Laraine Astle continues: 'After the inquest David Davies took over as acting chairman of the FA and he said he would like to come and see me. I told him all about what had happened to Jeff.

'He wiped a tear from his eye and said, 'I've got two daughters Mrs Astle and I'm the same age now as Jeff was when he was diagnosed. I can't imagine how difficult this must be for you.'

'He said, 'I'm going back to the FA now and I'm going to tell them everything you have just told me and I promise you I'm going to do something. I'm going to help.'

'A few weeks later a letter arrived from David Davies saying, 'Thank you for seeing me, would you and one of your daughters like to attend an England friendly at the City of Manchester Stadium?' They couldn't even ask all my daughters. Was that all my Jeff's life was worth? Two tickets to an England friendly. I didn't even bother replying.

'I've never heard another thing from them other than a solicitor's letter. I think it's absolutely disgraceful how the FA has behaved. They've lied and lied to us over all these years.'

However much the FA may wish Jeff Astle's story to disappear from the history books and for his family to be less outspoken about their fervent belief his dementia was caused by heading footballs, they are refusing to go quietly.

Last week Dr Ian Beasley, head of medicine at the FA, admitted at a Parliamentary meeting the game's governing body still have no clear protocols in place on how to deal with footballers who have suffered head injuries on the field.

A cursory search by The Mail on Sunday last week discovered more than 30 former professional footballers who have been diagnosed with motor neurone disease or other associated dementias in the past 20 years. Jeff Astle was just one of them.

The clock is still ticking.

Dawn was seething and the interview, coming as it did in the midst of a Parliamentary cross-party investigation into concussion in rugby, lifted the campaign to a new level.

We now had proof the FA was acting in the same malign manner as the NFL, kicking research studies down the road and burying bad news. With my own doubts about rugby's intention to get to the bottom of the issue, the story had suddenly taken an unexpected twist.

I felt desperately sorry for the Astles. They had been betrayed by those in power in football who once again had swept the issue under the carpet. A cover-up in plain sight no less with senior figures at the FA and PFA complicit. But anyone who thought the Astle family would lie down a second time was sorely mistaken.

Within days, the Astle family had set up the Justice for Jeff campaign and the following Saturday, rather than covering a rugby game, I found myself on a train to Hull, ostensibly to cover Hull City v West Bromwich Albion but really to cover the campaign's launch.

Nine minutes into the game, representing Jeff's shirt number, a 12-metre-long blue banner was unfurled behind the goal proclaiming 'Justice for Jeff' and the entire West Brom contingent applauded continuously for a minute. I felt a rush of emotion. The hairs on the back of my neck stood up and I choked back tears. It was to prove the beginning of a relentless campaign for justice for the forgotten victims of brain damage in football.

Dawn had the bit between her teeth and has never let go since. At times, her determination to get justice for her father and the countless thousands of other former footballers suffering early onset dementia has been truly staggering.

A few weeks later, in June 2014, after I'd introduced him to the Astle family, Professor Willie Stewart re-examined Jeff's brain and found he'd had CTE.

Just as I'd been inundated with telephone calls and messages from rugby players when I ran the 'Rugby's ticking timebomb' feature, now I was inundated with messages from former footballers and their families. It is to my eternal regret that I was so bombarded at the time, I was unable to reply to even a third of them. Here are just a sample:

On 17 March 2014, Keith Davies wrote:

I was very interested to read your article on page 17 of the *Mail on Sunday* regarding Jeff Astle.

My brother Eric played for Crewe Alexandra at centre half for over 10 years in the 1960s and 70s as a professional.

Approximately 9–10 years ago he was diagnosed with Parkinson's disease which resulted in his death on the 3rd January this year with resultant pneumonia after spending the last 3–4 months in hospital in Crewe.

I have always wondered whether the constant heading of the heavy leather footballs used in those days would have had cause to bring on Parkinson's.

Whilst we have had good deal of help financially from the PFA office in Manchester, who kindly contributed to his consultants fees, treatment and funeral costs.

Even so his widow, two daughters and myself never managed to establish a connection between whether him heading the ball would have caused or brought on his condition which obviously cut short his life.

I would be grateful if you would add this information to your dossier and should anything result from your enquiries perhaps you or the FA would contact us.

Whilst his widow, Beryl, does not want any publicity I am sure if further proof of the details I have given you is required this can be given you.

Good luck with your investigations.

On 30 March 2014, Joy Cruickshank wrote:

I have been reading with personal interest the articles that have appeared in your column regarding the number of professional footballers that have been diagnosed with dementia over the years. I would like to add the name of Frank Cruickshank, my husband, to the list of those who have this truly distressing illness.

Frank played for Notts County from 1953 to 1960 when Jeff Astle was there as a young professional. He had been signed by Burnley shortly prior to him joining Notts County but didn't settle and spent the rest of his professional career with the club. Joining Cheltenham Town as player manager and then to Cambridge Town again as player manager and then to Newmarket Town. Football has been his life.

In 2006 he was diagnosed with dementia with Lewy Body's and early Parkinson's disease, but signs of slowness and forgetfulness were showing sometime earlier.

Frank is now in long-term care as it became increasingly more difficult to care and cope with his illness. So, so sad to see the slow deterioration of such a fit sportsman who loved the game.

So I, of course, am a great supporter of your campaign and wish Jeff's widow Laraine success in her mission.

On 9 April 2014, Maria Ashton wrote:

I read your article in the *Mail on Sunday* 6 April 2014 newspaper regarding the unusually high dementia rates among professional football players.

My father (Robert McIlvenny) was a professional footballer, who will be 88 years of age in July and is now in a Home suffering from Alzheimer's. The first signs started to show approx. 6 years ago.

My mother and I have often discussed how this disease has affected his playing peer group of similar age, namely:

Verdi Godwin (now deceased)

Don Hunter (now deceased)

Harry Boyle (now deceased)

Albert Cheesebrough

These gentlemen all suffered dementia (Albert still living at home with his wife but now showing dementia signs). With the exception of Albert who is younger, they all played alongside my father and have been lifelong friends.

It does question the safety of continual heading of a football. Especially in my father's day when they said balls were so heavy.

The Justice for Jeff campaign gained extraordinary traction, fast. The FA were bang to rights and they knew it. After a period of procrastination from football's governing body, to his credit FA chairman Greg Dyke accepted his organization had badly failed the Astles and all Jeff's fellow players and their families.

And on 11 April 2015, Dyke apologized in person to the Astle family at the launch of the Jeff Astle Foundation, as I watched on with fellow patrons comedian Frank Skinner, Professor Willie Stewart and others in a hospitality box at the Hawthorns, home of West Brom.

Dyke looked me straight in the eye and said:

We promised the Astle family we would do some research and we didn't and that is a failure by the FA and yes, we are now going to do it.

It's going to be done. There will be a piece of work about head injuries and football. We want to get FIFA involved as well because if we draw some profound conclusions we'll need to get everyone involved.

We'll help fund the research and we'll put together a working group and we'll help fund it too. You need to separate the emotion and do the research and ask, 'What do we understand?' The suggestion of the Astle family is that head injuries are more likely to lead to early onset dementia and that is to do with heading the ball or physical contact. That's what we need to investigate and understand.

Let's see what the research finds and get FIFA involved too because this isn't going to be a British-only phenomenon, it's going to be a worldwide phenomenon. It won't disappear, that is for certain. That was a bad mistake by the FA [to not carry out research].

For what it's worth, I believed him. Football, it seemed, was waking up to concussion. It was another significant victory for our campaign.

14

Going rogue

A few weeks after handing in my notice at the *Mail on Sunday* I received a phone call from Stephen Jones at the *Sunday Times*. Now the highest-profile rugby union journalist in the world, Steve had been one of the trio of reporters – alongside Stuart Barnes and Paul Morgan – I had sat in front of with my dear friend Matt on that bleary-eyed flight from Brisbane to Canberra following the Lions' epic first Test win in 2001. He had since become a rival, travelling companion and, most importantly, a trusted friend. I respected him equally as a journalist and a human being.

A very different reporter to Peter Jackson, Steve is one of just a small handful of specialist sports writers who is not an ex-player whose opinion matters more than his ability to gather news stories. But to observe him phone in a 1,000-word match report to the desk within seconds of the final whistle is to observe a master at work. His sometimes intentionally provocative style is not to everyone's taste. But I had been lucky enough to get to know him as a friend. And my world was richer for it.

So when Steve told me another man I respected enormously, Steve Bale, the former *Independent* and *Daily Express* rugby correspondent who had also been a trusted travelling companion over the years, was retiring as a rugby writer at the *Sunday Times* and I should apply immediately, my ears pricked up.

Our daughter Ella was only a few days old and Debs and I had been talking seriously for months about setting up our own business away from sports journalism. And having fought so hard to improve player welfare over the years, often feeling like the lone voice in the room, I was also jaded and scarred by all the battles I'd fought.

For family reasons, I knew I'd made the right call to quit the *Mail on Sunday*. But the nagging doubt persisted that I'd walked away at the very point the problems I'd warned about for years were beginning to manifest. Deep down, I knew there was still work to do.

Since the start of the campaign in 2013, concussion numbers in professional rugby had gone through the roof. From the absurdly low figure of just 20 recorded concussions in English professional rugby in 2005/06, the year before Lewis Moody was twice allowed to play on after being knocked unconscious against Tonga in a World Cup pool game, to 41 the year before we launched our campaign to 86 the year of launching (2013/14).

As the attention remained, so the numbers continued to go up. In 2014/15, 110 concussions were recorded, then 113 in 2015/16, and by 2016/17 this figure had shot up to a jaw-dropping 169 recorded concussions in one season. A staggering 312 per cent increase in recorded concussions since the RFU's head of medicine had calmly said in a video supposedly aimed at raising awareness of the issue: 'Do I believe concussion is a problem within our game long term? No. Not at the moment.'

From one concussion being recorded every 6.85 matches in 2003/04, there was now one being recorded every 0.79 matches. In other words, more than one every match.

Matchday injuries were now also demonstrably worse than ever before, while perhaps most alarming were the figures I was seeing in training where the injury landscape, not just with concussions, was getting worse season by season. Eddie Jones' coaching methods had seemingly contributed to a significant rise in the figures, although they were tracking up anyway with an eye-watering 429 training ground injuries sustained by professional rugby players in England in 2016/17, up from 159 in the first year of the audit in 2002/03. Of these, 10 could be classed as 'career-threatening' including the unfortunate Sam Jones, who announced in March 2018 that he would never play rugby again following his ill-advised judo session with Maro Itoje in Brighton in 2016. A year later, that figure rose to 12.

By 2018/19, the frequency of training ground injuries would rise again to 528, and by 2019/20, an astonishing 551 injuries were suffered by professional rugby players in training in England alone.

My emotions were mixed. On the one hand I could at least take comfort from the fact I was not going mad. My predictions and worst-case forecasts were all coming true. But my overall sense was one of bitter frustration and anger that it had taken so long to recognize the problem which had been playing out before our very eyes.

Concussion was now the most likely injury for a professional player to suffer and the data was undeniable.

By the end of 2017, and with the CISG still insisting there was no proven 'cause and effect relationship' between concussion and CTE, Kemp was calling for government support to help solve rugby's burgeoning crisis and a 'major public health initiative to increase awareness of concussion'.

In an interview with the *Neuro Rehab Times* in October 2017 he said:

> Sport in general needs to answer the question of whether there is an association between playing sports and neurocognitive decline.
>
> It's a difficult question to answer because, as we age, we all see neurocognitive decline, which is one of the reasons for the limited amount of evidence around to date. We acknowledge that there may be an association [between rugby and CTE] but the reality is that the available evidence is limited and conflicting.

Unlike some other sports, we do actually have a long-term study underway, involving 205 ex-rugby players, most of whom were England internationals. Rugby has been pretty upfront about this issue.

The article also revealed that 'The RFU is working on the study with the London School of Hygiene & Tropical Medicine and researchers from Queen Mary University of London, The Institute of Occupational Medicine, University College London and Oxford University. It is backed by £450,000 in funding from The Drake Foundation, which supports sports concussion research. Results are expected to be published next year.'

Completely overlooking the massive spike in training ground injuries, and the rise in career-threatening injuries, which in 2017/18 would rise to a record 12, Kemp's failure to face facts continued, when he said: 'In the professional game, reported concussions have been going up dramatically over the last five years but all other contact injuries have remained stable. We think the rise is because we are much better at recognizing it.'

I was also not alone in being seriously concerned about the trickledown effect of professional rugby into schools and attempts to replicate the HIA and return to play protocols lower down the game. Worryingly, this was something Kemp seemed comfortable with.

'Some independent schools with big rugby programmes have even developed an approach to player recovery that looks very similar to that of professional clubs.'

So schoolchildren were being treated like professionals and this was somehow OK? Not just OK. Actively promoted.

And, just as the NFL's Elliott Pellman had with new helmet technology, Kemp continued to present completely unproven technologies as some kind of concussion panacea which would magic away the problem.

In August 2017, shortly after the worst concussion figures in the history of professional rugby had been published, a story appeared in *The Times* suggesting 'two millilitres of saliva may soon be all that is required to determine whether or not a rugby player has suffered a concussion.' Kemp was quoted as saying this supposedly revolutionary saliva test, being developed by Professor Tony Belli at Birmingham University, would be 'game changing'. The problem, like so many of the technologies promoted around this time, was that it was still nowhere near close to being proved reliable, safe or effective. But it got a headline, sating the media's appetite to show something was being done when in fact the problem was just getting worse.

There was no doubt rugby was ahead of football in its management and implementation of concussion protocols by now, although hardly a high bar to judge itself by, and I was prepared to give credit to the sport for finally getting ahead of the curve on that front.

At the start of 2017 I'd written several articles contrasting rugby union's position with football, with one praising the sport for 'moving decisively' on concussion. It was all relative. In reality, both sports had dragged their heels for decades and continued to do so. Rugby could barely keep the lid on the truth any longer.

Importantly for me, my friends and colleagues in the media were beginning to recognize the value in the work that I'd done and I was hugely flattered by Steve Jones's approach regarding the imminently vacant position at the *Sunday Times*.

Steve told me he wanted me to be his No.2. I would gather news stories and keep the pressure on the authorities, building on the work I'd done at the *Mail on Sunday* and taking the lead on player welfare-related issues. Over the past five years I'd established myself as the leading authority on concussion in sport across the English media and, as friends who'd both been routinely shortlisted as rugby journalist of the year at the Sports Journalists Awards over the past few years (Steve always won, I never did), neither of us doubted we could forge an effective and influential double act.

I applied for the position and before I knew it Alex Butler, the long-standing sports editor, invited me for an interview.

We got on well and Alex appeared interested in the work I'd done to that point. We devoured a plate of sandwiches in the hotel across the road from the *Times* building on the South Bank and discussed, among other things, the *Mail on Sunday*'s concussion campaign.

'Good campaign that,' Alex said. 'I often think it's one we should have run.'

He was charming and engaged and the conversation flowed, covering everything from concussion in rugby to me smuggling Richie Benaud out of the Lord's press box during the Pakistan spot-fixing scandal, which is a story I'll keep for another book. Overall, I felt the meeting couldn't have gone any better.

'Really good to meet you, Sam,' Alex said as I left. 'I'll let you know about the job in the next few days.'

Within two hours, he rang to offer me the job and I accepted.

I was elated. The idea of being No.2 to the highest-profile rugby writer on the planet in a paper with a reputation for brilliant sports coverage and a stable of superb writers including football correspondent Jonathan Northcroft, cricket correspondent Simon Wilde, rugby writer and good friend Stuart Barnes and, of course, David Walsh, was beyond my wildest dreams.

If I could build on the work I'd delivered at the *Mail on Sunday* in a paper so many rugby fans turned to for their coverage, the pressure for change I'd been calling for – including strict limits on contact training and fewer matches for the top players – would go up a gear.

But I was sorely mistaken. Literally within seconds of starting I knew I'd made a mistake. In the weeks leading up to my start date, I emailed Alex Butler several times to enquire about coming in to meet the team, discuss a plan of attack and generally acquaint myself. But he ignored every email. With a few days to go, I began to wonder if I'd imagined getting the job.

Then, just a few days before I was due to start, an email popped up from Butler inviting me to the office with the promise of lunch thrown in. I breathed a sigh of relief.

I turned up as agreed. Suited and booted. But Butler didn't. I was mortified. No excuse, no reason. Just a no show. It was the worst possible way to begin.

Over the course of the next few months I felt in complete limbo, realizing very quickly Alex had no interest in developing me as a journalist or using the network, knowledge and experience I'd built up over a decade to maintain pressure on rugby's authorities. I was an afterthought and felt completely undermined, and although I maintained an excellent relationship with Steve and Stuart Barnes, who remain friends to this day, few others on the paper gave me so much as a second glance or asked me to share my experience about concussion with them.

One Six Nations match, Wales v England at Cardiff, David Walsh, chief sports correspondent, sat alongside Steve, Barnes and myself in the press box. He never even asked me my name, let alone acknowledge the concussion movie I'd done. I didn't get a single word in the next day's paper. All the experience I'd built up, all the knowledge I had, all the battles I'd fought were for nothing. I was 40 years old but may as well have been a trainee back at the Press Association again. I had so much more to give but clearly no one – bar Steve and Barnesy – had the first clue what I was capable of.

'Life is too short,' I thought to myself that night. And I began to plot my escape.

*

Thankfully, the contract I had with the *Sunday Times* permitted me to work elsewhere.

*

Around the same time I'd been approached by the *Independent*'s sports editor Ed Malyon and asked to write a twice weekly column for them. Malyon, still in his early thirties, was energized, open minded and sharp as a tack. Reassuringly, he could not have been clearer about where he saw my strengths and said he wanted concussion and player welfare stories. And lots of them.

My relationship with the *Indy*, where I felt valued and respected, slightly offset the deep frustration I had at being ignored on the *Sunday Times*. They gave me a platform to write about the real issues in rugby.

Rugby's media had come a long way, no doubt, with many who had initially been hostile and sceptical about my message now supportive.

'The sport, to be fair, has reacted before to safety issues,' the *Telegraph*'s rugby correspondent Mick Cleary wrote in an article headlined 'Is rugby too dangerous for our kids?' in 2018. 'Perhaps it took too long but it has at least started to focus properly on concussion, albeit it took media lobbying from journalistic stalwarts such as Sam Peters to keep highlighting concerns.'

Meanwhile, World Rugby's attempts to empower referees by taking a 'zero tolerance' approach to head high tackles, which I largely supported, saw a predictable spike in red cards as players and coaches proved surprisingly slow to adapt.

Former players who had suffered dozens of head injuries themselves, now media pundits, were also still sometimes even slower to realize why the sport needed to change and why World Rugby was now attempting to do so. The 'rugby's gone soft' line bore no serious scrutiny but did not stop some who should have known better trotting it out.

In late 2017, Leicester's Manu Tuilagi was cited for recklessly making contact with the head of Munster's Chris Cloete, prompting former Ireland captain Brian O'Driscoll to tweet: 'I think the game has gone soft if we're picking up on marginal collisions like the Manu Tuilagi tackle he's been cited for.'

The citing commissioners agreed. 'It was found that Tuilagi had committed a reckless act of foul play in that his shoulder had made contact with Cloete's head but the committee was not satisfied that the offence warranted a red card,' a statement issued by the tournament organizers said.

Having such high-profile figures pushing back against change undermined what World Rugby was trying to achieve and I had some sympathy for them as a result. But the finding begged the question: was there zero tolerance of head contact or not?

The concussion and player welfare issue was now hotter than ever but almost every time I offered the *Sunday Times* a story they either weren't interested or didn't understand the nuance. Whereas Alison and Mike on the *Mail on Sunday* were able to grasp the issue through a combination of empathy, intellectual capacity and rugby knowledge, no one at the *Sunday Times* seemed to get it.

Eventually, more than six months after starting, I managed to convince them to let me run an article when the 2016/17 injury audit was published, several months later than normal.

The report made for seriously difficult reading for rugby fans, players and administrators alike. Concussions were up for a seventh year, with a record 169 concussions seeing the frequency rise to 20.9 per 1,000 playing hours.

Injury severity was also now outside of the expected range of year-on-year statistical variations while training ground injuries also stood at record levels with 429 injuries accounting for 36 per cent of all rugby injuries. It was astonishing to read.

By anyone's measure, even the most ardent of defenders of rugby union's injury risk profile, there was now an undeniable problem.

Perhaps the most telling line in the report read: 'While there has been a continued focus on improving concussion awareness and promoting behavioural changes among players, coaches, referees and medical staff, together with the introduction of real-time video into the Head Injury Assessment process, a change in the frequency and nature of game contact events cannot be excluded as a possible contributing factor to this increase [in concussion] and will be investigated.' Well, you don't say?

Finally, 23 years after the game turned professional, here was acknowledgement from the game's authorities that relentlessly speeding up the game 'cannot be excluded' as a factor in more frequent and severe injuries, including those to the brain.

The report continued:

> The incidence of training injuries rose during the 2016/17 season, having fallen in the two previous seasons. The average severity rose to its highest recorded level at 33 days. As a result of the increase in both incidence and severity of training injury the overall burden of training injury rose substantially for the 2016/17 season. In total, 36% of all injuries were sustained during training.
>
> There was a significant increase in the incidence and injury burden during full contact training. The most commonly occurring injury in these sessions was concussion. Determining training volume, intensity and activity involves balancing performance preparation with injury risk. In the 2016/17 season we saw increases in training injury burden, match injury burden and match contact injury incidence.

Even Kemp, the most vocal defender of rugby's safety record, finally had to concede action was needed: 'We need to look at identifying an effective but safe tackle technique to ensure that players can consistently deliver impactful tackles, while reducing the risk of inadvertent contact with an opponent's head, hip or knee.'

Tellingly, no one suggested reducing fixtures or introducing mandatory limits on contact training, even though it was clear World Rugby's move to tighten sanctions imposed for high tackles had done nothing to reduce concussion rates.

The RFU and Premiership Rugby's panic in the face of what I'd been telling them for years was evidenced by them copying the smoke and mirror PR tactics deployed by World Rugby a year earlier when they attempted to head off Patria Hume's report which found former rugby players who'd reported more than four concussions had poorer neurological function and reported worse health outcomes later in life. Before the official injury report findings were released, they issued an eight-point Professional Game Action Plan on Player Injuries.

Phil Winstanley, Premiership Rugby's long-standing rugby director, who along with CEO Mark McCafferty had only recently helped initiate the fixture landgrab which had so enraged almost every single professional player, said:

> Clearly the report has identified some significant challenges for us in relation to injury and player welfare.
>
> Player welfare has to and will remain at the centre of everything Premiership Rugby do as an organization and working with the RFU and RPA we have identified immediate actions which we have to take in addition to the work that we are already doing in this area.
>
> It is clear though that this is not just a Premiership issue: this is also a world game issue and we look forward to engaging with World Rugby to identify solutions which benefits [*sic*] all.

But rugby could no longer hide the truth. I'd been the canary down the mine, as one observer would later describe me as, screaming 'gas, gas, gas' for more than a decade and only now did the authorities accept there was a problem. They absolutely could and should have seen it coming.

Shockingly, the players were still being asked to play more rugby while injuries in training, despite us being told this was an area which had improved radically since the early days of professionalism, continued to rise rapidly.

In an interview with the BBC's Jamie Lyall, another who had written extensively about the issue, Willie Stewart gave his take.

> I know some former professional players who looked forward to the weekend match because it gave them a rest. During the week they were just getting destroyed.
>
> We're talking about diagnosable, recognisable brain injuries – there's more and more evidence coming that it's not just the ones that produce symptoms that are the problem, it's the cumulative effect of all the smaller ones as well, the ones that don't necessarily produce symptoms.
>
> If, during the week, instead of having several days of contact training with more and more impacts on top of each other, you do away with that, you're going to phenomenally reduce the number of impacts over the season and that can't be a bad thing.
>
> There's a whole lot of unnecessary exposure. Professional rugby players don't forget by Monday or Tuesday how to play rugby, how to tackle, how to go into a ruck…
>
> There comes a point where you have to say this is not an acceptable level and rugby reached that point several years ago. Rugby needs to change and cannot continue exposing people to a brain injury every match.

The neuropathologist also drew a comparison with boxing.

> If we think of boxing being a sport people shy away from because of the risks of brain injury then we're putting rugby in that league – that's why it has to change.

They're getting better at spotting the injury but that doesn't take away from the fact that the injuries are happening.

The bottom line is, we think brain injury is a problem and may pose a long-term problem for people who participate in these sports. Wouldn't it be better if we had the benefits and reduced the risks?

It was hard to disagree. Many still did.

But by the end of 2018, the absurdity of the position taken by the 'rugby's gone soft' brigade or those who had claimed the game was 'safer than ever' was illustrated in the most appalling terms.

In May, 17-year-old French rugby player Adrien Descrulhes did not realize he had suffered a brain injury on the field playing for amateur side Billom, where his father was the club secretary.

Adrien attended the club barbecue that evening but had a headache and felt nauseous and returned home to go to bed. He died in his sleep.

The coroner found he had suffered a fractured skull resulting in a catastrophic brain haemorrhage.

In August, Stade Aurillac wing Louis Fajfrowski, 21, was on the receiving end of a hard but legal chest-high tackle in a friendly against Rodez. He was treated on the field for several minutes but appeared to be recovering after going off.

But Louis soon became sleepy and nauseous and was taken to the changing room where he suffered three cardiac arrests and died.

'I don't know where rugby is going,' his heartbroken former team-mate Maxime Fucina would later say. 'I hope the league, federation and World Rugby will do something because it is scary. Louis was on the pitch. He asked nothing of anyone. He enjoyed rugby. One match and he is dead.'

Dr Jean Chazal, a French neurosurgeon, told Stuff.co.uk: 'The injuries we see today are more like road traffic accidents. The man who plays rugby today is heavier and runs faster. The shocks are stronger. It is a very big inflated engine on a chassis that was not designed to support it. These muscular players have the same bones, joints, tendons, internal organs, rib cage, brain and heart. It's a public health problem.'

An autopsy later recorded a verdict of accidental death from 'lethal fibrillation' following 'precordial chest trauma'.

In November, 23-year-old Nathan Soyeux, an engineering student in Dijon, also complained of nausea and losing consciousness after a tackle and was admitted to hospital, where he was placed in an induced coma. He died in January 2019.

In December, Stade Français youth flanker Nicolas Chauvin, 18, was hit by a two-man tackle playing against Bordeaux Bègles. He suffered a broken neck, brain damage and a cardiac arrest. Nicolas underwent emergency surgery but died three days later.

Nicolas's father, Philippe, gave a speech at Université Paris Descartes the following year where he warned rugby had given way to what he called 'the show'.

'The death of my son, following a fracture and tearing of the second cervical, is not normal,' he said. 'It is similar to a road accident or paragliding.'

In response to Chauvin's death, French sports minister Roxana Maracineanu called for rugby authorities to work towards making the game safer.

In December, the French Rugby Federation confirmed it would put together a global forum alongside World Rugby in March 2019 to discuss how to achieve this. To my surprise, I was invited.

'We were devastated by the series of fatal accidents,' World Rugby chief executive Brett Gosper said. 'For us it was a highly unusual spike. Deaths do happen from time to time in rugby, as they do in all sports, combat or otherwise, but we certainly haven't seen a run like this in a major rugby market, any rugby market actually.'

The use of the word 'market' when describing these tragedies summed up to me a sport whose administrators now knew the price of everything, but the value of nothing.

And it was against this backdrop that I fell out spectacularly with Steve Diamond.

The Sale Sharks director of rugby and former Russia Sevens coach had been on my radar since his 'slap on the head' comment in 2016. I'd also made it my business to keep close tabs on the Cillian Willis story and in doing so heard some stories about the culture within the Sale dressing room which made me extremely uncomfortable. Largely, I kept these stories to myself and will continue to do so in order to protect the individuals involved.

But despite my misgivings about Diamond, I certainly didn't travel to the AJ Bell Stadium on 22 September 2018 for Wasps' visit with the intention of writing the most provocative article of my career by some distance.

Sitting just a couple of rows away from Diamond in the press box, I could clearly hear him directing his medical team to keep Ben Curry on the field after the young flanker had suffered a neck injury just before half time.

'There's six minutes until half time, he's staying on,' Diamond shouted into his microphone. And stay on he did.

Then again, in the second half.

'What's wrong with him? Get him up,' he demanded when another Sale player with a facial injury was being tended by medics.

I'd witnessed some pretty grim stuff over the years but I honestly thought rugby had got past this sort of callous attitude towards medical staff and players. I was wrong.

The *Sunday Times* asked me for just 250 words on the match so there was no way I was going to get this sort of detail into it, but having witnessed Diamond's behaviour, I lit the blue touch paper on the train home.

Over the course of a two-hour journey from Manchester Piccadilly to London, I didn't hold back, reporting what I'd witnessed while also cataloguing a list of misdemeanours Diamond had committed over the past few years. It was a long charge sheet.

Despite what many including Diamond would later claim, there was actually very little of my opinion in it. Just a historical account of events which I believed reasonably represented his attitude to player welfare and concussion protocols at the time.

The previous week he had described referee Craig Maxwell-Keys as 'weak minded' and I felt it was time for someone in rugby to call him out.

'This was the same Diamond,' I wrote, 'who, in 2011, was given a 12-week suspended ban after admitting a charge of pushing Northampton Saints performance director Nick Johnston and making inappropriate comments in a TV interview.

'The same Diamond who was banned for 18 weeks for abusing match officials the following year and the same Diamond who publicly criticized the player welfare driven Head Injury Assessment (HIA) in 2016 when he was forced to move scrum half Mike Phillips to the wing in the second half of a game after concussed fly half Dan Mugford had been removed by medics.'

The article was published on the *Independent*'s website on Sunday morning and quickly went viral. My phone notifications immediately went ballistic. I was deluged with supportive messages from people within rugby, many who'd had to deal with Diamond first hand, including one former club press officer who claimed Diamond had pinned him to a wall because he was incensed by the changing facilities his team had been offered.

Unsurprisingly, Sale's fans were less enamoured with the article, as were Diamond and his son Sam, who was the club's media manager and who lodged a formal complaint with the Rugby Writers' Club, who immediately dismissed it.

If Diamond or anyone else at Sale had identified a single factual mistake in my copy they could have contacted me or the *Independent* and we would have taken steps to address it. But we never heard directly from anyone at Sale. Until the next game I covered with them in late December at Gloucester's Kingsholm Stadium, when Diamond was at it again, marauding around the press box screaming abuse at officials and Gloucester's players while also managing to have a row with a disabled spectator when she asked him to curb his language.

After the press conference finished, which I'd listened to but had declined to ask a question, Diamond made a beeline for me.

'You not asking me any questions?' the 50-year-old director of rugby demanded as he stood over me at my work desk.

'No, I don't need quotes,' I replied.

'You not asking me any questions?' he repeated.

'No, I don't need quotes,' I said again.

'No? No? What a pack of lies you wrote about me,' he stated as he loomed over my desk.

He was ticking. I asked him which part of the article was false or a lie.

'Where was the lie?' I asked.

'Loads of them,' he replied.

'Where? Go on, name one,' I said.

'Loads of them. Talking about HIAs,' he said.

Before I knew it he was offering me to go outside for a 'proper chat'.

I recalled the last time I'd felt physically threatened by a director of rugby: almost 10 years previously when Dean Richards had taken exception to an innocuous question in a press conference.

This time, at least I knew why Diamond was so incensed.

After initially declining the offer, and completely against my better judgement, I agreed to go outside into the stairwell by the lifts.

As soon as we were outside the media centre, Diamond turned to me. 'You fucking shithouse,' he growled, before realizing I was recording the incident and attempting to snatch my Dictaphone out of my hand while shouting 'get off me, get off me' as I stood by. He wanted it to sound as if I was attacking him on the tape.

'Get your hands off me,' he cried, as I tried to retrieve the property he'd ripped out of my hands a few moments before.

I remembered a comment a friend at Wasps had made to me once. He told me Diamond was a typical bully on the field who would be more than willing to take a cheap shot at the bottom of a ruck but if you squared up to him he'd always relent.

Verbally, I went on the attack, calling him a few choice names including a 'fucking bully', repeatedly.

It felt like I was venting years of frustration at a sport which had largely stood by and allowed players to be routinely abused without a thought for the longer-term consequences.

After a couple of minutes of verbally abusing each other, Diamond and I were parted bv freelance reporter Roger Panting, but not before Ben Coles, a staff reporter at the *Telegraph*, had recorded the tail end of the incident on his phone.

Afterwards, as we all caught our breath, Ben asked me what he should do with it, realizing the news value in footage showing a Premiership director of rugby involved in a heated verbal altercation with a reporter.

'Send it to your desk, mate,' I said. 'I've got nothing to hide.'

As I said this, my phone rang. It was the *Sunday Times* desk asking where my match report was. I apologized and told them I'd nearly been in a fight with Steve Diamond and would be late filing.

I was put on to Alex Butler and I told him what had happened.

'I'm sure you'd have taken him down,' he joked, but did not ask for any additional copy or a first-person account, which came as a surprise to me.

On the drive home my phone started ringing. A lot. The *Guardian* and *Telegraph* were running it as their lead story, complete with Ben's video footage in the latter's case, and the *Indy* wanted to know what the hell had happened.

I explained it was all to do with the original piece I'd written a few months earlier when I'd criticized Diamond's 'old school' methods. They asked me for a first-person piece to include 'every cough and spit' to be filed as soon as I could.

I'd fallen into the trap all journalists want to avoid. I had become the story. And I soon found out it was not a great place to be. Many no doubt felt I'd brought it on myself, which in several ways I had. I had dared to poke a bear who felt threatened and reacted pretty much as I'd expected.

But I was damned if I was going to be intimidated into not reporting what I'd seen with my own eyes. My first-person piece headlined 'I knew Steve Diamond was a bully – and now I know for sure' didn't exactly pour water on the flames. Ed Malyon would later tell me the article was the most read non-football story ever on the newspaper's website.

With the story dominating the sports agenda, Butler had obviously got it in the neck for hardly having a line about the incident in the paper and sent me a snotty email that Sunday night, as I was in the middle of the storm, demanding to know why I hadn't reported it and questioning my relationship with the *Independent*.

I replied immediately asking to speak with him in person. He never responded.

*

There's no doubt part of the reason I'd decided to write the original article was due to the intense frustration I'd felt at not being given any space in the *Sunday Times*. I'd already decided before writing it I was going to resign when the time was right, such was my lack of fulfilment in the job I was being asked to do.

Knowing I would soon be leaving the industry unquestionably influenced the tone of my reports. By removing any future commercial interest, I basically no longer cared whose cage I rattled. It was a very liberating feeling.

Again, I was reassured by the support I got from within the media, to my face at least, but the abuse I received from Sale's fans on social media was intense, highly personal and in some cases pretty extreme. It became, in social media terms, a pile on.

The story ran for several days and took a bizarre twist when, five days after the incident, former England winger Austin Healey, who I'd only ever met once when he broke wind in front of me and my friend, the severely injured war veteran Neil Heritage, on the set of BT Sport's *Rugby Tonight*, wrote a column in the *Telegraph* demanding I apologize.

I called Healey out on social media, asking why I should apologize and asking if he had more to reveal about his ties to Diamond. Within a couple of days Healey phoned me while I was in the car with my two-year-old daughter and started screaming abuse while on loudspeaker.

'Hold on, Austin,' I said after repeatedly being called a 'fucking wanker' by the former England star. 'My two-year-old is in the car, let me put you on to her, so you can speak to someone with the same mental age.' Then I hung up.

It was all getting a bit wearing. My case was not helped by another BT Sport interview conducted pitchside by Martin Bayfield, who I liked immensely and had always got on extremely well with, at Sale's next televised game. Diamond was given an extraordinarily easy ride with none of the accusations I'd made about his methods put to him and he accused me of being a 'rogue journalist'. I could live with that, I suppose, but I was disappointed Bayfield failed to press him on any of the charges.

The next time I saw the 6ft 10in former England lock, at Saracens' Allianz Park a couple of weeks later, Bayfield sought me out to apologize for not holding Diamond to account. I appreciated this and of course accepted the apology.

I write all this not because I have any interest whatsoever in restarting a war which, in truth, left neither Diamond nor me in much credit. But it hopefully gives some context to an incident which left neither of us in credit. I could feel myself drifting away from rugby.

*

Far more importantly, World Rugby were trying to work out how to respond to the tragic deaths in France which rocked the sport to its core in 2018 and early 2019.

With serious pressure now on them to act from the top of the French government, all playing out amid the backdrop of an attempted aggressive takeover of the sport by venture capital firm CVC Capital Partners, the sport's governing body were under intense scrutiny from all sides.

They decided to convene the first ever player welfare symposium, held at the French Rugby Federation's headquarters in Paris in February 2019. To my immense surprise, I was invited alongside Alex Lowe of *The Times* and Murray Kinsella from Irish website the42.ie.

A few days before the three-day symposium, the latest RFU and Premiership Rugby injury audit report – now rebranded the Professional Rugby Injury Surveillance Project – was published. And it was not good news.

Training injuries had continued to skyrocket, now sitting at a record 438 in the 2017/18 season, although concussion rates had dropped slightly from the previous year's record figures to the second highest ever recorded figure of 140 (17.9 per 1,000 playing hours). Career-threatening injuries were also the highest ever recorded with 12 in one season.

The overall burden of injury, combining incidence and severity, also stood at the highest level since records began in 2002.

A decade after rugby should have recognized what was coming down the track, even the staunchest defenders of the sport had to admit there was an issue.

'The data suggests that more significant changes to the game might be needed to reverse these trends,' said Kemp.

It was now clear to see the inadvertent impact Eddie Jones's methods were having on what was already a bleak picture when it came to training and injury risk.

Extraordinarily, RFU acting chief executive Nigel Melville attempted to justify this by arguing 'international rugby is played at great intensity so obviously they train at greater intensity.'

The previous October I'd written a piece for the *Independent* spotlighting the heightened injury risk of playing on artificial pitches, in which the RFU had in December 2015 announced they were to invest £50 million, rolling out 100 new plastic pitches. I'd witnessed several players rupture ankle and knee ligaments on the plastic pitches in what initially appeared completely innocuous incidents as their studs got caught in the fake turf. With stories of an increased risk of viral transmission and significant burns if pitches were not adequately watered, I felt more than justified in raising the issue.

My article sparked a sharp riposte from the RFU whose communications department climbed all over me, insisting the story had no merit and denying any evidence of a heightened risk.

So I was more than a little surprised to read this in the RFU and Premiership Rugby's own report:

> After five seasons it is also possible to describe the pattern
> of injuries on different playing surfaces in more detail. The
> incidence of injury was not different for any specific body
> region, but both severity and burden were greater for the lower
> limb on artificial turf compared with natural grass. Average
> severity for injuries to the lower limb on natural grass was

37 days compared with 50 days for injuries on artificial turf. Given that some lower limb injuries may be influenced by the traction between a player's boots and the pitch surface, with increased traction on artificial turf compared with natural grass under some conditions, this might contribute to the higher severity of lower limb injuries observed.

It was an astonishing admission. All those millions spent with no prior research carried out into the small matter of whether the pitches were more dangerous to play on.

Yet again, my concerns had only been met with derision and disdain from rugby's authorities.

I arrived at Charles de Gaulle airport with the same sense I was walking into the lion's den I'd had when I was summoned to interview Kemp at Twickenham in the early days of the campaign and the subsequent IRB medical conference in Dublin when Gosper told me his organisation was 'not a cigarette company'.

I expected my fellow symposium attendees to be hostile towards me and I was ready to have to justify a lot of what I'd written over the previous decade.

But almost as soon as I arrived, having shared an interesting taxi ride from the airport with former Scotland director of rugby Australian Scott Johnson, it seemed they were going to on a charm offensive.

Most of the great and the good in rugby were present including World Rugby president Bill Beaumont, CEO Brett Gosper, chief medical officer Martin Raftery and his newly appointed deputy Eanna Falvey along with senior representatives from the RFU and Premiership Rugby led by Kemp, Winstanley and Ryan, who was by now head of player development at the RFU. Hopley was also there, along with several high-profile former players and medics employed by the respective unions.

Beaumont sought me out early on, welcoming me with a big smile and vicelike handshake.

'Eh up, Sam. How's Dimes?' he quipped with a grin, referring to Steve Diamond.

Everyone was friendly, even Raftery and Kemp, and there were times when I felt relaxed in the esteemed company. I had to check myself not to fall into the trap of getting too cosy and too used to the lavish amounts of food and alcohol on offer.

I did, however, fall into the trap of muting my beliefs when at short notice I was invited onto a panel on the first morning alongside former All Black captain Conrad Smith and Springbok captain Jean de Villiers who were representing the International Rugby Players' Association. Without a clear brief, I felt hijacked and seriously out of place on stage alongside two rugby legends as Dominic Rumbles fired a succession of leading questions implying rugby safety had improved and media attitudes had too. To the best of my recollection, nothing was said about the four French players who'd died.

We were not permitted to record proceedings, so I cannot relate what precisely was said, although I acknowledged some of the good work I believed World Rugby had done while also accepting how difficult it could be to effect changes purely for safety reasons.

I listened intently and was especially interested in recent research showing coaches and directors of rugby were the least educated of all rugby's shareholders when it came to concussion. Now why didn't that surprise me?

I also listened intently to a presentation from Kemp and Ryan on why a tackle trial undertaken in the English Championship the previous season attempting to lower concussion rates had been cut short when data emerged showing it was having the opposite effect.

Kemp explained that players struggled to adapt to different laws in different competitions, while the 'below shoulder' directive had not been clearly enough explained to enable them to continue 'soak' tackles close to the breakdown which had not previously been penalized. By attempting to adhere too strictly to the new law, Kemp argued, players were ducking in too low to make tackles, getting their heads into awkward positions, and a spike in concussions occurred next to the breakdown as a result. The law of unintended consequences.

Some ideas were thrown around about how to make the game safer and, following fairly loose discussions, a couple seemed to get traction. One being Scott Johnson's '40–20' kick, which he argued would remove defenders from the line to defend deeper. The following year this was enacted into law.

France seemed ready to go it alone and soon after the event announced they would be carrying out a 'below waist' tackle trial effectively outlawing double tackles in the process. The move was not popular among any of the delegates I spoke to, with Kemp pushing for the reinstatement of the 'below armpit' trial which had failed in the Championship the previous season.

There were undoubtedly lots of good intentions but there was also a self-congratulatory air about the event and, to my mind anyway, a distinct lack of solemnity considering the four tragic reasons we were there.

And that sense of levity continued in the bar on both nights when an impressive amount of the European Champions Cup sponsor's product was consumed, all paid for by World Rugby, with boisterous evenings culminating in Hopley playing the piano while leading a rousing rendition of 'Leaving on a Jet Plane'. The party continued into the small hours. Considering why we were there, this felt in poor taste.

Having been among a tiny handful of journalists present to witness first hand what had been billed in some quarters as 'the most important gathering in rugby history', I felt sure I would be asked for the inside track by the *Sunday Times*. But I wasn't.

Instead, it was left to David Walsh, who hadn't previously shown much appetite for the concussion story, to write the 'definitive' piece on a symposium he hadn't even attended. Perhaps if he'd sought my view, I could have told him the event took place in Paris, not Dublin as he wrote in his article.

That was the final straw for me at the *Sunday Times* and, within a few weeks, I'd handed in my notice. Steve tried to convince me otherwise but I'd made my decision.

It was a huge relief leaving. I had put in a shift on the concussion front line and it was time to hand over the reins to someone else.

The following year, the last one reported on before the Covid-19 pandemic shut down the world and disrupted all data collection, concussion rates in English rugby remained staggeringly high with 159 recorded cases in the 2019/20 season, representing a 695 per cent increase in 14 years. In the same season there were a record 551 training ground injuries, representing 44 per cent of injuries sustained by professional players.

15

The bomb goes off

From the moment I started reading about former NFL stars suffering serious neurodegenerative problems in their forties and fifties, it began to concern me we'd see the same picture emerge in professional rugby union. Still in its relatively early days of professionalism, it was obvious to me rugby was now absolutely on a par in terms of the speed and size of collisions witnessed in American football. But with some players playing more than 40 games a season, as opposed to a maximum of 18 in the NFL, and the volume of collisions far higher per match in rugby, there was a strong argument that the American sport was actually far safer to play. Add to that the strict limits on contact training and face to face exposure to coaches, thanks largely to a robust and properly funded independent players' union, NFL stars now enjoyed levels of protection their rugby league and union counterparts could only dream of. They were also incredibly well payed.

But even when I started writing about the possibility of rugby union facing a dementia crisis, I obviously never wanted it to come true.

So, it was a chilling moment when former England players Steve Thompson and Michael Lipman, along with former Wales No.8 Alix Popham, publicly stated they'd been diagnosed with early onset dementia and probable CTE caused by the head injuries they suffered during their careers.

The trio, along with five other players all aged under 45, were part of a legal test case being brought against World Rugby, the RFU and the Welsh Rugby Union which could, and most probably would, change the face of the sport forever.

I'd known about these cases for several weeks, if not months, before the story broke, but, having been contacted by the legal firm representing the ex-players in the summer of 2020, I did not write about them, having signed a non-disclosure agreement before sharing what I knew – all of which is in this book – with the players' solicitor, Richard Boardman.

There wasn't much I hadn't heard by now when it came to concussion and its after-effects on players and their families, or so I thought, but even to me the testimonies the players gave were harrowing.

Thompson, who I'd cheered on when I was a fan and got to know when I'd become a journalist, was the first player to 'go public' when he spoke to Andy Bull of the *Guardian*.

'You see us lifting the World Cup and I can see me there jumping around. But I can't remember it,' Thompson said.

'I'd rather have just had a normal life. I'm just normal. Some people go for the big lights, whereas I never wanted that. Would I do it again? No, I wouldn't. I can't remember it. I've got no feelings about it.'

A World Cup winner in 2003 alongside the likes of Wilkinson, Moody, Johnson and Dallaglio, Thompson, who used to pride himself on his ability to remember myriad complicated lineout calls, was capped 73 times including the World Cup final, of which he has no recollection.

'I can't remember at all being there. Honestly, I don't know scores from any of the games.'

Thompson also spoke of the sense of despair he felt at forgetting basic directions, leaving his car running with keys in the ignition and, perhaps most upsetting of all, his wife's name.

'I could look at Steph sometimes. And she says it's like I'm a complete blank. And she'll go: "I'm Steph." The name's gone. Gone.'

Thompson also talked about suffering anxiety, mood swings and extreme fatigue.

Even with all the work I'd done in this space and knowledge of the risks I'd built up by now, I still couldn't quite bring myself to believe this was true.

A few months later I'd sit down with Thompson to film the BBC's *Head On* documentary. After we'd stopped filming in the office I sometimes use adjacent to my parents' house, I took Steve inside to meet my dad, an avid rugby fan, and my mum.

Mum chatted away merrily with Steve as Dad stood back in awe and at one point Mum asked him: 'So how many kids have you got, Steve?'

Thompson, who up to that point had been lucid and coherent, stopped in his tracks. He paused, waited, took a deep breath and paused again. His face had taken on a completely blank expression.

'Sorry, what did you say?' he asked.

'How many kids have you got, Steve?'

'I'm really sorry, I've got no idea,' he replied. It was a sobering moment. His dementia was evident.

The revelations from Thompson, Lipman and Popham rocked the sport to its foundations.

'There is no doubt this is the biggest situation in the history of our game, after some very distressing news about Steve and the other players last week. The challenge is how we move the dial forward,' said Damian Hopley, at that stage still chief executive of the RPA.

A spokesperson for World Rugby said: 'While not commenting on speculation, World Rugby takes player safety very seriously and implements injury-prevention, management and education strategies based on the latest available knowledge, research and evidence.'

A few weeks later I would visit Popham at his home in Newport, south Wales, where I spent two hours in the company of him and his wife Mel. Like so many of the players and their families who I'd spoken to over the past decade or more, they struck me as honest, determined, rugby-loving people who had become increasingly distrusting of the motives of the sport's authorities.

The worst predictions from the campaign were coming true. Young men, my age, suffering dementia in their forties. I'd asked so many doctors – Simon Kemp and Martin Raftery among them – in the early stages of the campaign if we were not better off erring on the side of caution in case the reported link between repetitive head injuries and early onset dementia proved stronger than they said they believed it to be at the time. Their response, Kemp's especially, was to accuse those of us who wanted to rein the sport back in of wanting to turn it into a non-contact sport. Here we were, less than 10 years later, witnessing the ticking timebomb we'd talked about going off. The players and their families were collateral damage in professional rugby union's greedy obsession with growth.

Predictably, there were doubters, Thompson's former team-mate Lawrence Dallaglio among them. Former rugby league star John Devereux was vociferous on social media where he insisted players 'knew what they had signed up for', which of course was complete tripe when it came to long-term brain damage but played well to the 'game's gone soft' brigade and anyone else who believed employers had no duty of care to employees.

Meanwhile, I was made aware of a number of current players' WhatsApp groups who were actively bad-mouthing the claimants, and Thompson himself suffered vicious abuse on social media including accusations of being an 'ambulance chaser', and 'rugby hater', while one woman on Twitter accused him of 'ruining rugby for her son'. After a decade out of the public eye, and following a diagnosis of early onset dementia, the abuse and hostility were understandably difficult to deal with for Thompson and his family.

The day after the news broke I was invited onto the *Times* podcast The Ruck with my old friend Stephen Jones, respected colleague Owen Slot and Lawrence Dallaglio, Thompson's former England team-mate.

Being at the height of the pandemic, the podcast was recorded via Zoom and as soon as the screen came up it was very obvious to me from his body language Dallaglio was hostile. A shareholder and board member at Wasps, as well as a media pundit with a host of rugby-related business interests, Dallaglio was one of the tiny handful of professional rugby players who had managed to stay relevant and maintain his profile in the sport after he retired.

And with multiple ex-player media pundits by definition still having commercial interests in the sport, most are compelled to defend it, warts and all. A rare few, and I'd include David Flatman and Monye in this group, are prepared to speak with more honesty. Others choose to toe the party line , or play down the reality of an issue which came with reputational risk for the game.

Owen opened proceedings and it was all convivial, despite Dallaglio's body language, which the listeners couldn't see, and it was humbling when Owen, who described the dementia revelations as 'bringing the future of the whole game very much under threat', gave me a special welcome in his introduction.

'I'm joined by Stephen Jones, Lawrence Dallaglio, who of course played in that 2003 team with Thompson, and Sam Peters. Sam is a journalist who has done more than anyone to forewarn the game of the possible dangers. He was writing about this stuff almost a decade ago. Unfortunately, we now know that he was right.'

Dallaglio was given the first opportunity to speak and I was taken aback by his lack of empathy for what his former team-mate was experiencing.

Well, to be honest with you, it's the first I've heard of it, which is a worry. I mean, Steve is not someone I've spent a lot of time with, since he retired and since I retired, primarily because he moved out to Dubai…

But I mean, listen, first of all, you know, very sad, really sad to hear and to read, you know, quite graphically, the struggles that he's had. I mean, I guess, as I said, I don't think myself or any of the team were aware of it. So, he's either on the other side of the world, or just keeping his thoughts to himself, until he's got together with some of the other people, and one of the lawyers.

As Dallaglio was a firm fixture in rugby's establishment, perhaps I shouldn't have been as surprised as I was that he was so determined to defend the sport's authorities while insinuating Thompson and his fellow dementia sufferers were complaining about nothing. He continued:

Clearly, concussion has always been a bit of a threat. It's got bigger and bigger because of the number of collisions and the size of those collisions in the last 10 or 15 years. But I think, as an ex-player, that a lot has been done by rugby to try and come to terms with concussion and deal with concussion. I think the sport could still continue to do a lot more, but there's no doubt that when the NFL came out with their commission, I think rugby moved quite quickly, to put together a series of protocols, and have those protocols in place, so the players can safely be taken away from the field of play.

But my fundamental understanding is when the NFL report was commissioned into American football, and the head collisions and the concussion, what they deduced, what they found was that the sport had already commissioned a lot of research into head injuries, and they knew the dangers and the inherent risks of what was going on, and they failed to do anything about it.

Which is fundamentally very serious, you know. If you as an employee are participating in a sport, where there's been a ton of research done on the laws of that sport, and on the collisions of that sport, and then the information is withheld from you as a player, I think you have a massive case to answer as a governing body. In which the NFL, you know, very quickly moved to get rid of, by settling out of court, you know, quite substantially in America.

As I understand this, Sam, and please correct me if I'm wrong, but the governing bodies of the RFU, World Rugby and the WRU, once that report was read, and the information was taken on board, maybe they started to take the whole subject of concussion much more seriously. And I think they didn't withhold information there, they actually implemented a series of protocols from that moment onwards, which continued to be reviewed on a regular basis.

Because I really do understand it's a serious matter, but it does have a whiff of 'have you been injured at work' about it.

Dallaglio's last line took my breath away but unquestionably remains a strongly held view within the game. In some people's eyes, these former players pursuing legal recompense are little more than ambulance-chasing money grabbers. Dallaglio as good as said it and I have subsequently viewed private WhatsApp comments on players' forums and public comments directed at Thompson via social media which suggest he is not alone in that view.

Stephen Jones picked up on Dallaglio's tone.

First of all, the reason we are all here is because of the real journalism Sam has done. I put Sam's campaign in the same orbit as David Walsh with Lance Armstrong. Marie Colvin's war reporting, people who just almost gave up their lives and certainly popularity to follow the story. And Sam followed it through when it was lonely.

To my shame, until Sam and I worked together on the paper, I hadn't really gone into anything. When we did work together, I thought this is a great campaign. I don't think we ever did in our paper, that's my paper, about the debates. But you know, I think that ambulance chasing is when people jump on the bandwagon. Well, at the top of this pile, eight people have been officially diagnosed with early onset dementia.

And I really give you credit, Sam, for battering through, and I hope you feel a bit now like David Walsh felt, when he had Lance Armstrong at his feet.

In truth, I didn't know how I felt. It was hard to feel elated when I knew the long-term consequences of the concussions I'd been reporting on were becoming reality. I was also saddened by the hostility I continued to face from many within the game, even now when players were coming forward in their thirties and forties with dementia.

I was critical of the RPA during the podcast, searching for some common ground between Dallaglio and myself where we could agree more should have been done to protect the players, rather than leaving the burden all on them. But he was reluctant to state what everyone in the sport knew at the time: the organization had let their members down. It baffled me why he wouldn't go there.

The following summer an RPA press release dropped in my inbox:

The Rugby Players Association is proud to announce our new partnership with specialist foreign exchange consultants Elite FX. The new three-year partnership with the RPA will not only include first-rate financial consultancy, but Elite FX will also be sponsoring an award at the annual RPA Awards as well as supporting our charity efforts with Restart.

Lawrence Dallaglio, former England rugby captain and an Elite FX director, said: 'Most players just want to focus on their sport and too often lack expert help to navigate the markets, making them vulnerable to negative movements. With Elite FX on your side you can make sure your money is protected.'

I groaned. Of course.

And Dallaglio was far from the only former team-mate of Thompson's to provide a lukewarm response.

Speaking on the BBC's Rugby Union Weekly podcast, Matt Dawson said it was his choice to play the game, and he 'knew what he was getting into'.

No one forced me to do this. In my era they [the authorities] acted with their best knowledge of the scenario.

I don't feel the game has let me down. The whole of my life is because I chose to play rugby, I'm a big boy, I made that decision.

I picked my vocation and I will take the consequences, I'm owning up to them, I'm having them so I've got to deal with them.

If they're bad then I've got to deal with them. But I'm not going to sit here and blame anyone, say it was anybody's fault. Whether I've got dementia now or whether I have it in 20 years.

Others were at least able to admit rugby's failings, especially those who were less commercially bound to the sport through media work.

Seven years after being knocked out and playing on in the Premiership final, Toby Flood, soon after the litigation was announced, told the *Telegraph*:

The sport is unrecognizable from when I started. The physiques of kids coming out of school is unbelievable. They can lift such massive weights. They are such athletes. No wonder there is such little space on the field. Every blade of grass gets covered.

You used to be able to study an opposition and figure out where there might be a defensive frailty. Not any more. The game is at a crossroads. The concussion issues are terrifying. There is real violence in the hits we see on the field.

One of the reasons I'd been able to gather so much information through the early stages of the campaign was because I'd stepped away from sport and the media's cult of celebrity. Guys like Nic Berry, Andy Hazell, Will Skinner and Dave Jackson were hardly household names away from their own clubs' fanbases, and without the need to leverage their media profiles for commercial gain, they were able to speak with real honesty and integrity about their concerns for the sport.

I realized those with the highest profile had most to lose from being seen to criticize the game, and it was after the legal case was announced that I spoke with another journeyman player, the 44-year-old former Rotherham and Gloucester flanker Neil Spence, who told me he received bangs on the head 'pretty much every game'.

'Day to day is a bit of a struggle,' he told me in a typically staccato and clipped speech pattern I'd become accustomed to when talking to people suffering from brain injuries.

Just general confusion. General tasks. I feel a bit slow with everything I do. I have to think meticulously about where I'm going, what I'm doing, what I need to take. I'm working as a schoolteacher. Have I got my laptop bag? Have I got all my pens and everything else?

'I've become very hesitant in a car. I live on an estate and I'll drive to the top of the road where there's a roundabout and Sarah will have to say pretty much every time we get to it where we need to go. Even though I know exactly where I'm going when I leave the house, by the time I get to the roundabout I'm completely blank. No idea whatsoever where I'm meant to go. Do I turn left or right? No idea.

I'll leave things in the wrong places and not notice. My fiancée Sarah has found dirty dishes in the fridge and food items in the dishwasher. I'll leave things on. The oven. The iron.

The main thing that made me think everything wasn't OK was when I went to pick up my two children from nursery one afternoon but drove past their nursery completely and went to set up for a coaching session. I was working as an RFU community coach at the time. I was meant to be picking my kids up from nursery but by the time I realized, the school had closed. It was only 500 yards down the road but I was in completely the wrong location.

But, with head still firmly in the sand, RFU chief executive Bill Sweeney parroted the same lines I'd heard from Kemp almost a decade earlier.

'There is no scientific proof of the causal link between concussion and CTE, that is not a proven thing, and research is ongoing into that,' said Sweeney. 'There are differences between American football and rugby union.'

Others applauded the move to take legal action, including Sir Clive Woodward.

'After the stand taken by Steve Thompson, Alix Popham, Michael Lipman and others, rugby must address the issues and take the initiative,' Woodward wrote in the *Daily Mail*. 'In such a physical game, player welfare is everything and, if rugby is to thrive, we must acknowledge this fully, with a view to making the present and future much safer at every level of the game… Of course the physical nature of rugby is a huge part of its appeal but we have definitely gone so far down that path that "physicality" has overpowered the game.'

Since Thompson, Lipman and Popham first went public with their diagnoses more than 225 players have joined the case and I can only see that number going up as more players learn how rugby's authorities buried their heads in the sand about the mounting injury risk in a bid to grow the commercial base.

And it is not just professional rugby union which has an issue. In October 2022, 75 former rugby league players joined the class action suit, while in early 2023 another 55 former amateur union players joined the legal case against the RFU, World Rugby and WRU.

Richard Boardman, of Rylands Legal, said:

> We are seeing the same worrying symptoms in numerous cases across both codes of rugby. These symptoms include chronic depression, aggression, significant memory loss, incontinence, drug and alcohol addiction, and, in some cases, suicide attempts.
>
> This claim isn't just about financial compensation; it is also about making the game safer and ensuring current and former players get tested so that if they are suffering a brain injury, they can get the clinical help they need. The players we represent love the game.

And, despite what Dawson, Devereux and others say, it is simply not true to suggest players knew what they were getting into in the early days of professionalism because so few doctors at that time were prepared to discuss or relate the information about long-term neurodegenerative diseases which was available to them. Many doctors didn't even know, in part because they weren't told by those privy to some of the historic research. Others chose not to relate what they knew or mispresented current data or previously accepted science and research to the point of devaluing it completely.

In March 2022, Paul McCrory, this century's most influential sports doctor, who once described CTE as 'all that hoo-ha going on in the States' and spent much of his working life denigrating independent research, both old and new, while on sport's payroll, was exposed as a plagiarist.

Nine months earlier, researcher Steve Haake had emailed editors at the *British Journal of Sports Medicine* complaining that an article they'd published in 2005, written by McCrory and titled 'The Time Lords – Measurement and Performance in Sprinting', included large sections of his own research which had originally been published in *Physics World* in 2000 and titled 'Physics, Technology and the Olympics'.

'I put the articles side by side and compared them: of 1,106 words in McCrory's article, 560 were mine (50.7%). Not only that, but the narrative arc of the article was exactly the same. I was outraged,' Haake would later write on his blog.

'I sent an email to the editor of the *BJSM* notifying them of plagiarism by McCrory. They got back to me the same day to say it would be investigated by the parent company, the *British Medical Journal.*'

After six months of waiting, Haake was notified that the investigation had found McCrory guilty of committing an 'unlawful and indefensible breach of copyright' and the offending article would be retracted.

This alone was hugely damaging for McCrory's reputation. Plagiarism, in the world of research, along with misrepresenting previous work, is about as egregious as it gets. McCrory emailed Haake apologizing profusely while blaming the error on accidentally uploading the incorrect draft of the manuscript.

His email to Haake on 1 March 2022 stated:

I was unaware this problem had happened until I was
contacted by the editor of the *BMJ* in December 2021 and
once I realized this terrible error I requested that the paper be

retracted formally. The *BMJ* editor told me that any retraction would likely result in adverse media for me and possible academic sanctions. Nevertheless I felt it important that the retraction should be made as soon as possible. This episode reflects extremely poorly on my due diligence in this regard.

Once again I offer my sincere and humble apologies for this episode and would emphasize that this was an isolated and unfortunate incident.

It was, in fact, nothing of the sort. Sending off a series of emails, McCrory embarked on a desperate face-saving exercise. But it was too late. Within an hour of receiving McCrory's first email, Haake received another, this time from Nick Brown of Linnaeus University in Sweden, 'telling me that he has already found two further editorials by McCrory in which 80–90% of the words have been copied from elsewhere'.

Australian newspaper the *Herald Sun* ran a story headlined 'AFL's key concussion advisor accused of "inventing research" after plagiarism storm' in which concussion campaigner Peter Jess was quoted as saying: 'This is a scandal. The fundamental basis of research is integrity and honesty. And he's been found guilty of taking something that is not his and saying it is.'

But it got worse. Much worse. With Brown, a relentless data sleuth, now on his case, the true extent of McCrory's corrupt practice was exposed with Brown uncovering no fewer than 10 plagiarized articles within a matter of days. With nowhere to turn McCrory resigned from the Concussion in Sport Group, upon which he had sat as the single most powerful figure for almost two decades. Without fanfare, he also exited stage left from Michael Turner's International Concussion and Head Injury Research Foundation, which had championed its association with McCrory, using a picture of him alongside Turner at Croke Park in the launch press release in April 2016, which stated: 'The Scientific Committee is chaired by Professor

Paul McCrory, widely recognized as a global leader in the field of concussion research.'

The fact McCrory had published no credible research into CTE, as exposed by Australian investigative reporter Wendy Carlisle in 2018, was conveniently overlooked by many.

Gradually, other organizations began to distance themselves from McCrory; his biography on the University of Melbourne website disappeared overnight. The Australian Football League also moved to disassociate themselves from him.

And as with so many things related to concussion, the more people dug, the more they found.

By September 2022, the *BMJ* had admitted there was now an 'ongoing effort' to identify all the articles of which McCrory was sole author after all 10 articles initially identified by Brown in March were retracted.

'Dr McCrory has been churning out very similar stories for 20 years, while, as far as I have been able to establish, performing very little original empirical or other research in that time,' Brown said. 'If you're saying exactly the same thing about this topic as you did a decade ago, what kind of research are you doing?'

With McCrory having reserved much of his ire for the work of the Boston Group and the Concussion Legacy Foundation, led by Professors Ann McKee and Bob Cantu along with Chris Nowinski, who had done so much to expose sport's links with CTE, the group understandably had plenty to say when their adversary's wrongdoing was exposed.

Nowinski wrote on the Foundation's website:

McCrory has been perhaps the most influential voice
representing professional sports organizations in their
organized efforts to minimize and dismiss the evidence
that repeated hits to the head – like those in American and

Australian football, soccer, and rugby – can cause CTE. He
famously belittled CTE as 'all the carry on and hoo-ha you get
from the United States' in a 2016 lecture at the University of
Melbourne Florey Neuroscience Institute...

These new revelations of McCrory's plagiarism, along with
the knowledge that he has been misrepresenting the research
of others for years, is troubling. People are dying every day of
CTE. Families are suffering. It was just announced that CTE
was diagnosed in 12 of the first 21 Australian athletes whose
brains were studied at the Australian Sports Brain Bank.

Yet many sports minimize the risk of CTE because they've
been listening to Paul McCrory tell them that CTE is hoo-ha.
In my opinion, this is more than just a question of ethics and
academic integrity, it has harmed athletes.

Every sports organization that has relied on McCrory's
denial of the link between head trauma and CTE must start
fresh. Perhaps they should start with the US Centers for Disease
Control and Prevention 2019 fact sheet, which states:

'The research to-date suggests that CTE is caused in part by
repeated traumatic brain injuries, including concussions, and
repeated hits to the head, called subconcussive head impacts.'

Whatever comes next, the future of the Concussion in Sport
Group is in question.

A few months later, the *BMJ* said in a statement: 'Trust in
McCrory's work, specifically articles he published as a single author,
is broken.'

It is hard to overstate the damage done to the quality of the
conversation around brain injury in sport and blocks put in the path of
change caused by the ripple effect of McCrory's misrepresentation of
research, published via the hugely influential *BJSM* where he was editor
between 2001 and 2008 and editor at large until as recently as 2019.

In 2022, a *BJM* and *BJSM* investigation found, on top of 10 retracted papers, nine cases of plagiarism and countless other serious concerns about McCrory's conflicted ethics, that McCrory's paper 'When to retire after concussion?' had been retracted for misrepresenting the findings of Augustus Thorndike's 1952 paper, which the editors said amounted to 'an attempted erasure of a warning about the potentially foreseeable and worrying consequences of head impacts'.

This prompted the *BJSM* to ask: 'Did a misquotation warp the concussion narrative?' while finding the effect was to 'distort' previously accepted concussion research which 'may have altered the interpretation of concussion science and thus shaped the content of consensus statements on concussion'.

This distortion can be seen in plain sight. I have a paper in my possession published around 2001 titled 'Rugby Football Union and CogSport Concussion Management' written by McCrory and with 'specific modifications for use in England rugby by Simon Kemp'. The paper stated that among footballers who had been found to be suffering neurocognitive decline in Scandinavia, which researchers had linked to 'repetitive trauma linked to heading', 'the pattern of deficits is equally consistent with alcohol related brain impairment.' It went on:

> Similarly, there is little evidence that sustaining several concussions over a sporting career will necessarily result in permanent damage. The anecdotal approach originally proposed by Quigley in 1945 and adopted by Thorndike suggested that if an athlete suffered three concussions which involved loss of consciousness for any period of time, the athlete should be removed from contact sports for the remainder of the season. This has no scientific validity yet

continues to be quoted to this day as the main rationale in most return to play protocols.

By undermining and misrepresenting Thorndike and Quigley's work McCrory, and by extension Kemp, legitimized CogSport and prepared the ground for shorter return to play times.

This was further emphasized by highlighting a 1992 paper by D. Parkinson titled 'Concussion is completely reversable; an hypothesis', which, according to McCrory and Kemp's paper, found that 'In animal studies of experimental concussion, animals have been repeatedly concussed 20 to 35 times during the same day and within a two hour period. Despite these unusually high number of injuries no residual or cumulative effect was detected.'

Rugby players, it seems, were comparable to laboratory rats. As one of the most prolifically published researchers – in total McCrory had 530 published research articles and 34,502 citations on Google Scholar – he could reach a massive audience, while as editor of the *BJSM* and lead author of the CISG, he had the power to favour research which suited his agenda while refusing to publish research which didn't.

As lead signatory on the CISG McCrory held enormous sway as time after time they denied a causal link between repeated head injuries and CTE, when in fact there was one. By doing so, this enabled sport to take a less urgent approach. Wait and see. Time will tell. More research is needed. The same lines continue to be pushed today as a barrier to change.

In the meantime, former players including Steve Thompson and his family continue to suffer.

'In my mind Paul McCrory is little better than a murderer,' Thompson told me, in an allegation he would later repeat on BBC's *Newsnight*. 'It's disgusting how sport has allowed him to peddle his nonsense for so long. I'm living proof CTE exists.'

Former Leeds Rhinos captain Stevie Ward, who I met at a

Parliamentary roundtable chaired by Chris Bryant in October 2022, and who was forced to retire after suffering multiple concussions in his career, agreed.

'That culture around concussion comes from the top. At the end of the day, a lot of doctors and people who work in the game, they're just, they're doing what they believe is science, you know. And that's the worrying thing. You get someone who's at the top of these issues, and they're not telling the truth. I think it's disgusting, criminal to be honest.

'Paul McCrory has played puppet master with our lives.'

Dr Judith Gates, one of the founding trustees of Head for Change whose husband Bill is a former professional footballer now suffering from dementia, which she believes is connected to his career, said:

> The Concussion in Sport Group has been immensely influential, along with Paul McCrory. Since the early 2000s they have published every four years a consensus statement that has controlled the narrative on sports related head injuries. So therefore, they controlled litigation in America. They controlled the views of the governing bodies in the United Kingdom. They literally controlled the story that was told and the beliefs that were held.

With McCrory and the CISG now under more intense scrutiny than at any point in its history, their grip on the narrative is slipping. The NHS website, which in 2013 had no mention of CTE, now states: 'If you've had repeated blows to the head or concussions over many years, you may have a higher chance of getting chronic traumatic encephalopathy.'

In October 2022, the world's largest biomedical research agency, the US National Institutes of Health, rewrote its official guidance on the dangers of repetitive head impacts following research published by Harvard University, Oxford Brookes University and 11 other academic institutions, alongside analysis from the Concussion Legacy Foundation, which applied what is known as the Bradford Hill Criteria for Causation, which was the accepted method used to link smoking with lung cancer.

The new NIH guidance noted: 'CTE is a delayed neurodegenerative disorder that was initially identified in postmortem brains and, research-to-date suggests, is caused in part by repeated traumatic brain injuries.'

It is, of course, high time we ended speculation about whether or not head injuries cause CTE, historically only diagnosable post-mortem but, thanks to improvements in scanning techniques and equipment, increasingly diagnosable in living people. The NIH in America and the NHS in the UK say they do and so does more than a century of science, dating back way before Harrison Martland found significant neurodegenerative pathologies in the brains of 'punch-drunk' boxers. To suggest anything else is disingenuous at best, downright dangerous at worst.

This sport-wide cover up, playing dumb to and undermining science which had long been established, was led by McCrory, the CISG and other complicit medics. This amounted, in my opinion, to a concerted and sophisticated attempt to muddy the science and create doubt where previously none existed.

In his 2020 book *The Triumph of Doubt: Dark Money and the Science of Deception*, David Michaels, who served as Assistant Secretary for Labor under President Obama, cites climate change, opioids, obesity, air pollution and concussion as battlegrounds for truth where huge corporations have spent vast amounts to create confusion, spread doubt and avoid tighter regulation or litigation.

> It is public relations disguised as science. The companies' PR experts provide these scientists with contrarian sound bites that play well with reporters, who are mired in the trap of believing

there must be two sides to every story equally worthy of fair-minded consideration. The scientists are deployed to influence regulatory agencies that might be trying to protect the public, or to defend against lawsuits by people who believe they were injured by the product in question. The corporations and their hired guns market their studies and reports as 'sound science' but actually they just *sound like* science. Such bought-and-paid-for corporate research is sanctified, while any academic research that might threaten corporate interests is vilified. There's a word for that: Orwellian.

Sound familiar?

16

If in doubt, sit them out

The 'debate', if indeed there ever really was one, over whether or not repetitive head trauma increases the risk of developing neurological problems in later life is over. How big those problems are and who is most susceptible to them remains unclear. But an overwhelming body of evidence now exists – including research published by the Drake Foundation in 2021, which found 23 per cent of elite adult rugby players had abnormalities in brain structure, while half showed an unexpected change in brain volume – to highlight an uncomfortable truth. Rugby union has a brain injury problem. The problems it faces today are largely because it spent the best part of two decades following the onset of professionalism pretending it didn't.

When their findings were published, Drake Foundation founder James Drake said:

> Common sense dictates that the number and ferocity of impacts, both in training and actual play, need to be significantly reduced. These latest results add further support to this notion, particularly when coupled with existing findings across sport and anecdotal evidence.

Since rugby was professionalized in the 1990s, the game has changed beyond all recognition. Players are now generally bigger and more powerful, so we have to be mindful of all the ramifications that increased impacts will have on their bodies.

There is a causal link between repeated head injuries and neuro-degenerative problems in later life and those who suggest otherwise are akin to those denying climate change.

In 2020, RFU chief executive Bill Sweeney said: 'It is very hypothetical, the science is not black and white. There is no scientific proof of the causal link between concussion and CTE, that is not a proven thing.'

During the course of researching this book, I spoke to many old contacts, friends and some adversaries. Some were encouraged by the changes sport had made while others remained deeply cynical.

Dawn Astle and Rachel Walden, both daughters of former footballers who died from CTE, now work alongside the Concussion Legacy Foundation's executive director Adam White in the Professional Footballers' Association's Brain Health Department.

'It does feel very different now to 10 years ago,' Dawn told me in late 2022. 'The PFA and FA now accept there is a link between head injuries and CTE, which means we can get on with working out what we are going to do about it. I'm definitely feeling more positive about the way football is going. The fact the PFA have brought people like myself, Rachel and Adam "in-house" shows they are prepared to hear some tough home truths. I'd rather be shouting from the inside, out, than the other way around.'

With the Scottish Football Association acting upon Willie Stewart's 2019 FIELD study by banning children under 12 from heading the ball the following year, the FA now looks set to follow suit after initiating a trial in 2022.

However, resistance to change at the top of football remains steadfast, with the Premier League in February 2023 rejecting FA proposals to introduce concussion substitutions which would have brought them into line with professional rugby union and cricket.

Culturally, football still has a very long way to go.

Rugby, unquestionably, has taken steps in the right direction. Commentators no longer laud the 'bravery' of players carrying on with brain damage, and medics are more empowered, while players look out for each other on the field and no longer see concussion as the joke it once was. Damian Hopley has left the RPA, which has improved its governance and structure, and now appears more like the trade union it was set up to be.

The Head Injury Assessment remains deeply flawed, despite recent claims by World Rugby that it is 90 per cent successful in detecting on-field concussions, but it should at least be credited with highlighting to those who hadn't previously been inclined to look, or indeed care, just how many brain injuries occur on a professional rugby field.

Decisions to remove players from the field are now widely accepted by players and fans alike, with commentators less inclined to describe a player's 'warrior spirit' and more inclined to praise medics when they do the right thing by taking the player off.

Clearly, this is a good thing. But it does not mean rugby is safer. Far from it.

All the evidence shows rugby union has become significantly more dangerous over the past three decades. And much of the evidence we have gathered since then indicates it was already more dangerous than we previously believed. The trends in the data are there for all to see. Just type into Google 'Professional Rugby Injury Surveillance Project' and see what the data says. Severity of injuries? Up. Training ground injuries? Up. Concussions? Up.

From the 1993–97 research by Edinburgh University which showed a doubling in the number of injuries suffered by professional players during that period, to the RFU's own injury data, from what

I have seen with my own eyes, it is impossible to conclude anything other than that professional rugby union's injury risk profile has radically increased over the past 28 years.

But even though rugby's authorities are in possession of this information, they continue to allow more demands to be heaped on players. Rest periods between seasons remain woefully inadequate and poorly policed; training injury rates are higher than ever before; squad sizes are being cut as rugby's commercial reality bites; and concussion rates are higher than at any point in the history of the sport.

If player welfare truly was ever really rugby union's number one priority, how on earth have we got to this point?

The corporately organized attempts to deny the growing risks, led by senior figures from within the RFU and World Rugby, and aided and abetted in some instances by a complicit media, have caused more injuries to players than was necessary and intolerable subsequent reputational damage.

By denying what was obvious to see, rugby union delayed action being taken earlier to protect the sport's image. Players have suffered directly as a result. And rugby union is not alone in this regard. The same could be said of several other contact sports, notably rugby league, American football, Australian rules football, association football and ice hockey. By amplifying the voices of conflicted doctors, most notably Paul McCrory, professional sport allowed a toxic culture to take hold, built upon harmful notions of masculinity – the Muscular Christian 'man up' culture – which facilitated and enabled environments where mismanagement of brain injuries became acceptable.

Only in the past decade, largely due to the work of people such as Willie Stewart, Adam White, Dawn Astle, Peter Robinson, Chris Bryant and those journalists who have also picked up the baton, has sport's governing bodies' ultimate authority and control of the narrative been questioned.

In recent times, organizations including the Concussion Legacy Foundation, Headway, Progressive Rugby, Head for Change, the Jeff Astle Foundation and the Drake Foundation, to name just a few, have invested time, money and vast amounts of human resource into gathering the evidence and providing support to players and their families denied for decades by governing bodies more concerned with protecting reputations than doing the right thing.

Rugby has come a long way, no doubt, but it still has a long way to go. There remain many in the sport deeply resistant to change. Even though the evidence that it is needed now goes far beyond reasonable doubt.

World Rugby's decision in November 2022 to provide a platform at their medical symposium, attended by many of the most senior medics and administrators, to Dr Rudy Castellani was in my opinion a grievous error of judgement. It spoke of retrenching, not opening up.

Dr Castellani, professor of pathology at Northwestern University Feinberg School of Medicine, and self-confessed 'unabashed denier' of the Boston Group's research, in my opinion parroted many of the same lines we had heard in previous years from men like McCrory. A man who no longer has any credibility in sports medicine.

At World Rugby's conference in Amsterdam Dr Castellani explained that, among other reservations he has about the Boston research, there is insufficient evidence to describe CTE as a 'neurodegenerative' disease. It is also his view that there are 'factual inaccuracies' in the guidance issued by the US National Institutes of Health, which acknowledges a causal link between CTE and head trauma. As Andy Bull wrote with typically acerbic understatement in the *Guardian*, this is 'something of a fringe view'.

For as long as there are those prepared to die on a hill saying it really doesn't matter how many times you batter your brain, there will be athletes in contact sport who die prematurely with dementia.

As long as these people exist, the professional rugby juggernaut will carry on unchecked, and to hell with the consequences.

Perhaps that is all governments and commercially driven sports bodies want.

Giving evidence to an Australian Senate Inquiry into concussion in sport in February 2023, Queensland University researcher and historian Dr Stephen Townsend gave evidence focused on the history of concussion in Australian sport and compared the cultural and legal landscape around brain injury and contact sport to smoking.

'I think that's an apt comparison, because Australia in many ways is addicted to contact sport,' he said. 'We love it even though it kills us. I think the smoking comparison is also apt because it prompts us to consider the availability of health information to athletes and parents.'

Townsend added that Australia had seen 'periods of major public concern about sports concussion' in the 1930s and early 1980s but in both instances the concerns of doctors, athletes and researchers were 'suppressed by sporting leagues and their supporters' because sport was 'too culturally and economically important to change'.

Clearly there is nuance, but citing alcohol, drug abuse, lack of physical activity and other 'lifestyle choices' as risk factors for dementia, as World Rugby did in 2021, again risks muddying the waters when it comes to CTE. The solitary common denominator in all 345 cases of CTE found among the 376 brains (91.7 per cent) of retired NFL players by Ann McKee's team at Boston has been repetitive head trauma.

There is no suggestion 91.7 per cent of all those who play contact sport develop CTE, for there are not always symptoms, but all the Boston evidence points to one single causal factor: repetitive head injuries. The Boston Group are transparent and open about their studies having selection bias as those brains donated are almost always donated by families of players who have died with symptoms of the disease. But it also puts into stark perspective the absurdity of

McCrory's position, and others, who have sought to promote a false narrative that CTE cases are 'vanishingly small' or even non-existent.

And while the Boston Group are open about the weakness in their study, I should be open about the weakness in mine: women. I fully acknowledge this book does not appropriately represent women's experience of concussion, other than through the valuable and powerful testimony provided by mothers, wives and partners of male athletes affected by brain injury. Women such as Althea Trayhern, Jen Cudmore, Karen Walton, Mel Berry, Dawn Astle, Mel Popham, Judith Gates and latterly Linda O'Leary, whose son Nic was forced to check himself into a psychiatric unit in 2016 after a serious brain injury he'd suffered on the rugby field eight years earlier, aged 16, went undiagnosed. Nic, a hitherto happy-go-lucky young man, has since attempted suicide on a number of occasions and says thoughts of suicide will 'never leave me'.

It has been clear for many years that women are more susceptible to brain injuries than men, although the precise reasons remain unclear, while the suicide of Scotland No.8 Siobhan Cattigan in November 2021, which her parents, Morven and Neil, say resulted from two separate head injuries sustained playing rugby, has brought the issue to the top of the news agenda.

'Something catastrophic had happened to Siobhan's brain,' her parents told the *Sunday Times* in 2022, adding 'it had got to the point where she could no longer live with the pain in her head and Siobhan succumbed to an irrational thought and impulsive action.'

The SRU's refusal for almost 18 months to acknowledge Siobhan's death in a public tribute, before finally relenting in March 2023 ahead of Scotland's home Six Nations encounter with Ireland, demonstrated precisely the same a lack of empathy and humanity I first detected in professional rugby union in the early days of covering the sport.

Meanwhile, former England centre Kat Merchant is another brave woman who has spoken publicly about her struggles with the brain injuries which forced her premature retirement in 2014.

'Everybody says "oh it's one of those things". I had 11 concussions, some of my early ones I'd feel OK afterwards, but then the two that I had were a year apart, they set me back for maybe three or four months,' Merchant told the Rugby Wrap Up website in 2015.

'I didn't feel right. Mentally things are a lot more taxing and physically every time I tried to train I'd get another setback. I don't want players to ever get to that point, but that's what made me become a lot more serious about it.'

I am a huge fan of women's sport and am thrilled that football, rugby and cricket are all now firmly established as viable television spectacles in their own right after decades of being dismissed. But with the welcome growth in all these sports, there needs to be a renewed focus on safety to ensure commercial temptation doesn't blinker the authorities to their moral duty to protect their athletes.

And all the while, Paul McCrory's toxic legacy lives on. As recently as March 2023, I was shocked to attend a Parliamentary roundtable discussion led by Chris Bryant, where one of those formulating the UK's co-ordinated response to acquired brain injury in sport said that 'some doctors still question whether second impact syndrome exists'.

It was yet another jaw-dropping moment further illustrating the viral effect of McCrory's work.

I also learned from that meeting of a plan to publish UK-wide protocols – or guidelines as many insist they should be called – relating to concussion in sport which will adopt the SRU's 'If In Doubt, Sit Them Out' message created by Peter Robinson, Willie Stewart and James Robson. It has taken almost a decade for this to happen. Bryant's tireless work has been central to delivering this.

However, there will be no mention in the guidelines of CTE or the long-term risks of repetitive brain injury, while the data will be gathered, processed and presented by Bath University and largely funded by the RFU, where Simon Kemp, the man who said concussion 'wasn't a problem for rugby in the long-term' in 2013, remains head of medical services at the time of writing.

It would be churlish not to list some of the good things which have happened during Kemp's extraordinarily long tenure. These include a massive upgrade in Twickenham's medical facilities to rival the best stadiums in the world and latterly, following the announcement of legal action against the RFU, significant investment in a post-retirement mental health clinic for concerned ex-players to have their brains assessed. But Kemp, in my view, has been a central part of the problem.

Meanwhile, there has been an undeniable reduction in the number of concussions missed on the field by doctors, although this needs to be placed in context because the actual number of brain-injured players has skyrocketed by almost 800 per cent. And that is just in the time concussions have been recorded. And remember that the Scottish research showed injury rates doubled between 1993 and 1997.

In 2020/21, concussion rates in English professional rugby hit 22.2 concussions per 1,000 playing hours, the highest figure since records began. Whatever the unions might say, this is simply not just down to better identification. And even if it is, which I dispute, why did it take a media campaign to get them to sit up and take notice? It was already happening in plain sight.

And the cynicism of their communications continues. The same day that record high concussion figure was announced, World Rugby moved the mandatory stand-down following a diagnosed concussion from six days to 12 days, following the decision to abolish the three-week stand-down in 2011.

World Rugby's chief medical officer Eanna Falvey said: 'It is going to be a new mindset for coaches and players. Our approach means it is now overwhelmingly likely a player diagnosed with a concussion won't play in their team's next match. World Rugby firmly believes that scientific evidence supports our protocols, but we are continually monitoring and testing them to ensure that they are fit for the modern game.'

And all the while, despite a deluge of statistics pumped out by World Rugby and the RFU's powerful PR machines supporting the HIA's effectiveness, brain injuries continue to be mismanaged.

For example, in May 2021, Exeter Chiefs hooker Luke Cowan Dickie was knocked unconscious in the Premiership final. The next day he boarded a flight to South Africa and appeared on the bench for the British and Irish Lions against Sigma Lions a week later.

The incident sparked fury among campaigners, including former England scrum half Kyran Bracken, who just two months earlier provided damning testimony to an inquiry by the Department for Culture, Media and Sport into concussion which criticized sport for 'marking its own homework', found governing bodies 'unaccountable' and criticized the government for 'failing to take action on player welfare'.

Bracken tweeted: 'Luke is unconscious for over 20 seconds. Possibly 40-60 secs. How can he play the following week? I am absolutely disgusted that the powers that be allow this to happen. A stain on our great game.'

The following year, in February 2022, Wales prop Tomas Francis suffered a brain injury midway through the second half against England, demonstrating several obvious symptoms which meant he should have been immediately removed. Instead, Francis was allowed to play on after passing an HIA he should never even have undergone. A Six Nations Head Injury Review panel comprising, among others, Kemp, World Rugby's head of medicine Martin Raftery and the WRU's medical manager Prav Mathema, found there were no grounds for disciplinary action.

This was despite concluding 'in this instance one or more criteria one indications had been present that should have resulted in Francis being immediately and permanently removed from play'.

In April 2022, England Under 20 doctor Simon Rayner became, to my knowledge, the first medical practitioner in the history of professional rugby union to be sanctioned for errors contributing to mismanagement of a concussed player.

At a severely delayed hearing, Rayner received an eight-week ban, reduced to four for his previously exemplary record, for 'grave' and 'unacceptable' conduct late on in England's Six Nations encounter with Italy the previous February.

The incident occurred when Rayner attempted to overrule the independent matchday doctor, who judged that England winger Deago Bailey needed to leave the field for an HIA. Rayner's interaction with referee Aurélie Groizeleau was also deemed 'unacceptable' and 'not in the spirit of the game'.

In November 2022, Australia scrum half Nic White was allowed to play on against Ireland after appearing unsteady on his feet – one of the category one criteria for immediate removal – following a blow to his head. He passed an HIA and returned to the field.

Lobby group Progressive Rugby tweeted:

> Progressive Rugby respectfully require answers from
> @wallabies after a player who exhibited category 1 symptoms
> of brain injury (Nic White) was not permanently removed
> from the game between Ireland and Australia. White, clearly
> unsteady and dazed, instead underwent a HIA and was
> returned to the field. This is unacceptable and further deepens
> our concern about the HIA protocol and whether it is fit for the
> purpose of properly protecting players.

A review panel cited problems with accessing television footage but found no case for the Wallaby medical team to answer.

In January 2023, I asked Kemp, following the White case, if he still had faith in the HIA, which to my mind drew comparisons with the George North case in 2016.

'Sam. George North does not happen any more,' Kemp told me emphatically. As so often in the past, he was wrong.

The following month, playing for Wales, North went limp after being smashed in the head by Scotland hooker George Turner's shoulder while attempting a tackle. Turner was shown a yellow card but North, despite displaying obvious symptoms and with a long concussion history, played on before eventually being removed shortly before half time to undergo an HIA.

At half time, BBC commentators John Barclay and Jonathan Davies criticized the decision not to remove him permanently before the break.

'I don't understand why he hasn't been dragged off straight away,' said Davies in the BBC studio.

Barclay added: 'The good news is they saw it. He can't come back on the pitch. If you're looking at the process, he's shown a clear sign of concussion as he's gone limp. Whether he's lost consciousness or not is irrelevant. He can't come back on the pitch.'

After half time, North returned to the pitch and played the entire second half.

It was, to my knowledge, the fourth time the player had been allowed to play on in a live televised game, having visibly suffered a brain injury. Three of those incidents were on the WRU's watch.

'How does rugby keep getting this so wrong?' asked *Times* rugby journalist Will Kelleher.

I began this book by stating that I love rugby union. Nothing will change that. But it's also pretty obvious that I, along with countless others, have found it increasingly difficult to love a sport whose administrators have lost their capacity for compassion.

Money has distorted the game's values, and conflicts of interest have crippled the sport and prevented it having an honest conversation with itself. Player welfare has suffered as a result and it is now reasonable to argue that playing professional rugby really isn't very good for you.

Players deserve to be told the truth so they can make an informed choice. Yes, there are myriad good reasons to play rugby. Not least its ability, when run the right way, to bring communities together and provide children with a fun, aerobic and skills-based game. Lasting friendships are made through rugby, and sport more broadly, but if we are going to cheer on the collisions, we have to admit they come at a price.

Would you choose a job which requires you to repeatedly and routinely bash your head? Participants in contact sport, just like those of us who choose to smoke the occasional cigarette or drink a pint of beer, need to be able to make an educated choice. Contact sport should come with a health warning. I have no doubt many, probably even the majority of players, would still choose to play, even if they knew the risks.

To a degree, that has always been the case. Even once the risks of playing professional rugby were beginning to be revealed, England and Leicester prop Dan Cole, having uncomplainingly played 41 matches in the 2012/13 season and requiring spinal surgery as a direct consequence, told the BBC: 'My grandfather worked down a coal mine. The seam collapsed on him and he broke his back. He was left injured by his job and I will possibly have the same consequences. But I enjoy my job a lot more than he enjoyed his, so it's a pay-off.'

I doubt this would change significantly even if they were given an informed choice, as I have argued so vociferously they should be. In fact, a number of players have come forward since rugby's legal case was announced declaring they would do it all again in a heartbeat.

Shortly before this book went to print, England No.8 Billy Vunipola, whose family originate from Tonga but who gained a rugby scholarship to elite English public school Harrow, was asked by former Scotland lock Jim Hamilton on the Rugby Pod if he was worried about what life would be like when he is 50.

> No, this is the life I chose. And this is my mindset, for me personally. I've got a kid now, I understand that risk, but my parents sacrificed to come over to England, to a country that is obviously very foreign to them. Different language, to give me an opportunity to grow up in such a privileged country.
>
> And that is my role for my son, and that's what I'm trying to play. If that means something might happen, I can't… I just can't live my life thinking like that. You know, I've got to be present in the now, and whatever happens in the future, you know I don't want to say anything now that I could regret in the future.
>
> But… in terms of you know 'yeah I'll be fine, don't worry about me', but this is the life I chose, this is what I signed up for. I would love to be like the healthiest person in the world but, that's just the way it is and you've got to accept it. And that's the only thing, that's all I can say about myself.

Hamilton said in response: 'And this is what I've been sat on, Bill, for the last year or two since everything came out. Mate, I grew up on a fucking council estate in Cov. I had nothing. Right, rugby gave me everything. And I can't go, "oh well I didn't miss it, miss a game for concussion that's so-and-so's fault, or you know they covered something up." I don't even know. I don't even know what happened, all I know is I had the best fucking 15 years of my life.'

Often, it is left to those who have retired and not pursued media careers for whatever reason who are best placed to be honest about the reality of life as a professional.

'My hip's f**ked,' Dylan Hartley told the *Mail on Sunday* in October 2022.

I've got arthritis so I'm getting a replacement. It's pretty debilitating. I can't walk properly, I don't sleep well, can't tie my shoelaces, struggle to play with my kids, struggle to sit on the toilet.

I know I've had some knocks on my head and now I'm doing my rehab so I'm in the best possible place in 10 years' time. I wouldn't call it fear, I'd call it awareness. The reason I refused to have my brain scanned until this month is because, deep down, I didn't want to know. If I'm told my brain's damaged – and I've had brain injuries so there probably is some damage – then all I can do is be proactive.

Lewis Moody, who lost his father to Alzheimer's in 2021, recognizes change needs to happen across the sport. 'I love the game of rugby,' he said.

My kids love it, they absolutely obsess about it. And they would do contact every waking second of every day if they could. So it's up to us to take the power out of their hands. The technical work around the contact area, the tackle technique, the scrummage, you can do that without putting the bodies in a position where you're going to sustain a head injury.

People may go 'that's really hypocritical of you, Lewis Moody, Mad Dog Moody, because you used to play like an idiot, you were insane'. Well, I wasn't insane. I loved playing the way I did, I loved the contact element of the game, I loved the hours we spent battering each other on the training field. I played the game within the parameters, and in the way that I could, at a time that I could. And I would do it differently now.

Moody was speaking to the lobby group Progressive Rugby, an organization formed in 2021 and whose aims align closely with what I've been calling for for more than a decade. I support their position on player welfare and believe they have the best interests of rugby and its players at heart.

They have called for a number of urgent changes to be made to improve player welfare which include:

- Minimum 21-day non-negotiable blanket stand-down after a brain injury, irrespective of elite player's concussion history

- Failure of in-game HIA to trigger minimum 21-day period

- Mandated weekly 'bone on bone' contact training limit of 15 minutes

- Game limit reduced by 20 per cent to 25 games (or match equivalent minutes) and mandated

- Stiff punishments including Club/Country fines and points deductions for non-compliance

- Minimum eight-week protected annual rest including at least two weeks in-season, with a further five-week break between seasons and additional one week to be used at any time

- Injury replacements only to eliminate collisions between fatigued and fresh players

Progressive Rugby has done an excellent job continuing the critical work of keeping pressure on rugby's authorities to act on their player welfare rhetoric. A series of truly shocking articles on their website, including one with former England and Leicester full back Tim Stimpson, which I read during the course of writing this book, still stopped me in my tracks, despite my experience in this field.

Stimpson, formerly Leicester's RPA representative, spoke of a Boxing Day fixture against Harlequins in 2001 where he was allowed to play on despite suffering 20 fractures of his cheekbone eight minutes into the game when he was inadvertently head butted by his own player, Alesana Tuilagi.

'I didn't regain consciousness until I was off the pitch,' Stimpson told Progressive Rugby.

'One of the Harlequin's medics felt around the socket and determined I was ok to go back on. I told them no way – I could hear Niagara Falls in my head, there was clearly a lot of blood.'

The next morning, Stimpson awoke in his parents' house in Wakefield and looked in the mirror, only to see his eyeball had sunk into his skull as a result of the facial fractures. He required 24 hours of surgery to insert metal plates to stabilise the injury, some of which remains in his face today. His testimony today provides yet more compelling evidence of a culture in rugby completely at odds with the presentation of a sport which placed player welfare at the top of the agenda.

> At Leicester we prided ourselves on kicking the shit out of each other at training – and it worked too, we had a pretty awesome record,' Stimpson said.
>
> But the evidence we got it wrong is starting to mount, and I have numerous teammates suffering life-changing consequences from repeated concussions including depression and memory loss.

This has nothing to do with us being a more risk-averse society but everything to do with responding to a risk threat which has increased radically in less than three decades and which was denied for much of that time. It is not perception that rugby has got more dangerous or that more high-speed collisions and more games being played have caused more concussions. It is a fact.

I didn't want the predictions I made in 2013 about professional rugby players in the their thirties and forties developing dementia to come true. But the timebomb has gone off. How rugby union responds will define its future.

Those who claim the 'game's gone soft' are the flat earthers. It is simply a flawed argument. Rugby is a tougher sport to play today than at any point in its 150-year codified history.

Meanwhile, those who say nothing can or should be done are akin to climate deniers. Shifting baselines make them think everything has always been this way. It hasn't and it can be different again.

Denial will kill rugby, not concussion. It has always been there and always be. But rugby union, and all contact sports, need to accept the risk to convince parents their children are in safe hands when they take to the field. The most dangerous thing to do now would be to do nothing.

And the idea rugby will die if new tackle laws are effectively implemented is nonsensical. Who remembers the hit at the scrum now, or pines for tip tackles? American football had its concussion reckoning and is as commercially vibrant today as ever.

Rugby needs to put any idea of global domination to one side and look after its own. Endless growth is the enemy of good. Because commercial sustainability in the sport can only ever be achieved if enough players actually want to play the game. And at the moment, participation numbers in the amateur rugby union are nosediving.

Less can be more for the game's top stars, those most at risk of developing problems in later life because of the volume of sub-concussive and concussive hits they are exposed to. They should play less rugby in front of bigger crowds in smarter, more technologically interactive stadiums. They could reduce contact training and be fit for matchday.

And while they are at it, rugby's authorities could make significant savings by cutting out the nonsense around internationals including environmentally damaging pyrotechnics and eardrum-destroying blaring music all designed to falsely force an atmosphere. Cut that budget and put it all into a slush fund for players, who should also pay into it during their careers via a players' union completely independent from the RFU and Premier Rugby.

Those seeking to milk more money and serve their own interests will continue to promise unicorns are on the horizon. Saliva tests, mouthguard technology, magic helmets, more research. It's always just over the horizon. Tweaking the laws is also, in my view, a false dawn, although clearly reducing head-on-head contact makes sense. But be careful of the law of unintended consequences. Whatever happens, rugby's great global experiment appears set to continue, using its players as crash test dummies when the onus should be on the clubs, unions, medical staff and administrators to ensure their protocols are adhered to, exposures reduced and players properly protected from a threat which has increased dramatically since rugby union turned professional.

Many current and former professionals will completely disagree with me, especially those carving careers in the media. That is fine. The shifting baseline theory applies to the current players, while many former players who remain in the public eye, for reasons I have examined, are too conflicted to give an honest assessment. I've been fortunate, or unfortunate depending how you look at it, to be able to see the wood for the trees.

Sadly, change is only happening now because people at the top of rugby, and sport more broadly, fear being held legally accountable. If that happens, I will willingly provide my testimony. In truth, it should never have got to this stage.

Do I still love the game? Always. Would I let my kids play now? Yes, if I could trust that the coaches cared more about their wellbeing than winning. Does rugby union require radical change to survive? Unquestionably.

Rugby union has more difficult decisions to make. And it needs to make them fast. Decisions about tackle height, training load and rest. Decisions about whether money should drive sport or people. Decisions about whether winning is more important than protecting players' brains. Decisions which define the viability of rugby.

But, ultimately, what is a difficult decision? I recall the words of my friend Peter Robinson.

People talk about hard decisions and taking a kid off during a game is supposedly a hard decision. But for me a hard decision is whether to switch a life support machine off or donate your kids' organs after they've died. They're the real hard decisions.

If in doubt, sit them out.

Appendix

All data from the RFU Professional Rugby Injury Surveillance Project (2002-2020)

Research and Graphs by Tom Sansom

While there is no official RFU injury data before 2002, other peer-reviewed studies, notably one carried out by the University of Edinburgh, indicate an approximate doubling of rugby union's injury profile in just a few years after the sport turned professional in 1995.

The following graphs clearly show that between 2002 and 2020, while the overall frequency of injuries in English professional rugby remained largely stable, the severity of injuries, as well as the frequency and severity of concussions all increased across this period, notably in training.

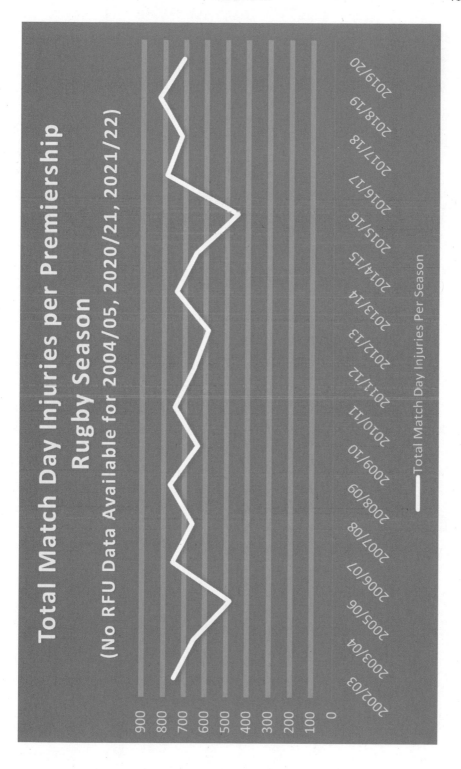

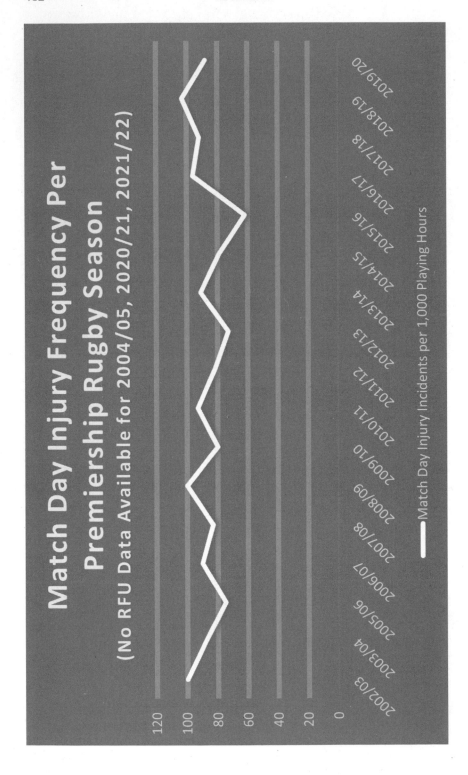

Match Day Injury Frequency Per Premiership Rugby Season

(No RFU Data Available for 2004/05, 2020/21, 2021/22)

Match Day Injury Incidents per 1,000 Playing Hours

Match Day Injury Incidents per 1,000 Playing Hours

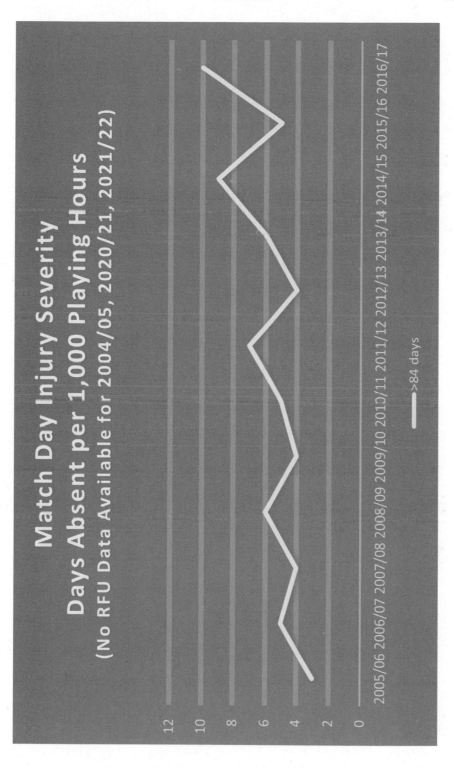

Match Day Injury Severity
Days Absent per 1,000 Playing Hours
(No RFU Data Available for 2004/05, 2020/21, 2021/22)

>84 days

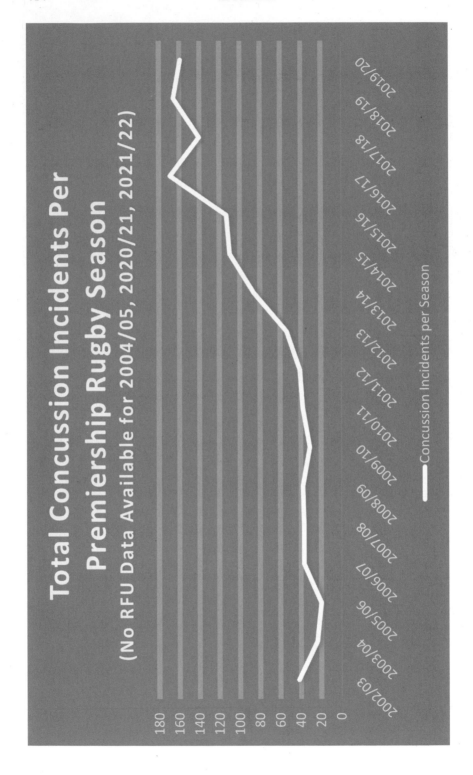

Total Concussion Incidents Per Premiership Rugby Season

(No RFU Data Available for 2004/05, 2020/21, 2021/22)

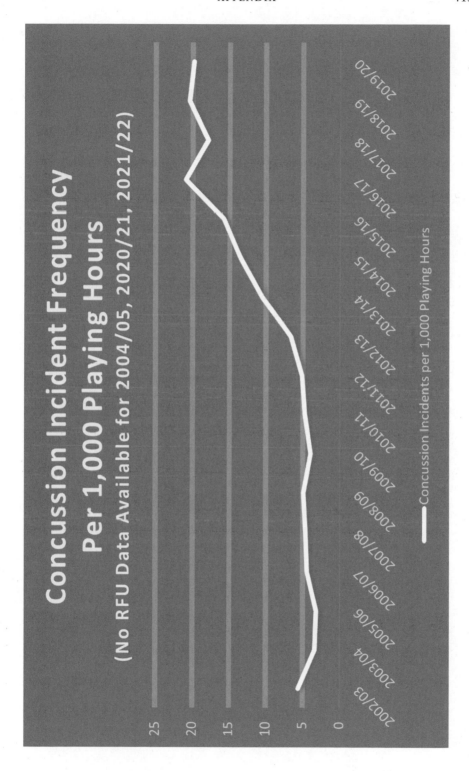

Concussion Incident Frequency Per 1,000 Playing Hours

(No RFU Data Available for 2004/05, 2020/21, 2021/22)

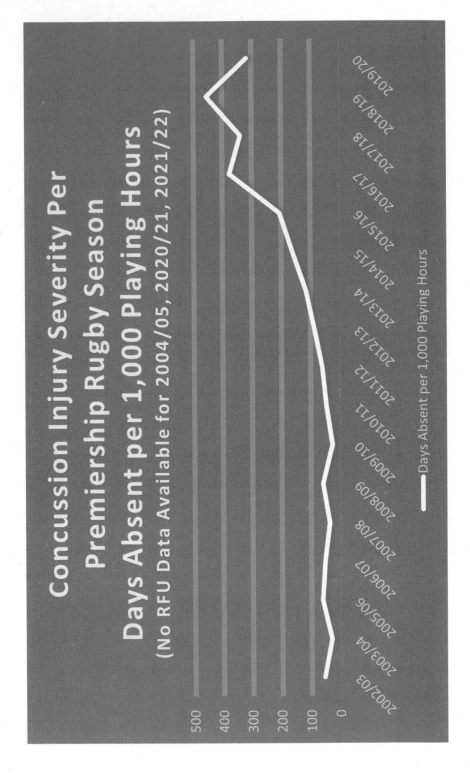

Concussion Injury Severity Per Premiership Rugby Season

Days Absent per 1,000 Playing Hours
(No RFU Data Available for 2004/05, 2020/21, 2021/22)

—— Days Absent per 1,000 Playing Hours

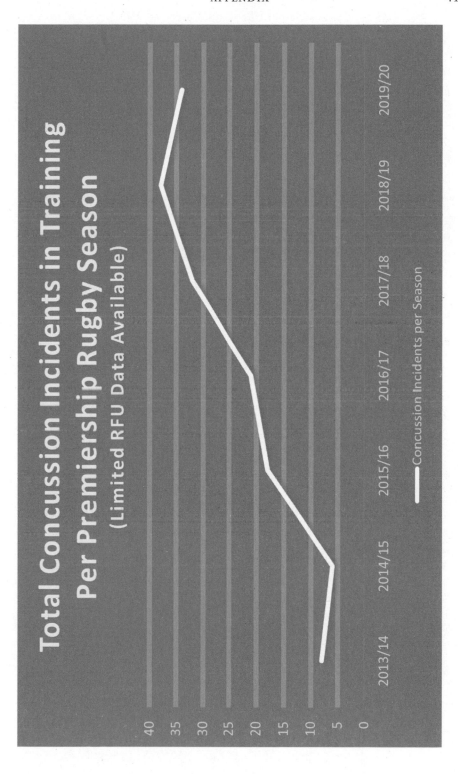

Total Concussion Incidents in Training Per Premiership Rugby Season
(Limited RFU Data Available)

—— Concussion Incidents per Season

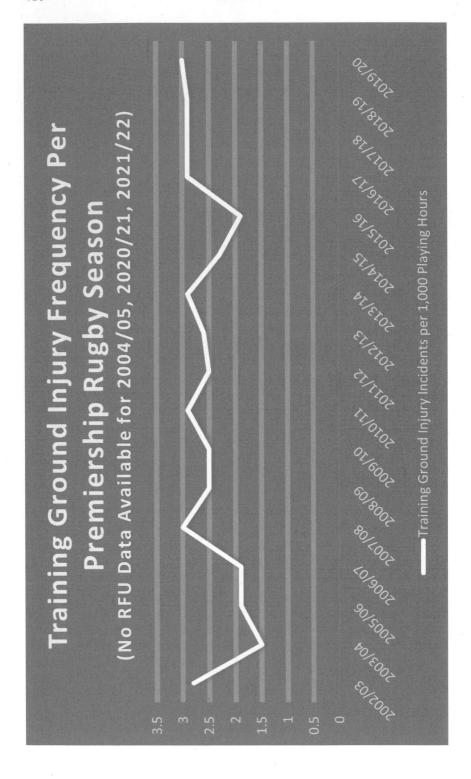

Training Ground Injury Frequency Per Premiership Rugby Season

(No RFU Data Available for 2004/05, 2020/21, 2021/22)

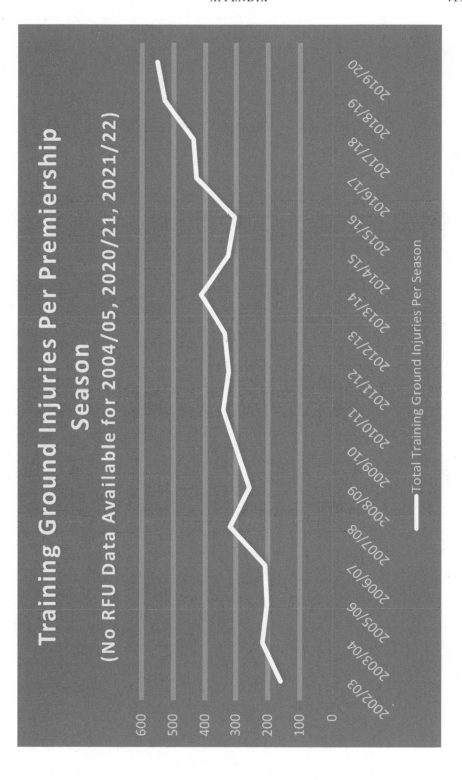

Training Ground Injuries Per Premiership Season

(No RFU Data Available for 2004/05, 2020/21, 2021/22)

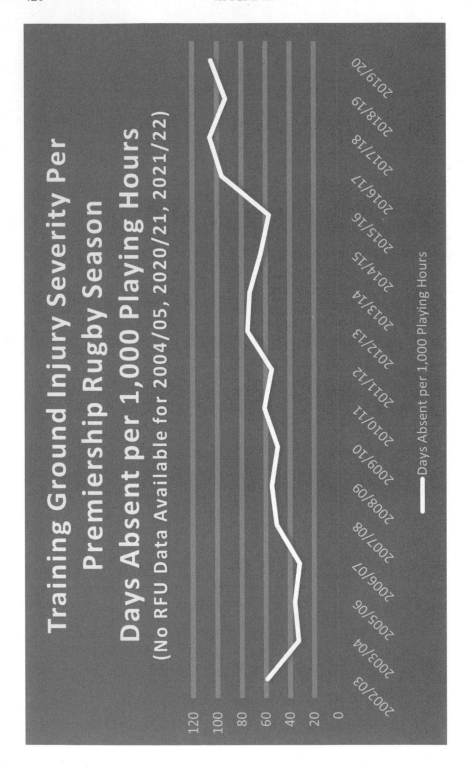

Acknowledgements

Writing this part of the book was the bit I dreaded most because so many people have helped me along the way that I have no doubt whatsoever I will miss someone out as an oversight. So let me please begin by stating now that if you have been part of what has been an extraordinary journey in sport for me, and I have not mentioned you either here or in the pages of the book, I am hugely grateful for your support and would like to thank you.

However, there are some people who have played such a prominent part I cannot forget them, starting with my wife Debs and parents Roy and Jennie, who have afforded me the time and space to deliver a book of which I am truly proud. I'm going to say now that's enough book dedications.

To my big brother Tom, thank you for being there all the way and for sharing your love and passion for sport over the years. My determination not to let this concussion story drop is in no small part down to the competitive instincts you instilled in me as I tried to survive your left-arm fast bowling in the nets growing up.

To the publishers at Atlantic Books, especially editor Ed Faulkner and copy editor Tamsin Shelton, I would like to thank you for having faith in my story and belief I could deliver this book. It is far better than I could possibly have hoped when I began work on it. One day I'll go back to the first draft and cringe with embarrassment.

Thanks also to Sir Clive Woodward, who wrote such a magnificent foreword to this book, and for all my friends and former colleagues who have provided extraordinarily generous and supportive quotes to help promote it.

To my literary agent and old friend from Edinburgh University, Oliver Munson, thanks for finding me the deal.

And to everyone on the sports desk at the *Mail on Sunday*, notably Alison Kervin, Cara Sloman and Mike Richards, thank you for all your support during my time on the paper and for having the bravery to run a story which so many others backed away from. I truly believe we achieved a great thing together and I will always cherish the time we spent working together on such an important campaign.

Thanks also to Chris Bryant MP, and all the other politicians who have followed his relentless lead in recent years, in attempting to get the Aquired Brain Injury Bill across the line. It is good to know integrity can still flourish in some sections of UK politics.

To all the charities and brain injury campaigners, notably Ben's mum and dad, Peter and Carole Robinson, Professor Willie Stewart, Luke Griggs at Headway, Dawn and Laraine Astle at the Jeff Astle Foundation, Judith Gates at Head for Change, Dr Adam White (now PFA) and Nathan Howarth at the Concussion Legacy Foundation and Tom Morris at Progressive Rugby, thank you. I look forward to working with all of you again in some capacity in the future. To Drs Barry O'Driscoll and James Robson, thank you for being the 'canaries down the mine' and warning of rugby's mounting injury risk while working within the confines of the sport. In my eyes, you are both heroes and rugby players across the world have much to thank you for.

To the players who had the bravery to talk openly about concussion in those early days when it was still taboo, in particular Lewis Moody, Nic Berry, Jamie Cudmore and Al Hargreaves, latterly Steve Thompson and Alix Popham, thank you. You are all leaders of men and I'm proud to call you friends.

Thanks in equal measure to all the families of players I have spoken to over the years who trusted me to tell their stories with sensitivity and respect. To Althea Treyharn, Mel Popham, Mel Berry.

I'd like to thank Dr Barry O'Driscoll, recently described to me as being my 'fellow canary down the mine', and who had the courage and moral fortitude to resign his position on World Rugby's medical advisory board in 2012 and in doing so confirm to me there was a very serious problem which needed investigating.

And to my old friends, the crew of the Row2Recovery, a group of British war veterans who never complained about their lot, but who fundamentally helped inform my take on concussion in professional rugby, where I believed players unfailing loyalty, trust and bravery was being abused by those who stood to benefit without accountability. Thank you to all the rugby journalists – The Jacks – who helped me researching this book, especially my friends Dan Schofield, Peter Jackson, Alan Dymock, Stephen Jones, Steve Bale, Julian Guyer, Alex Lowe. Adam Hathaway, Nic Simon and Hugh Godwin and photographer Graham Chadwick who all contributed to this book in some way shape or form.

I would also like to pay tribute to the journalists who have picked up the concussion baton in recent years and held power to account. Notably Jeremy Wilson, Hannah Walker-Brown, Kieran Gill and more latterly David Walsh and Heather Dewar.

To the team at Planted – especially Paul Rae – thank you for filling in so effectively in my absence to work on this book. You knew how important this is to me and we share the same values. Thank you my friend.

Last, but absolutely not, least, I would like to thank a young sports journalist with a brilliant future: Tom Sansom who helped me compile much of the data and interview transcriptions for this book. Tom, I could not have asked for more from you and while not all of your excellent work made it into the final edition, I could not have done this book without you. You are a credit to the University of Gloucester's media department, and I would readily work with both of you again in the future.

There you have it, I told you I'd forget someone. And if that someone is you, thank you.

Index